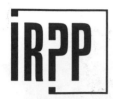

**Institute for
Research on
Public Policy**

*Institut de
recherche
en politiques
publiques*

Founded in 1972, the Institute for Research on Public Policy is an independent, national, nonprofit organization.

IRPP seeks to improve public policy in Canada by generating research, providing insight and sparking debate that will contribute to the public policy decision-making process and strengthen the quality of the public policy decisions made by Canadian governments, citizens, institutions and organizations.

IRPP's independence is assured by an endowment fund, to which federal and provincial governments and the private sector have contributed.

Fondé en 1972, l'Institut de recherche en politiques publiques (IRPP) est un organisme canadien, indépendant et sans but lucratif.

L'IRPP cherche à améliorer les politiques publiques canadiennes en encourageant la recherche, en mettant de l'avant de nouvelles perspectives et en suscitant des débats qui contribueront au processus décisionnel en matière de politiques publiques et qui rehausseront la qualité des décisions que prennent les gouvernements, les citoyens, les institutions et les organismes canadiens.

L'indépendance de l'IRPP est assurée par un fonds de dotation, auquel ont souscrit le gouvernement fédéral, les gouvernements provinciaux et le secteur privé.

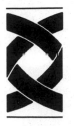

The Institute of Intergovernmental Relations is the only organization in Canada whose sole objective is to promote research and communication on the challenges facing federal systems of governance. We pursue our objective through research and a publication program, seminars and conferences. The Institute links academics and practitioners of federalism in federal and provincial governments.

THE INSTITUTE OF
INTERGOVERNMENTAL
RELATIONS

L'INSTITUT DES RELATIONS
INTERGOUVERNEMENTALES

'Institut est le seul organisme canadien à se consacrer exclusivement à la recherche et aux échanges sur les questions du fédéralisme.

Les priorités de recherche de l'Institut portent présentement sur le fédéralisme fiscal, l'union sociale, la modification éventuelle des institutions politiques fédérales, les nouveaux mécanismes de relations fédérales-provinciales, le fédéralisme canadien au regard de l'économie mondiale et le fédéralisme comparatif.

L'Institut réalise ses objectifs par le biais de recherches effectuées par son personnel et par des universitaires de l'Université Queen's et d'ailleurs, de même que par des conférences et des colloques.

L'Institut sert de lien entre les universitaires, les fonctionnaires fédéraux et provinciaux et le secteur privé.

MONEY, POLITICS
AND HEALTH CARE

RECONSTRUCTING THE
FEDERAL-PROVINCIAL PARTNERSHIP

EDITED BY
HARVEY LAZAR AND FRANCE ST-HILAIRE

THE INSTITUTE FOR RESEARCH ON PUBLIC POLICY
AND
THE INSTITUTE OF INTERGOVERNMENTAL RELATIONS

Printed in Canada
Dépôt légal 2003

National Library of Canada
Bibliothèque nationale du Québec

Cataloguing in Publication

Money, politics and health care : reconstructing the
federal-provincial partnership / Harvey Lazar, France
St-Hilaire, editors.

Includes bibliographical references.
ISBN 0-88645-208-2 (bound).--ISBN 0-88645-200-7
(pbk.)

1. Medical care--Canada--Finance. 2. Medical policy--
Canada.
3. Federal-provincial relations--Canada. 4. Transfer pay-
ments--Canada. I. Lazar, Harvey II. St-Hilaire, France
III. Institute for Research on Public Policy.

RA410.55.C35M65 2003   362.1'0971
C2003-904622-2

PROJECT DIRECTORS
Harvey Lazar (IIGR)
France St-Hilaire (IRPP)

RESEARCH ASSISTANT
Jennifer Love (IRPP)

EDITORIAL ASSISTANT
Francesca Worrall (IRPP)

COPY-EDITING AND PROOFREADING
Jane McWhinney

DESIGN AND PRODUCTION
Schumacher Design

PUBLISHED BY
Institute for Research on Public Policy (IRPP)
Institut de recherche en politiques publiques
1470 Peel Street, suite 200
Montreal, Quebec H3A 1T1
Tel: 514-985-2461
Fax: 514-985-2559
E-mail: irpp@irpp.org
www.irpp.org
AND
The Institute of Intergovernmental Relations
L'Institut des relations intergouvernementales
Queen's University
Kingston, Ontario K7L 3N6
Tel: 613-533-2080
Fax: 613-533-6868
E-mail: iigr@qsilver.queensu.ca
www.iigr.ca

CONTENTS

T he Commission on the Future of Health Care in Canada undertook a number of in-depth research initiatives and analytical studies to inform its deliberations. One of these initiatives related to the role of federal-provincial relations, and especially fiscal federalism, in the development of publicly insured universal health care. In November 2001 the Commission asked the Institute of Intergovernmental Relations in the School of Policy Studies at Queen's University to undertake this major research activity.

Prior to asking that we undertake this work, the Commission identified the following issues as items needing to be addressed in the proposed project.

1) What mechanisms do or should exist for encouraging cooperation and managing conflict between governments (both federal-provincial and interprovincial) in the area of health care financing?

2) What are the strengths and weaknesses of the transfer instruments currently employed by the federal government? What alternative transfer instruments are available to the federal government? On what criteria would one evaluate the utility of those current and alternative instruments? How do those different instruments affect the operation of the principles that underlie the medicare pact?

3) What are the competing interpretations of the federal government's role in health care and how do those different interpretations conceive of its fiscal role in the financing of the health care system? How has the debate over the federal role in health care changed over time? What other role(s) could the federal government play (other than through transfers) that would be practicable and consistent with the constitutional division of powers and the principles of the medicare pact?

4) It is often argued that there is a vertical fiscal imbalance in the federation whereby the federal government has a greater ability to raise revenue, but that provinces have greater obligations for social spending (health care, social services, etc.). To what extent is the relative nature and extent of the apparent vertical fiscal imbalance relevant insofar as there are transfers

designed to equalize the fiscal capacity of provincial governments with regard to social spending (i.e., the CHST)?

5) The ability of individual provinces to raise revenue also varies considerably (what is commonly called a horizontal fiscal imbalance) and is ameliorated by equalization payments from the federal government. To what extent is it necessary to rethink the way in which the federation deals with this horizontal fiscal imbalance?

Over the following several months, the Institute for Intergovernmental Relations provided three background studies to the Commission in response to many, albeit not all, of the above questions. The Institute subsequently also prepared a synthesis report for the Commission, which integrated the key analyses from the three studies. This volume makes available these reports undertaken for the Commission.

We began our work with some assumptions, and it may be useful to highlight key ones here. To start with, we observed that there are a number of competing views within Canada regarding the nature of Canadian federalism and regarding the appropriate role of the state (and thus by inference for markets and the non-profit sector) in society and the economy. A particular focus for us was this divided opinion about the extent to which redistribution is appropriate and the geographic territory over which such redistribution should occur (all of Canada, within provinces only, or some combination of the two). These differences reflect a range of values in regard to the nature and scope of the Canadian sharing community. A discussion of three representative views of the sharing community is set out in chapter 1, and it is carried forward into the subsequent chapters of this volume.

Since there is considerable support for all three views within Canada, and since the question of which view prevails at any point in time is more a matter of societal consensus than of technical analysis, we saw our task as one of advising on the principles that might guide the use of intergovernmental mechanisms under each of the visions or models. The result is that we have not arrived at a single set of recommendations about how intergovernmental relations can be strengthened with a view to facilitating improvements in the quality or sustainability of universal publicly financed health care in Canada. Rather, we have laid out the kinds of principles and policy options that might help to improve medicare under alternative views of the sharing community. Our assessment overall is that there is room for major improvements in the role of intergovernmental relations under each of the alternatives.

In describing its research needs, the Commission drew attention to the issues of vertical and horizontal fiscal balance/imbalance in Canada and was interested in the extent to which they might affect its thinking about the role of the federal government in financing provincial health care programs. We chose to concentrate more heavily on the vertical balance/imbalance issues, since much of the controversy over the financing role of the federal government in health care in recent years has been linked to provincial criticism that Ottawa has more revenues than it needs relative to its expenditure responsibilities, whereas provinces lack comparable fiscal clout. We devote a full chapter here to unpacking the arguments and analysis. In so doing, we hope that we will help Canadians to better understand the positions of both orders of government on this issue and their relevance to questions about the nature and form of Ottawa's financial contribution to health care.

The Commission published its findings and recommendations in November 2002. We believe that there is much in the research and analysis of our preparatory work for the Commisson that is important grist for public policy debate. The question of the appropriate role for the federal and provincial governments in the financing of public health is an issue that is not likely to be resolved overnight. That is the reason that this volume is being published.

The chapters in this volume are not, word for word, the texts we submitted to the Commission but they are close to the originals. In a few places, we have provided updated numbers and clarified meaning. We also have divided one very long paper into two separate chapters in order to make the text easier to digest. The last chapter, which is based on the final synthesis report that was submitted by the research team to the Commission, provides an overview and summary of the main arguments, recommendations, and policy options derived from the analysis in the preceding chapters.

Since the Commission released its report, the first ministers have met and a new First Ministers' Accord on Health Care Renewal has been announced. In a number of respects, we consider this new set of arrangements a step forward when evaluated against the analysis that follows in this volume. But in several ways, it clearly falls far short. Thus, we were not at all surprised to observe the provincial and territorial premiers expressing their dissatisfaction with the new arrangements even as they were being announced. The timing of the First Ministers' meeting, following the release of two major reports (Romanow and Kirby reports) on the future of health care in Canada, had given rise to high

expectations. Indeed, it was hoped that this meeting would mark the beginning
of a process of renewal and fundamental reform based on a common vision and
solid financial commitment for the long term. Instead, there has been little evidence of a more collaborative stance between Ottawa, who more or less imposed
the rules of the game, and the provinces and territories, who begrudgingly took
what money was offered fully expecting to be back for more.

Disagreements about money are probably inevitable, and part of the normal jockeying for power in the federation. In and of themselves they are not necessarily a bad thing. In the case of health care, however, these disagreements are
symptomatic of an intergovernmental dynamic that is helpful neither to the cause
of health care reform nor to the well-being of the federation. As a result, the political will necessary to effectively meet some of the worthy goals laid out in the
accord may be lacking (for example on performance indicators). In the last chapter of the volume, we propose a set of principles that might guide the federal-
provincial-territorial relationship on health care. In our view, these principles
remain as appropriate in the aftermath of the February 2003 Health Accord as
they were before it was announced.

The team that undertook this work for the Commission initially included Professors Keith Banting and Robin Boadway of Queen's University, and
Professor David Cameron of the University of Toronto as well as the undersigned.
Before long, Jean-François Tremblay and Jennifer McCrea-Logie, former students
of certain team members, became part of the team.

We were helped in our work by three advisers : Stephen Bornstein of St.
John's, Newfoundland; Claude Forget, from Montreal, Quebec; and David Kelly,
from Victoria, British Columbia. All three have had rich experience in matters of
health policy from a number of different perspectives. They kindly read drafts of
the chapters and offered valuable comments that helped us immensely in our
work. As is usual in such matters, however, they are in no way responsible for
shortcomings in the final product. Tom McIntosh of the Commission staff, and
now at the University of Regina, also participated in our team meetings with the
advisers. He too helped us with comments and suggestions and ensured that our
work was sensitive to the research needs of the Commission.

The publication of this volume is a joint venture of the Institute of
Intergovernmental Relations, School of Policy Studies at Queen's University and
the Institute for Research on Public Policy (IRPP). In helping us prepare this volume, we want especially to thank Patti Candido of the Queen's Institute for her

role in helping to organize meetings of the research team while our work for the Commission was being prepared, Suzanne Ostiguy-McIntyre of the IRPP for overseeing the production process, Francesca Worrall for editorial assistance, Jennifer Love for research assistance, and finally Jenny Schumacher of Schumacher Design, who designed the book cover and was responsible for the desktop publishing.

Harvey Lazar
Director
Institute of Intergovernmental Relations
School of Policy Studies
Queen's University

France St-Hilaire
Vice-President, Research
Institute for Research on Public Policy

CONTRIBUTORS

Keith Banting is Professor at the School of Policy Studies at Queen's University, and holder of the Queen's Research Chair in Public Policy.

Robin Boadway is Sir Edward Peacock Professor of Economic Theory at Queen's University.

David Cameron is Professor of Political Science at the University of Toronto.

Harvey Lazar is Director of the Institute of Intergovernmental Relations at Queen's University.

Jennifer McCrea-Logie has completed a doctorate in political science with a focus on health policy at the University of Toronto.

France St-Hilaire is Vice-President, Research, at the Institute for Research on Public Policy (IRPP) in Montreal.

Jean-François Tremblay is Professor of Economics at the University of Ottawa.

CHAPTER 1 ▐▬▬▬▬

DEFINING THE SHARING COMMUNITY: THE FEDERAL ROLE IN HEALTH CARE

KEITH BANTING AND ROBIN BOADWAY

This chapter explores the considerations that underpin the role of the federal government in the provision of health care. Debates over federalism and
health care have been intense in Canada. This history of conflict in part
reflects different approaches to federalism in this country. For some Canadians, the
promise of federalism is that it unites citizens over a vast and fragmented territory
and creates a central government that can provide leadership in critical areas of
public policy. For others, the promise of federalism is that it can reflect the diversities of our regions and enhance the scope for governance at the provincial level.
And for still other Canadians, especially many from Quebec, the promise of federalism is that it can accommodate the distinctiveness of a particular province
through asymmetrical relations with the rest of the country.

The history of debate over health care also reflects distinctive features of
the health policy. The health sector has witnessed more dramatic clashes between
federal and provincial governments than other social programs. Although constitutional politics and energy policy may have strained the political fabric of the
country more seriously at different times, health policy has ignited a series of
intergovernmental sparks in recent decades. A number of factors accentuate the
sensitivity of health policy:

> The sector itself is very complex, operating as it does through networks of
hospitals, medical professions, regional institutions, and community organizations, all of which are capable of vigorous political action.

> Health insurance also represents Canada's most ambitious social pro-
gram, which can displace market mechanisms more thoroughly than
programs such as public pensions. It is therefore not surprising that

ideological conflict over the role of the state in health care policy often
flows through intergovernmental channels.

> The federal government maintains a stronger role in program definition
in health care than in other programs financed by the Canadian Health
and Social Transfer (CHST), despite its reduced financial transfers.

> Health care is very important to the population and has taken on sym-
bolic dimensions well beyond those of a mere public program.

Given the controversy over Canadian federalism and the pressures on health policy, it is perhaps understandable that the role of the federal government in health
care has been the subject of recurring and difficult debates.

Our purpose here is to examine the choices that must be made in defining the role of the federal government in health care. A comprehensive interpretation of a role for the federal government in health care inevitably incorporates
three distinct dimensions of choice. The first dimension concerns the general role
of the state. The second concerns the particular role of the central government in
a federal state. And the third concerns the instruments through which the federal
government pursues its role. These three dimensions of choice are distinctive: as
we shall see, they involve different sets of considerations. However, they are also
cumulative. For those opposed to a state role in health care, the second and third
choices do not arise. And for those who accept the case for a public role in health
care but oppose federal involvement in the sector, the choice of instruments is
irrelevant. Accordingly, any comprehensive interpretation of an active role for the
federal government in health care inevitably represents all three dimensions.

What types of considerations are inherent in these judgments, and what
types of rationales have been advanced for an active federal role? The argument
advanced here is that the primary rationale for the extensive public intervention
in health care that one sees in OECD countries is one based on arguments of
redistributive equity, especially those founded on principles of social insurance.
Social insurance refers to the public sharing of the risks of ill health that would
otherwise go uninsured in a purely market-based system. Certain inefficiencies
of the private provision of health insurance can also reflect market failures. While
these inefficiencies point to the need for public intervention, efficiency considerations alone do not justify full public insurance. In the final analysis, the logic of
social insurance is its compelling rationale. Given this equity-based argument for
public intervention, decisions about the role of the federal government revolve
primarily around the extent to which the relevant sharing community for social

insurance purposes is seen to be the country as a whole rather than individual provinces and territories. The extent of the federal role and the mix of preferred instruments depend upon the societal consensus about the sharing community, suitably tempered by efficiency considerations.

In this chapter we develop this argument in distinct steps. First we set the context of the discussion by providing a brief overview of the setting for the debate, focusing on the constitutional framework and the current federal-provincial balance in health care. We go on to examine the general rationale for a public role in the health care sector, emphasizing especially the area of health insurance. Building on this analysis, we consider the role of government in a federal state, and in particular the role of the federal government in health care. After discussing the choice of instruments through which the federal government conducts its role, we pull the threads of the discussion together by examining the ways in which judgments on each of the three dimensions of choice may be combined in the debate over the federal role in health care in Canada.

A word of caution is in order at the outset. Our concern is the role of the federal government in health care, not health policy or the management of the health sector *per se*. This both limits the extent of our inquiry and requires that we take as given certain features of the policy environment, while recognizing that these could change. As a consequence, our discussion of federal policy instruments is presented at a level of generality so as to encompass the possibility of evolving policies.

FEDERALISM AND HEALTH CARE: THE CONTEXT

I n this section we present a brief survey of the context of federalism and health care in Canada, examining the constitutional division of powers in the field, the evolution of the role of the federal government in health care, the structure of financial transfers to the provinces which have underpinned that role, and the growing controversy that has surrounded federal-provincial relations in recent years.

The Constitutional Framework

The emergence of the modern social role of the state posed a constitutional dilemma for Canada. The *Constitution Act, 1867* was very much a document of the nineteenth century, reflecting nineteenth-century conceptions of the appropriate role of government. The health and social needs of Canadians in 1867 were very much a private matter for the individual, the family, the church, and charitable institutions, and the state's role was largely confined to rudimentary forms of relief for the poor administered through local agencies. Not surprisingly, such a minor function of government did not attract a lot of attention either in the debates that preceded Confederation or in the constitution itself, and twentieth-century words such as "health care" or "income security" or "social services" did not appear in the list of jurisdictions allocated to the two senior levels of government. When the social role of the state began to expand in the twentieth century, Canada had to resolve the division of responsibility in new domains of state action. This resolution came slowly through a variety of mechanisms. In part, jurisdiction was inferred from other powers in the constitution; in areas such as unemployment insurance and pensions, the formal division of powers was altered through constitutional amendment. In other areas, more informal means of adjustment were employed.

In the case of health care, the constitution gives important powers to both the federal and provincial governments. As constitutional expert Peter Hogg observes: "Health is not a single matter assigned by the Constitution exclusively to one level of government"; rather, it is "an amorphous topic which is distributed to the federal Parliament or the provincial Legislatures depending on the purpose or effect of the particular health measure in issue" (Hogg 2000, 18.4; Lajoie and Molinari 1978, 579). Section 92 of the *Constitution Act, 1867* gave the provinces a central role in the field, and section 92(7) specifically grants to the provinces authority over hospitals. In addition, jurisdiction was inferred from other more general provincial powers, especially section 92(13) dealing with property and civil rights and section 92(16) dealing with matters of a local or private nature. In the early decades of the twentieth century, the courts held that these sections empowered provincial governments to regulate the medical professions and commercial insurance plans. This authority was extended to the new instrument of social insurance during the late 1930s. In striking down the 1935 federal New Deal legislation, the courts determined that social insurance programs financed in whole or in part by premiums paid by or on behalf of the potential beneficiary fall within provincial jurisdiction. The majority of the Supreme Court declared: "Insurance of all sorts, including insurance against unemployment and health insurances, have always been recognized as being exclusively provincial matters under the head 'Property and Civil Rights,'" or under the head 'Matters of a Merely Local or Private Nature in the Province'." And the Judicial Committee of the Privy Council, the final court of appeal at the time, concurred: "In pith and substance this *Act* is an insurance Act affecting the civil rights of employers and employed in each Province, and as such is invalid." Although subsequent amendments to the constitution gave the federal government jurisdiction over unemployment insurance and contributory pensions,[1] no such amendments took place in the case of health insurance. As a result, provinces have control over the medical professions, hospitals, and health insurance; these responsibilities clearly place them at the centre of health services.

The constitution also provides footing for a federal presence in health care. Authority over criminal law gives the federal government a role in the protection of public health through legislation such as the *Food and Drug Act* and the *Tobacco Products Control Act*. In addition, the federal *Narcotics Control Act* has been upheld under the "Peace, Order and Good Government (POGG)" clause.[2] Other sections of the constitution give the federal government responsibility for the welfare – including health care – of specific classes of people, including "Indians," "aliens," inmates in federal prisons, and members of the armed forces. In addition, the federal tax powers are the basis of extensive federal involvement in the financing of health care expenditures through the various tax credits allowed under the personal income tax system and GST exemptions; and the federal role in research gives federal agencies a major role in health research and information.

However, the federal government's primary role in health services for the population as a whole has developed through financial transfers to provincial governments. These transfers find their constitutional footing in section 36 of the *Constitution Act, 1982* and the doctrine of the federal spending power. Section 36(1) commits the federal and provincial governments to "promoting equal opportunities for the well-being of Canadians," and "providing essential public services of reasonable quality to all Canadians." Section 36(2) then commits both levels of government "to the principle of making equalization payments to ensure that provincial governments have sufficient revenues to provide reasonably comparable levels of public services at reasonably comparable levels of taxation." There is a debate about whether section 36 is simply a statement of principle that is non-justiciable, or whether it constitutes a distinct grant of authority to the federal government, especially in the case of equalization grants. As we shall see, however, the principle of equalization articulated in this section is fundamental to debates about the role of the federal government in health care.

The doctrine of the federal spending power has also been critical. This doctrine holds that "the federal Parliament may spend or lend its funds to any government or institution or individual it chooses, for any purpose it chooses; and that it may attach to any grant or loan any conditions it chooses, including conditions it could not directly legislate" (Hogg 2000, 6.8a). This power is not specified explicitly in the constitution but is inferred from federal powers to levy taxes, to legislate in relation to public property, and to appropriate federal funds. The idea of a federal spending power is not unique to Canada. In one form or other, other federations also recognize as constitutionally legitimate a federal spending power in areas of state or provincial jurisdiction (Watts 1999). In Canada, however, the use of the spending power has been controversial, and has been challenged both politically and judicially. In the mid-1950s, for example, Quebec's Royal Commission of Inquiry on Constitutional Problems (Tremblay Commission) asked: "What would be the use of a careful description of legislative powers if one of the governments could get around it and, to some extent, annul it by its taxation methods and its fashion of spending?" (Royal Commission on Constitutional Problems 1956, vol. 2, 216). Nevertheless, court decisions on the constitutionality of the spending power have repeatedly sustained the federal position, and federal transfers finding their constitutional footing on this power have played a central role in the evolution of health care in Canada.

The Evolution of the Federal Role in Health Care Services

The federal government plays a number of critical roles in health policy in Canada. It has a direct presence through a number of important programs that it delivers directly or through wider partnerships. These programs focus on research and evaluation, health promotion and protection, and support for health care information systems and infrastructure. In addition, the federal government is responsible for the direct delivery of the full range of health services to First Nations and the Inuit communities, and for some health services to the RCMP, Correctional Services, the Armed Forces, and veterans. Table 1 indicates the level of federal expenditures under these programs. Table 2 also shows the scope of federal support to health care spending through tax expenditures available to individuals and institutions in Canada.

Table 1

HEALTH CANADA'S SPENDING BY TYPE OF ACTIVITY, 2000/01

	Actual Spending (millions of dollars)	Percentage of Total Spending
Health care policy	112.6	4.8
Health promotion and protection	634.4	27.3
First Nations and Inuit health	1,266.5	54.6
Information and knowledge management	126.7	5.5
Departmental management and administration	180.3	7.8

Source: Health Canada, Departmental performance report (2000/2001), p. 25.

Table 2

PERSONAL INCOME TAX EXPENDITURES AND GST TAX EXPENDITURES RELATED TO HEALTH, 1996-2001 (millions of dollars)

	1996	1998	2001
Personal income tax expenditures			
Non-taxation of business-paid health and dental benefits	1,490	1,650	1,560
Disability tax credit	265	265	385
Medical expense credit	330	405	465
Medical expense supplement for earners	-	42	63
Sub-total	2,085	2,362	2,473
GST tax expenditures			
Prescription drugs	210	230	270
Medical devices	85	90	105
Health care services	490	545	630
Rebate for hospitals	235	265	325
Sub-total	1,020	1,130	1,330

Source: Department of Finance Canada, Tax expenditures and evaluations, various years (accessed October 10, 2003). www.fin.gc.ca/purl/taxexp-e.html

In addition to its directly delivered programs, however, the federal government has had a pervasive influence on the health services enjoyed by Canadians generally through its financial transfers to provincial governments, and it is this dimension of the federal role that constitutes the primary focus of this study (Standing Senate Committee 2001b). Historically, federal transfers to provinces helped define the basic parameters of the Canadian system of health care. While most of the key innovations emerged first at the provincial level, the federal government played a central role in the process. In the early stages, it played a *transformative* role by extending innovations that emerged in individual provinces across the country as a whole; in more recent decades, it has played a *sustaining* role, maintaining and reinforcing the pan-Canadian model.

In 1945, the federal government set the agenda for the postwar era by proposing a national program of health insurance as part of the policy package it presented to the Dominion-Provincial Conference on Reconstruction. When the larger package collapsed because of the rejection of the associated proposals for federal-provincial fiscal relations by Ontario and Quebec, initiative shifted to the provinces. In 1947 Saskatchewan introduced hospital insurance, and British Columbia and Alberta followed in quick succession. These governments repeatedly pressed for federal support of their programs, but Ottawa was initially reluctant. It introduced National Health Grants in 1948 to assist provinces with hospital construction and public health services, but insisted that it would support provincial health insurance programs only when a majority of the provinces representing a majority of the population was ready to join a nationwide scheme. In the mid-1950s, however, Ontario and Newfoundland joined the list of provinces demanding federal action, and the federal government introduced the *Hospital Insurance and Diagnostic Services Act, 1957*. The legislation passed unanimously in the House of Commons.

Under the 1957 legislation, the federal government shared the costs of provincial hospital insurance programs that met federal conditions. Provincial plans had to provide universal coverage to all residents of the province on uniform terms and conditions, include specified diagnostic services, and limit co-insurance or "deterrent" charges so as to ensure that an excessive financial burden was not placed on patients. In addition, provincial plans were subject to stringent federal auditing. Despite the federal controls, by 1961 all provinces had signed agreements to join the federal plan. Quebec was the last to join, and did so only with the advent of the new provincial Liberal government led by Jean Lesage. By 1964, however, the Hall Commission found fit to describe the program as a remarkably successful example of "cooperative federalism" (Royal Commission on Health Services 1964, 413).

Soon, however, negotiations for the introduction of medicare, which covered physicians' services, created more federal-provincial sparks. The medical profession and the insurance industry were strongly opposed, and ideological differences intensified intergovernmental conflict. Once again, Saskatchewan took the lead by introducing a universal model in the early 1960s and pressing for federal support. However, conservative governments in Alberta, British Columbia, and Ontario were committed to the principle of private health insurance for the majority of the population, and they implemented programs that limited the public role to hard-to-insure groups such as the elderly and the poor.[3] In 1965 the federal government chose to act and, prompted in part by the report of the Royal Commission on Health Services chaired by Emmett Hall, opted for the universal model pioneered in Saskatchewan. Although the new program started with fewer administrative and reporting controls than in the case of hospital insurance, the *Medical Care Act* of 1966 did establish four conditions. To qualify for federal support, provincial plans had to provide for: public administration of medical plans; coverage of "all services rendered by medical practitioners that are medically required"; universal coverage of provincial residents on equal terms and conditions; and the portability of benefits. There is some ambiguity about whether "access" was viewed as a co-equal fifth principle or condition at the time. The prime minister's speech to the federal-provincial conference in 1965 had not treated "reasonable access" as a formal principle. The 1966 legislation did require that insured persons not be charged fees that impede or preclude "reasonable access" to insured services; but uncertainty later emerged about whether the legal effect of this provision was simply to preclude provincial government charges for physicians' services or whether it also applied to extra-billing by physicians themselves. Whatever the uncertainties surrounding its origins, however, reasonable access soon evolved to the status of a co-equal principle.

The decision to join the 1966 medicare plan was difficult for the conservative governments in the three provinces that had to undo their recently established programs. The long-serving Alberta health minister resigned in protest, and Premier Robarts of Ontario denounced medicare as "a Machiavellian scheme" that was "one of the greatest frauds that has ever been perpetrated on the people of this country" (Taylor 1987, 375). Nonetheless, all provinces had medicare programs in place by 1971, three years after the implementation of the federal legislation.

With a cross-country health care system in place, the federal role began to shift subtly toward system maintenance. The first phase of this evolution came in 1977 with the transition to Established Program Financing (EPF), which will be discussed more fully below. The second was the passage of the *Canada Health Act* (CHA) in 1984. This legislation was a response to the growing prevalence in a number of provinces of extra-billing by doctors and the introduction of hospital fees, both of which the federal government opposed as inhibiting equal access to health care. The issues had been discussed in federal-provincial forums for years and examined in several joint studies, but the differences proved unbridgeable. When the Alberta government pressed the issue in 1983 by introducing a hospital fee of $20 a day, the federal government announced that it would legislate. The CHA introduced several important innovations. It amalgamated the previously separate hospital and medical insurance legislations, and established a fully integrated set of five "principles" that provincial health care plans would be required to meet to qualify for federal support. To the four conditions set out in the 1965 legislation, the CHA added the principle of "reasonable access" in order to prohibit charges at the point of service. To facilitate enforcement, the legislation determined that such charges would lead to dollar-for-dollar deductions in the federal transfer. Although provincial government were angered by the legislation, as we shall see in more detail below they generally moved to compliance over the next few years.

From this review, it is evident that the federal government played a central role in defining the basic policy framework that guided the development of the Canadian health care system in the early postwar decades, and in sustaining that framework on a countrywide basis in the decades that followed.

Transfers to the Provinces

An appreciation of the structure and evolution of federal fiscal transfers is critical to understanding federal-provincial tensions in the field, and a closer look at these transfers is worthwhile.

The nature of federal transfers has evolved as Ottawa has shifted from a transformative to a sustaining role in health care. In the early stages, when the emphasis was on building a countrywide system of health care, the favoured instrument was the shared-cost program. However, from the outset, federal support for health services differed in important ways from the classic shared-cost program, which is perhaps best typified by the case of social welfare. Prior to

1996 federal transfers for social welfare were based on cost sharing under the Canada Assistance Plan (CAP). For every dollar of eligible provincial expenditures, the federal government contributed one dollar. This system had some important consequences, which ultimately led to its demise. Since costs were shared only for expenditures deemed to be eligible by the federal government, provinces complained that federal conditions constrained their capacity to reform and redefine their programs. But in addition, some critics argued that the 50:50 sharing rule provided an incentive for provinces to expand the generosity of their programs, and the federal government did impose a "cap" on CAP growth for the three wealthiest provinces in 1990.

The approach taken in financing health care had some similarities to social welfare cost sharing. Under the terms of the 1957 *Hospital Insurance and Diagnostic Services Act* and the 1966 *Medical Care Act*, financial support was dependent on provincial acceptance of federal conditions, and covered only specified services, creating an incentive for provinces to expand those services at the expense of others (for example, hospital services rather than extended care). But there were also important differences. Under the 1957 legislation, provinces received 25 percent of provincial per capita costs and 25 percent of national per capita costs. Thus, while the federal government covered on average half of the costs, only 25 percent of individual provinces' incremental costs were covered, so the incentive effects on provincial spending were less than under CAP. In the case of the 1966 *Medical Care Act*, provinces received 50 percent of national average per capita costs, so there was no cost sharing at the margin. As a result, the financial formula in health care was closer to a block grant than a traditional matching one, and subsequent transitions were less dramatic than in the case of social welfare.

The shift in federal emphasis from transforming to sustaining the pan-Canadian model of health care soon left an imprint on the transfer system. By the mid-1970s, the provincial programs could be viewed as "established," and perhaps did not require the same level of federal intervention to encourage the provinces to maintain them. Moreover, the federal government worried that its open-ended commitment to pay half of provincial expenditures in a number of programs, including health care, was eroding its capacity to control its own budget. Provincial governments also had frustrations with the traditional shared-cost model. They sought escape from the onerous negotiations about eligibility issues, such as the need to decide which hospital beds were acute care beds and therefore eligible for cost sharing under the health care arrangements, and which hospital beds were long-term care beds that were not.

After extensive federal-provincial negotiations, a compromise emerged in the form of the Established Programs Financing (EPF). The transfers for hospital and medical services, as well as for post-secondary education, were combined in one block grant. The federal government gained greater predictability over increases to its financial commitment, which was no longer based on provincial expenditures but now was to escalate according to a formula based on the rate of growth in the economy as a whole. The provinces gained a further reduction in the specificity of federal administrative controls. Although the conditions attached to medicare remained in place, federal officials no longer had to rule on whether particular provincial expenditures were eligible for cost sharing.

The EPF transfer was an equal per capita payment to each province, of which half was initially paid as cash and the other half as a tax point transfer, which included 13.5 percentage points of personal income tax room and 1 percentage point of corporate income tax. Since the tax points were ultimately equalized, they too amounted to an equal per capita amount for the provinces receiving equalization. At the time of introduction of the EPF, the federal government adopted two practices in accounting that have been important to the politics of federal-provincial recrimination ever since. First, Ottawa nominally divided the EPF transfer into components for health and post-secondary education, using the proportions that existed at the time EPF was introduced. Second, it calculated its contribution to health care financing to include not only the cash transfer but also the value of the tax-point transfer. There is considerable debate about whether this is a meaningful practice, since for all intents and purposes the tax points, once transferred, became part of provincial own-source revenues. But the federal government has maintained the practice, especially as the share of the EPF transfer consisting of cash has declined gradually, partly because the value of the tax points grew more rapidly than GNP, and partly because the federal government from time to time reduced the rate of growth temporarily for fiscal reasons. Table 3 tracks the resulting shift in the balance between the cash and the tax transfer.

The next significant change in the form of the federal transfers for health services came in 1995 with the introduction of the Canada Health and Social Transfer (CHST), which combined EPF and the previously separate transfer for social welfare into a single block transfer. The impetus for this change was more fiscal than structural. The federal government found itself in an untenable deficit

Table 3

HEALTH PORTION OF FEDERAL TRANSFERS TO PROVINCES

(billions of dollars)

	Cash Transfer	Tax Transfer	Total Transfer
1977/78	2.8	1.9	4.7
1982/83	5.0	3.6	8.7
1987/88	7.1	5.5	12.6
1992/93	8.2	6.7	14.9
1996/97	6.3	8.3	14.6
2000/01	8.1	10.4	18.5

Source: Department of Finance Canada, Backgrounder on federal support for health in Canada (March 29, 2000), p. 9.

and debt situation, and embarked on an expenditure-cutting strategy. Transfers to the provinces were cut as part of the exercise, with the severity of the cut depending on how one did the calculation. If one measured the cut in federal transfers using both cash and tax points as the basis (as did the federal government), the cut in transfers was in line with federal expenditure cuts more generally. However, as a proportion of federal cash transfers, the cuts in federal transfers to the provinces were significantly greater than those in other elements of the budget.

Although the impetus was fiscal, several features of the CHST should be mentioned. First, unlike the EPF and CAP systems, growth in the transfer under the CHST is no longer formula-based but is decided at the discretion of the federal government. This discretionary power reinforces concern that the federal government increasingly makes unilateral and unannounced changes to major transfer programs. Second, the CHST maintains the practice established with the EPF of breaking down the amounts, notionally intended for health, post-secondary education, and social welfare. Thus, 43 percent of the CHST cash component is attributed to health. This breakdown is purely nominal, however: there is no mechanism to ensure that provinces actually spend their allocations according to those ratios. Indeed, the funds once received are fully fungible, so it would be impossible to enforce the allocations.

Some lessons from this experience are relevant for subsequent discussions. The first is that federal transfers for health care have always been large-ly block transfers rather than matching ones. The exception is the 25 percent matching component in the original hospital grants. The 50:50 sharing rule applied more to the overall size of the grant than to its relationship with indi-vidual provinces' expenditures. The second is that similar general conditions have been maintained throughout important changes in the underlying struc-ture of transfers. As we have seen, the switch to EPF and the introduction of the CHST did not alter the conditions or principles associated with the health transfer at the time the changes were made. Third, probably the most signifi-cant historical shift was the introduction of the EPF, which produced an instantaneous splitting of the transfer into cash and tax point transfer compo-nents. This division was to become a slow-acting poison pill in federal-provin-cial relations, since there was no longer an agreed answer to the question of what proportion of provincial health expenditures was met by the federal gov-ernment. This poison pill began to take effect as the rate of growth in the trans-fer declined, and intensified its action when the formula-based rate of growth of block transfers for social programs was abolished with the introduction of the CHST. The fact that the size of the CHST is now at the discretion of the federal government is itself a cause of contention. In addition, the precipitous decline in the cash component has put the controversy over the tax point trans-fer component more fully in the spotlight.

The cumulative effect of these trends is that the transition from the use of health transfers for transformative to maintenance purposes essentially involved changes in the level of transfers but not necessarily to their basic form. Separate health transfers enabled the federal government to encourage the provinces to introduce public hospital insurance and public medical insur-ance sequentially. In each case, the transfer was largely a block payment, with the federal government contributing roughly half the *national* share of costs. Once the programs were established, they were amalgamated into a single block transfer along with post-secondary education and, later, welfare, and the size of the transfer was reduced, gradually at some points and more dramati-cally at others. The basic assumption was that the transformative role required more of a federal presence than the maintenance role. However, the question as to whether the federal financial commitment has fallen below the level need-ed to support this maintenance role is now a source of considerable intergov-ernmental tension.

The Growth of Intergovernmental Tensions

The recent history of federal-provincial relations in health care has been punctuated by dramatic political conflicts, and provinces have increasingly challenged the federal role in health care. In part, the challenge is a long-standing one. The government of Quebec in particular has consistently denied the legitimacy of the federal spending power and its role in health care. This orientation is based on its traditional interpretation of the constitution, and reflects a distinctive political identity and a desire to preserve a greater level of self-determination. In recent years, however, other provinces have also challenged the federal role in health care. In contrast to Quebec, their challenge flows less from constitutional doctrine than from frustration with a long series of federal program changes.

The fundamental issue is the growing gap between the policy role and the financial role of the federal government. On the policy side, the federal government has continued to defend the general parameters of the universal model of health care. Its most forceful step was the introduction of the *Canada Health Act* in 1984. This Act was opposed by all provincial governments and became a symbol of federal unilateralism. But the legislation was immensely popular with the electorate, and it passed unanimously in the House of Commons. Despite an unprecedented appearance by provincial health ministers before the Senate, approval in that chamber was also unanimous. The federal government proceeded to implement the legislation, withholding a total of $247 million from provinces that allowed extra-billing or user charges. Although these penalties were to be refunded when provinces came into compliance with the Act, it was the public support for the *Canada Health Act* that convinced provinces to comply. Provincial authorities often had to face difficult negotiations with the medical profession, which demanded higher fee schedules to compensate for the banning of extra-billing. Ontario had to cope with a twenty-five-day strike by a majority of doctors, and Saskatchewan doctors held a series of rotating one-day strikes. The final settlements with the doctors raised provincial costs in a number of provinces but, given the block nature of the federal transfer, provinces had to absorb the increase themselves (Tuohy 1994b). In the end, all of the federal withholdings were refunded, but the provinces had to cope with the larger financial fallout of federal policy.

In contrast to its forceful policy role, federal financial support for health care has been weakened by a long series of unilateral decisions. In 1986

Ottawa limited the indexation of its transfers to the increase in GDP less 2 percentage points; in 1990 federal transfers were frozen in absolute terms, a freeze that lasted for four years; and in 1995 the combined cash transfer for health, welfare, and post-secondary education under the new CHST was cut by approximately $6 billion. Although the government reversed this cut by increasing funding during the subsequent election campaign and several times since then, its contribution to health costs has clearly declined over time. How deep the erosion has been depends on how one defines the "real" federal contribution. The federal government insists that its contribution includes both the annual cash transfer and the value of the tax points. Provinces reply that the tax points are part of the general provincial tax base and that the federal contribution is limited to the cash transfer. From the provincial perspective, the key story is a continuous decline in the federal cash transfer as a proportion of provincial health expenditures.

Table 4 illustrates the difference between the federal and provincial views. As these data show, the notional cash contribution of the federal government as a proportion of provincial health expenditures has eroded continuously since the late 1970s, and especially since the advent of the CHST in 1995. At the same time, the proportion accounted for by the tax point transfer has held its own. In the federal view, the total transfer (cash plus tax points) accounted for almost 30 percent of provincial health expenditures in 2000 compared with about 40 percent in 1977, a decline of close to a third. From the provinces' perspective, the federal contribution over the same period fell from about 25 percent to about 13 percent, a decline of about one-half.

The tension between the policy and financial roles of the federal government embittered federal-provincial relations and made enforcement of the conditions of the *Canada Health Act* more politically difficult. The federal government has never penalized provinces for non-compliance with the five basic principles enunciated in the Act, despite concerns raised by the Auditor General of Canada and others about portability, comprehensiveness, and accessibility (Auditor General of Canada 1999). However, Ottawa has penalized provinces for permitting extra-billing and user fees, and its action against facility fees sparked a bitter controversy. The 1990s witnessed the growth of private clinics providing specialized medical services and charging patients a "facility fee," which in some cases was substantial. The federal government argued that such fees created differential access to medical care and thereby violated the *Canada Health Act*. In 1995 Ottawa

Table 4

FEDERAL GOVERNMENT TRANSFERS FOR HEALTH CARE AS A SHARE OF
PROVINCIAL GOVERNMENTS' EXPENDITURES ON HEALTH CARE, 1975-2000
(percent)

Year	Cash	Tax	Total
1975	41.3		41.3
1976	40.5		40.5
1977	25.2	17.1	42.3
1978	26.1	17.1	44.0
1979	27.0	17.5	44.5
1980	25.3	17.7	43.7
1981	24.1	17.2	41.3
1982	22.7	16.4	39.5
1983	24.1	15.1	39.2
1984	24.0	15.6	39.6
1985	23.8	15.6	39.7
1986	22.9	16.1	39.0
1987	21.6	16.8	38.4
1988	20.4	16.8	37.2
1989	19.1	16.8	36.1
1990	17.9	16.0	33.9
1991	17.1	14.7	31.9
1992	17.0	13.9	30.9
1993	16.9	14.2	31.1
1994	16.6	14.7	31.3
1995	16.4	15.8	32.1
1996	12.9	16.9	29.8
1997	10.6	17.9	28.5
1998	10.0	17.9	27.9
1999	12.7	17.4	30.1
2000	12.8	16.5	29.3

Source: Calculated using transfer data from the Department of Finance Canada and expenditure data from the Canadian Institute for Health Information (CIHI).

began to compute penalties under the Act for four provinces: Alberta, Manitoba, Newfoundland, and Nova Scotia (see Table 5). The conflict was sharpest with Alberta, where government support for private clinics was strongest.[4] Over several years, however, the provinces largely moved into compliance. Nevertheless, the coincidence of the unilateral introduction of the CHST, a large cut in funding, and the campaign against facility fees generated deep anger in several provinces and a broad-based provincial questioning of the legitimacy of the federal role.

The complexities of these debates are explored in the other chapters of this volume. However, the lesson is clear. It is time to step back from the day-to-day battles, and to reflect once again on fundamental questions about federalism and health care. What is the appropriate role of the state in health care? What are the basic principles and considerations that should inform debates about the federal role in health care? What are the choices, and what is at stake in choosing among them? These questions are taken up in the sections that follow.

THE GENERAL RATIONALE FOR STATE INTERVENTION IN THE HEALTH ARENA

As noted earlier, the case for federal intervention in the health sector presupposes some general rationale for government intervention in the first place. Moreover, different attitudes about the nature of the general role for government inform the debate over federal and provincial responsibilities.

Health care services are unlike most other goods and services used by persons in the market economy. Resources used in the health sector are not allocated solely, or even primarily, by the price mechanism. Governments are heavily involved in the various stages of their provision, including the training of professionals who deliver health care, the regulation or provision of various forms of health care services and products, the financing of health costs, regulation of health standards in product markets and places of employment, public education, research and development, and the prevention and eradication of various forms of disease.

In this section we outline the arguments for government intervention in health care. Policy analysts often find it useful to disaggregate these arguments into two main sorts – those concerned with efficiency and those concerned with equity. Although in the end the two sorts of arguments are interdependent, the

Table 5

DEDUCTIONS FROM PROVINCIAL TRANSFERS UNDER THE CANADA HEALTH ACT
IN THE 1990S (thousands of dollars)

	Nfld	PEI	NS	NB	Que	Ont	Man	Sask	Alta	BC	Can
1992/93										83	83
1993/94										1,223	1,223
1994/95										676	676
1995/96	46		32				269		2,319	43	2,709
1996/97	96		72				588		1,266		2,022
1997/98	128		57				587				772
1998/99	53		39				612				704
1999/00			48								48

Source: Standing Senate Committee on Social Affairs, Science and Technology, *The Story So Far*. Vol. 2 of *The Health of Canadians – The Federal Role. Interim Report* (Ottawa: Queen's Printer for Canada, March 2001), table 2.3, p. 39.

distinction remains a useful one, and we adopt it here. The outcome of this discussion and an evaluation of the legitimacy of the various arguments for state intervention will serve as important considerations for our subsequent discussion of the role of the federal government. We begin with efficiency considerations, since economists typically invoke these as the main source of market failure. However, as will become clear, the primary rationale for government intervention in health care is based on redistributive equity or social insurance grounds. Efficiency considerations are nonetheless important for selecting among policy instruments for achieving these social objectives.

Efficiency and Market Failure

Markets are efficient mechanisms for allocating resources to the extent that they result in all "gains from trade" being exploited. Well-functioning competitive markets have the feature that the market price reflects both the benefit to the user of the last unit purchased and the cost to the supplier of the last unit produced. At quantities below that, the benefit of an additional unit of product would exceed the cost of providing another unit, so mutually beneficial gains can be obtained by expanding output, and vice versa for quantities above that. A *prime facie* case for government intervention exists whenever the benefit to users of an additional unit consumed exceeds the resource cost of producing another unit.

Public finance economists have identified a number of situations in which markets may fail to provide certain types of goods or services efficiently. Some of the more important ones include the following:

> *The free-rider problem*: Persons cannot be easily excluded from obtaining the benefits of some goods (for example, public goods) so will not willingly pay a price for them.

> *Externalities*: The production or consumption of some products yields benefits or costs to third parties that are not reflected in market prices.

> *Increasing returns to scale*: Competition cannot be sustained, so the market ends up being served by a small number of firms who are able to restrict output and increase prices above marginal costs.

> *Asymmetric information*: One side of the market is better informed than the other side; the better informed party has a form of informational advantage analogous to a monopoly advantage, and is able to manipulate prices in its favour.

> *Coordination problems*: In a changing world, supply decisions and demand decisions taken at the same time are not always coordinated, so prices are temporarily out of equilibrium, and the amounts demanded and supplied are not equalized.

> *Transaction costs*: Trading in the real world can be a complicated matter, and resources must be used up in purely administrative costs (legal fees, advertising, record-keeping, and overhead).

Some or all of these elements are present in the markets for health services and products. In fact, health care consists of a wide variety of types of goods and services, including medical care, hospitals, diagnostic services, pharmaceuticals, prosthetics, immunization, preventive measures, and so on. Different aspects of health care may be subject to different forms of market failure. However, asymmetric information, economies of scale, and externalities in particular, inform debates about the role of government in health care, including especially the choice of policy instruments. We begin with the sources of market failure that have dominated much of the economics debate – moral hazard and adverse selection – before turning to those that might be more important in establishing a role for public provision of health care per se.

Asymmetric Information and Moral Hazard

Moral hazard is one consequence of asymmetric information. It occurs when one side of a transaction cannot observe actions or characteristics of the other side that affect the benefits generated from the transaction. It is especially prone to happen in insurance situations when an insurer cannot observe the behaviour or the state of persons being insured. Moral hazard can take two forms – an *ex ante* form and *ex post* form. *Ex ante* moral hazard occurs when preventive action cannot be observed. The existence of insurance provides an incentive for persons to reduce their level of preventive effort, thereby increasing either the probability of an insurable outcome or its magnitude. Thus, fire insurance may induce persons to be less vigilant, and automobile insurance may induce them to drive less safely. *Ex post* moral hazard occurs when the severity of insurable outcomes can be mitigated by compensating expenditures. Theft insurance may replace items that are stolen, but these are difficult to verify. In either case, the insurance providers will react by restricting the amount of insurance that can be purchased by devices such as co-payments or deductibles. This is inefficient in the sense that if preventive actions and *ex post* compensating expenditures could be perfectly monitored, insurance could be made contingent on them and full insurance could be provided.

Health care is prone to both types of moral hazard, especially to the *ex post* form. Once persons become ill, to the extent that health insurance covers the cost of curative expenditures, there will be an incentive to incur inefficiently large amounts of care. Health insurance may also induce lower levels of preventive expenditures. In these circumstances, insurance will again be inefficient, and in private markets this would be reflected in user charges either of the co-payment or the deductible form.

The extent of the inefficiency due to moral hazard depends upon the extent of discretion available to users of health care services. Clearly there are many forms of service over which the insured person has limited discretion. For medical, hospital, and diagnostic services, health care professionals have much more discretion than those being insured. In these cases, moral hazard applies more to the behaviour of these professionals than to the person using the health services. The moral hazard problem then turns into a problem involving incentives facing those who deliver the services. Various forms of payment can be used to mitigate the problem, such as capitation and salary components alongside, or instead of, fees for service.

For our purposes, however, the asymmetric information problems that give rise to moral hazard are not likely to be significantly different for public health insurance than for private health insurance. The implication is that, although moral hazard leads to inefficiency, it does so whether the insurance is provided by the public sector or the market. Market failure due to moral hazard does not imply an efficiency case for public provision. In fact, it does not even imply that public intervention in other ways (subsidization and regulation, for example) is justified. Private market responses to moral hazard using co-insurance or deductible provisions to limit the extent of insurance turn out to be efficient responses, given the information available, and there is no guarantee that public interference with these market mechanisms will improve efficiency.

Asymmetric Information and Adverse Selection

A second consequence of asymmetric information is adverse selection. Adverse selection occurs when persons face systematically different risks because of different personal characteristics. If insurers could classify persons according to their risk class, they would charge appropriately different insurance premiums to reflect the likelihood of claims. This would be an efficient thing to do. However, if households cannot be so classified, inefficient outcomes will prevail. There are two possibilities. If insurance companies cannot identify the total amount of insurance households buy, the best they can do is offer a uniform insurance contract — a so-called pooling contract — to all persons regardless of risk class. Such insurance will be inefficient because low-risk persons will face excessive premiums given their level of risk, and will therefore underinsure. On the other hand, if insurers can observe the quantity of insurance each person buys, they can make available different quantity/price combinations that induce households to self-select (referred to as separating contracts). Once again, this is inefficient because the package intended for low-risk persons cannot be generous enough to attract high-risk purchasers. More important, in this case there may be no equilibrium in the insurance industry. Insurers will attempt to cream off the low-risk persons, but in so doing they will force other insurers to make a loss and revise their policies. Notice that this adverse selection argument relies on persons themselves being better informed than insurance companies about their risk class.

Adverse selection problems might plague private markets for health insurance. If insurance companies cannot perfectly observe the risk of ill health for individuals as well as the individuals themselves can, they cannot tailor insurance policies efficiently. Private insurance markets will at best be inefficient, at worst unstable. Whether or not adverse selection is a quantitatively significant problem is an open question. In the case of health care, it is certainly conceivable that insurance companies can make themselves as well informed as persons seeking insurance. Indeed, this ability may well increase dramatically to the extent that DNA profiling becomes possible.

As in the case of moral hazard, however, it is not obvious that the government can do better than private markets. It is not likely to be better informed than insurance companies. The one possible form of intervention that might improve efficiency is to mandate compulsory insurance coverage. This at least avoids the problem of unstable insurance markets that never reach equilibrium outcomes. However, as in the case of automobile insurance, there is no particular reason why the mandatory insurance provided must be public rather than private.

It should be pointed out that from a pure efficiency point of view, the fact that persons are in different risk classes is itself not relevant. A fully efficient health insurance scheme would be one that charged higher premiums to those who are at greater risk of becoming ill. Indeed, there may be some persons who are virtually uninsurable because of their level of risk. And, those who are more at risk may well have fewer resources with which to purchase insurance.

In fact, it may well be that insurance companies can end up doing *too much* sorting of households by risk class, the opposite of an adverse selection problem. This might occur to the extent that insurance is for a limited term. Thus, after households incur an illness, it will be in the interests of the insurance company to change the terms of a policy once it comes up for renewal. If insurance policies are not long-lasting, persons who become ill may subsequently be uninsurable. To the extent that this occurs, insurance might be considered inefficient from an *ex ante* point of view since individuals are unable to insure themselves fully against all future health contingencies (Cutler 2002). One might have thought that markets would take care of this problem by offering very long-term insurance contracts. But insurance companies may be unable to do so because of the uncertainties that exist about future medical technologies and costs. It might be argued that the prevalence of occupational health insurance plans is a partial response to this problem, since they offer more permanent protection to employees who become ill. A full response might involve public provision, which effectively pools all risk types together whether they are privately insurable or not.

In fact, the case for public insurance based on the uninsurability of households that have become ill in the past is basically the same as the social insurance rationale for public insurance discussed below. Whether it is considered an efficiency or an equity rationale is an open question. In our discussion, we treat it as an equity rationale.

If moral hazard and adverse selection do not point to an efficiency case for public intervention, other considerations do raise relevant concerns.

Asymmetric Information and the Monopoly Power of Health Care Providers

Another form of asymmetric information is more relevant for the health care sector, and that is the imbalance among service providers, clients, and those financing health care. A significant feature of health care is that the providers are typically much better informed than the individuals being served or the institutions doing the insuring. Their skills ensure that they have effective control over the supply of health care. Moreover, in many cases, health professionals have collective control over the supply of their numbers as well as over other aspects of their behaviour (training, discipline, and remuneration). A substantial proportion of the costs of training health care professionals is either directly or indirectly borne by the public sector. These facts suggest that some collectivization of the demand or financing side is called for as a counterweight. In the absence of such collectivization, suppliers of health care would effectively be in a near-monopoly position, with the result that market prices would be excessive and supply inadequate.

In fact, some of this tendency to monopolization might be countered by the existence of large insurance companies, but that possibility gives rise to a category of problems considered next. The desire to have a collective institution acting as a counterweight to the inevitable existence of monopoly on the supply side of health care constitutes an argument for the single-payer system of financing health care. A single payer serves to ensure that the monopoly power of suppliers is not exploited by excessive prices for health care services and costs of health care professionals, which constitute the bulk of the costs of health care. Moreover, the obvious choice of a single payer is the public sector. The alternative would be to create a private monopoly representing suppliers, and that would have its own disadvantages.

Economies of Scale, Administrative Costs, and Cost Control

Economies of scale constitute another source of monopolistic tendency in addition to the information advantages just discussed. In industries characterized by economies of scale, it is hard to maintain the amount of competition required to generate an efficient allocation of resources. In such circumstances, governments might intervene by public ownership or by regulation in an effort to avoid the monopolistic tendencies that would otherwise arise. However, it is hard to maintain that scale is a determining issue in the health sector, since health services are typically delivered to individuals by small units such as doctors' practices and hospitals. The most likely candidates for non-competitive behaviour arising from economies of scale might be insurance companies. These must be large enough to be able to diversify insurance risks, so scale is obviously important to them. But a number of insurance companies offer supplementary health insurance plans at the moment, and entry into the industry is open. Given that the products they provide are reasonably close substitutes, it does not take a large number of firms to ensure competitiveness. Moreover, even if scale were a problem, it is not clear that public provision would be the best policy response.

Administrative costs, however, do represent a more compelling argument for a public role. There is evidence from the United States that the purely administrative costs of using private insurance as the primary means of financing health care are very high as a proportion of health care expenditures. There may be various reasons for this. One is that private insurers might be willing to incur costs of advertising and other measures to diversify their products in a world where products are otherwise very similar. Private insurance might lead to more litigation, with the ensuing costs of settling claims. Administrative costs are imposed on doctors and hospitals who must deal with several insurance companies. There are also costs associated with acquiring the kind of detailed information that is necessarily involved in providing insurance, as well as various legal costs. These considerations suggest that there may be significant economies to be gained from single-payer systems. Given that, there are also advantages in the single payer being the public sector in order to avoid the obvious disadvantages of a monopoly private insurer.

Finally, many analysts contend that a single-payer system provides for more effective cost control in health care for reasons that go beyond administrative costs and countering the potential monopoly power of health providers. It is often argued that, in the context of multiple payers in health services, attempts to contain health spending in one area simply shift the pressures elsewhere in the system, much as when a balloon, squeezed at one end, expands at the other. This tendency for cost containment to be weakened by cost shifting has been discussed extensively in the United States, where efforts to contain costs in public programs such as Medicare and Medicaid led providers such as hospitals to transfer more of the costs to private insurers. In contrast, a single-payer model provides more powerful levers of cost control. Canadian provinces approximate the single-payer model, and when they sought to limit their costs, especially between 1992 and 1997, service providers were left with nowhere to shift their costs. Presumably, more effective cost containment contributes to efficiency in a wider sense by containing pressures for upward movement in the taxes associated with health care.

Externalities and Public Goods

Many forms of health services have an aspect of public good or externality to them. Control of communicable disease is an obvious example. Others include sanitation, health safety regulation, water quality, and air quality. The provision of health-related information constitutes a health service in a broader sense. Examples include information regarding healthy activities and health promotion measures. In all of these cases, private provision would be inefficient because of the free-rider problem. There seems to be little dispute about the rationale for government intervention in these cases, although the form of the intervention may be in dispute (witness the debate over privatization of water provision and regulation).

Summarizing the Efficiency Case

In summary, there is an efficiency case for government intervention in the health care field. This case does not depend primarily on moral hazard, adverse selection, or economies of scale. Although moral hazard and adverse selection may well be present in the health sector, the public sector is not likely to be able to overcome the informational problems that give rise to these phenomena. At best, there might be arguments for mandatory health insurance, which might be provided either privately or publicly, to overcome the consequences of adverse selection. Nor are there arguments based on economies of scale. However, there are efficiency arguments for a single-payer system, to avoid what seem to be excessive administrative costs of operating private health insurance, to balance the collective organizations representing health care professionals, and to enhance the capacity for effective cost control. There is also a strong case for public intervention in areas of public health, public safety, and public information.

While the efficiency case for public intervention is important, it is sub-

ject to two qualifications. First, although the failures of the private sector constitute a necessary prerequisite for state intervention, they are not sufficient. There
may be shortcomings in public sector solutions as well. We have already referred
to the fact that the government may be no better informed than the private sector and therefore may not be able to overcome moral hazard and adverse selection any better. In addition, there may be various sources of failure that temper
the case for government intervention. One source of failure is that the public sector may be prone to its own forms of inefficiency. Since it does not have the discipline of competition, it is argued that there are not the same incentives for cost
effectiveness that exist in the private sector. This constitutes a caveat that might
be set against the advantages of a public single-payer system. However, there are
some substitute devices that may be used to enhance public sector efficiency. One
that is relevant in federations is decentralization, which may induce forms of
political competition conducive to efficiency. A second is the use of the private
sector to supply services even where they are being financed publicly. There may
also be various ways of enhancing the accountability of public health care, such
as the provision of full information to the public and the use of public audits.

Second, while these efficiency arguments are important, they may not
seem sufficient, on their own, to justify fully the kinds of state intervention that
one observes in almost all OECD countries (with the major exception of the
United States), the most apparent of which is the provision of more or less universal coverage of basic medical and hospital services. This is an outcome that
goes beyond a single-payer system and the provision of public health. It generates a much different allocation of health services to individuals than the market
system would entail. The case for this type of approach must be based on considerations other than economic efficiency, to which we now turn.

Redistributive Equity, Social Justice, and Sharing

Much of government policy is concerned with redistribution in favour of
those who are deemed to be deserving or in need. Modern redistribution theory
posits that individuals differ in a variety of characteristics, all of which affect the
outcomes they face in the market economy. A distinction is often made between
those characteristics for which differences ought to be compensated – the "principle of compensation" – and those for which the individual is deemed responsible
– the "principle of responsibility" (Roemer 1998). In the latter category one might

include individual preferences, such as the taste for leisure, the choice of automobiles, smoking, and the like. In the former category, one would include differences in income-earning ability, inherited wealth, and, more relevant for our purposes, differences in health status that are not fully under the control of the individual. Ideally, governments might be willing to compensate fully for differences over which the individual has no control, but not for differences that result from individual decisions, although in practice the two may not be perfectly distinguishable.

Debates about redistribution in the health sector are conditioned by two critical characteristics that set many forms of health care aside from other products and services. First, the need for health care is typically uncertain, or risky: it is only needed in the event of ill health. Second, the risk of ill health is unevenly distributed among the population as a whole. Markets can often be established to pool or share risk among members of the population at large, especially when outcomes are randomly distributed among the population. However, risks of ill health are not always insurable on the same terms among different members of the population. Some persons have a systematically higher risk of illness than others. Private insurance companies would offer appropriately different terms to persons with different levels of insurability, and those with a higher risk of illness could only be insured at much higher costs. Indeed, some may be virtually uninsurable in the sense that the chances of their falling ill are very high. Moreover, one's insurability can change over time as one's risk of illness varies. A person who acquires heart disease is unlikely to be able to purchase health insurance easily after that fact becomes known. Thus, the extent of insurability depends upon the extent to which one's susceptibility to ill health is already known. The extreme case of this change in insurability occurs at birth, since one is typically born with particular health characteristics, making some persons more insurable than others. However, one's insurability at birth is in some sense a matter of luck: some persons are born luckier than others.

The institution of social insurance is used to capture and offset this kind of luck. Social insurance is the term used by economists for schemes that compensate persons for bad luck even if it arises in an uninsurable form, as in the case of differing degrees of illness insurability. The notion that individuals ought to be compensated for their inherent difference in health status is a normative principle which incorporates a value judgment that not all will accept. However, it is a principle that is consistent with the observed tendency of governments to redistribute extensively through the health care system.

It is important to note that the meaning of social insurance as it is used here in the economic sense differs from that used in some other contexts, including legal ones. The key feature that makes it social rather than private insurance is that payouts are conditioned mainly by need rather than by purely actuarial, or insurance profitability, principles. In a sense, social insurance requires that the relevant risks be pooled across society as a whole, whether its members are insurable or not. Moreover, there is no need for social insurance to be financed by contributions, or if it is, for contributions to bear a close relation to expected benefits. On the contrary, full redistributive equity is better achieved if the system is financed out of general revenues. This differs from the definition of social insurance in constitutional jurisprudence discussed in the last section, which conceived of social insurance more narrowly as insurance delivered by the public sector but having important characteristics normally associated with private insurance. In that context, social insurance refers to public schemes in which there is some relation between contributions and expected benefits, albeit not necessarily fully actuarial (Myles and Pierson 1997). Contributors acquire an entitlement to some level of benefits in the future, as in unemployment insurance or public pensions such as the Canada and Quebec Pension Plans. As we saw, the challenge to the constitutionality of federal programs in these two areas in the 1930s turned in large part on their contributory nature. This is of more than pedantic relevance to the issues at hand. If schemes that are social insurance in the economic sense but are financed out of general revenues are not considered to be social insurance in a legal sense, the federal government might have wider latitude to implement them without running afoul of the constitution.

Even if one accepts the economist's notion of social insurance, its implementation is not straightforward. As with differences in productive ability, differences in health status – and therefore differences in illness insurability – cannot be readily observed by government. If they could be, transfers could be made contingent on health status to compensate different persons for differences in private insurability. These would be sufficient to allow everyone to buy full coverage of basic insurance at actuarial rates.[5] However, with health status unobservable, any compensation scheme must rely on actual usage of the health care system, which points to a larger role for public health insurance.

Several points should be noted about the sort of coverage that would be appropriate under a system motivated by social insurance rather than simply by efficiency:

> Since the idea of social insurance is to compensate persons, regardless of

their means, for differences in health status, basic forms of health care would be available universally to all persons. This would be like a universal pooling insurance scheme available equally to all individuals but also financed out of a common pool of general revenues that is structured with ability to pay (vertical equity) taken into account. This pooling can equivalently be viewed, along with other schemes of redistribution, as a form of *community sharing*. All members of the relevant community are treated uniformly by the social insurance system. What "relevant community" means is important in a federal context, and we shall return to that issue in the next section.

> The pattern of health expenditures across households would be far different from that found under a private insurance scheme. In particular, there would be a significant redistributive component implicit in the health care system (except in the very unlikely event that there was a perfect negative correlation between higher incomes and good health status). Lower-income households would obtain much higher benefits from the system than they could pay for – or would be willing to pay for – on the private market, and vice versa for higher-income persons. However, there would also be implicit redistribution among individuals within income groups since some would have better health characteristics than others. The point is that an income tax transfer system could not possibly be relied on to compensate deserving persons, given the inability of governments to target those with a higher risk of illness.[6]

> This inability in turn implies that the private sector could not be left to itself to provide social insurance. In principle, the public sector could fund the provision of basic health services through its general revenue-raising system and still allow the health services to be provided in a regulated manner by private providers. But, even in this case, there is no real role for private insurers, since the government does the financing out of general revenues. Notice that a social insurance system is effectively a single-payer system, so would capture some of the advantages of such systems noted in the previous discussion.

> A system of social insurance does not get around incentive problems, which arise precisely because individual health characteristics and behaviour cannot be perfectly monitored. The presence of possibly adverse incentive effects gives rise to an efficiency/equity trade-off that

might be addressed, for example, by user fees. A concern with user fees is that they would be a deterrent to lower-income households, and therefore violate the principle of social insurance unless they were somehow geared to income.

> The logic of social insurance itself does not reject a dual private/public system. As long as a public system is financed out of general revenues and makes health services uniformly available, the co-existence of a private system serving those who wish to opt out is not inconsistent with the principles of social insurance. Arguments to the contrary stem from judgments of political feasibility and the sustainability of a public system in the face of a parallel private one. Studies suggest that increases in private funding are associated with declines, over time, in allocation of public funds to health care (Flood, Stabile, and Tuohy 2002).

While the equity or social justice arguments are based on social insurance or community sharing, other related normative objectives are also relevant in the health context. One is equality of opportunity. In contrast with the standard notion of vertical equity, which concentrates on equalizing *ex post* market outcomes, equality of opportunity refers to equalizing the *ex ante* position of persons – equalizing the ability of different households to participate in the economic and social life of society. Good health, like education, contributes to this objective. Another social justice argument is economic security, which refers to offsetting the effects of unanticipated changes in one's economic circumstances. To the extent that ill health affects economic outcomes through lost productivity, health care contributes to economic security. This benefit is obviously of the same class of concerns as social insurance itself. Health care might also be seen as an important dimension of intergenerational equity. To the extent that there are arguments for redistributing from the current working generations to the elderly, the provision of health to the latter may be a particularly attractive means of making the transfer in a way that targets the most needy. Thus, even in the United States, where public health insurance is generally not available, it is available to retirees.

Finally, there is an argument, referred to as the Samaritan's dilemma (Buchanan 1975), which can be used to justify state intervention in insurance-type markets. The argument is that persons who expect to be cared for in the future will have less incentive to take measures to ensure their future well-being. Thus, they may acquire too little insurance, take too little care of themselves, engage in excessively risky activities, save too little for retirement, and undertake too little training. Government for its part is the Samaritan: it cannot help helping those in need in the future. Economists refer to this as the problem of time inconsistency. It has been used as an argument for state intervention in pensions, automobile insurance, unemployment insurance, and even education (Boadway and Keen 2000). It might also have some contributing relevance to state intervention in health insurance. If individuals do not insure themselves, in anticipation that they will be cared for by society in the event of major illness, the state might improve matters by instituting mandatory health insurance.

In weighing these various considerations of redistributive equity or social justice, however, the one based on social insurance seems to be the most convincing.

Summarizing the Case for a Public Role in Health Care

The case for a public role in the health sector is thus rooted in both efficiency and equity concerns. Efficiency considerations suggest that single-payer systems can reduce administrative costs, balance the collective organizations representing health care professionals, and strengthen the capacity to restrain the rate of growth in costs. Public action is also important to offset externalities in the field of public health. However, the scope and nature of government intervention in the health sector in most OECD countries, especially in the provision of health insurance, are also based heavily on concerns for equity and sharing. The most powerful rationale for state intervention in health care is based on the notion of social insurance. The core argument is that persons ought in principle to be compensated for differences in their risk of ill health, over which they have no control. This constitutes a form of community sharing, and in the final analysis, the equity argument for a public role depends on a collective sense of responsibility of citizens for each other.

It is worth re-emphasizing that the legitimacy of the social insurance role of government relies on acceptance of the values underlying it. Not surprisingly, therefore, debates over the appropriate role of public health policies are often controversial, and the level of consensus among the population is critical. Lack of unanimous consensus is a typical feature of redistributive policies. This is not just a matter of conflicting individual interests, but more importantly one of conflicting conceptions of the public interest. Some fear that policy will be determined more by special interests than by a broad consensus on the public interest. This problem has no easy remedy, and there will be those who take a more cynical view of government, and use it to argue against state intervention in health care. In the end, however, one must accept the legitimacy of decisions taken through our democratic institutions.

Recognition of the complex nature of the case for a public role in health care – and of the importance of a commitment to community sharing – is essential when considering the division of responsibilities for health care between federal and provincial governments. It is to this second dimension of choice that we now turn.

DEFINING THE SHARING COMMUNITY IN A FEDERATION

D eciding on the appropriate role for the state in the provision of health care is only the first step in mapping the public sector role in the area. The next dimension of choice concerns how the public role should be divided between different levels of government. Although this step faces all countries, it takes on a special significance in federal states, where constitutional authority is formally divided between federal and provincial or territorial governments.

We have seen in the previous section the part that equity and efficiency considerations play in staking out a role for the state. In a federation, these values take on an additional dimension. Given our earlier conclusion that it is equity – or, equivalently, social insurance and sharing – that supports the sort of comprehensive public health insurance systems found in most OECD countries, we begin with that value. Efficiency considerations, which condition the appropriate type and design of policy instruments, are taken up subsequently. Our aim is to consider the additional issues that arise in applying these values in a federal context, where citizens are simultaneously members of a province or territory and the national community.

Redistributive Equity and the Sharing Community

As we have seen, a commitment to the principle of social insurance depends on an underlying sense of shared responsibility of individuals for each other. However, this leaves open the question of the precise dimensions of the community within which sharing takes place.

Every country must define for itself the community within which sharing takes place and decisions about the extent of that sharing are made. In a unitary nation, one presumes that a common standard of redistributive equity applies for all citizens across the country, there being no particular reason to discriminate against citizens in one region as opposed to those in another. To use the terminology of economics, both horizontal and vertical equity ought to apply. Persons who are in like circumstances with respect to the characteristics being compensated ought to be treated identically, no matter where they reside.[7] Common standards of sharing apply nationwide, and the broad policy framework is set by the national government.

In a federation, matters are complicated by the fact that individuals are members of two political communities – the community of citizens across the country as a whole, and the community of residents within each province. The relevant community for sharing purposes can apply along a spectrum that spans two extreme possibilities. At one extreme, the entire country can be viewed as the relevant sharing community. We refer to this as the *exclusively countrywide* sharing case. In this case, redistributive equity would apply nationwide as in a unitary state, and decisions about the extent of that redistribution would be made by the political representatives of the country as a whole. The objective of redistributive or social insurance policies would be to compensate persons for differences in insurability by the same amount regardless of their province of residence. That is, horizontal equity would apply across the entire country: persons who are otherwise identical but reside in different provinces would receive identical treatment with respect to redistributive policies. In practice, there may be reasons why horizontal equity cannot be fully achieved, such as inequities that might arise if it is much more costly to provide relevant services in, say, distant locations or small centres. But that would not detract from the fact that, in principle, the sharing community is considered to be the country as a whole. The extent of redistribution from the more to the less advantaged, that is, the degree of vertical equity pursued, would depend upon the national political consensus about the amount of compensation for individual circumstances that is appropriate.

At the other extreme, the *exclusively provincial* sharing case, one might think of the province as being the sharing community. According to this view, redistribution occurs mainly among residents in each province. The extent of vertical redistribution and the concept of horizontally equitable treatment would both apply at the provincial level, and each provincial government would define the scope of redistribution separately. It is clear that if this were the case, there would be considerable variation among provinces. Different provinces have very different fiscal capacities for achieving redistributive goals: they have different demographic and geographic make-ups; and their citizens may well reach different consensuses about the appropriate degree of sharing. In this case, unlike that of a countrywide sharing community, horizontal equity would not apply across the country: otherwise identical persons would contribute different amounts or receive different benefits from the public sector (provincial and federal governments taken together). Moreover, the degree of vertical redistribution could vary significantly from province to province.

The exclusively countrywide and the exclusively provincial sharing communities are the two extreme cases of possible sharing communities in a federation. We can virtually rule both cases out as being irrelevant for the Canadian federation. The exclusively countrywide case would be incompatible with any provincial differences in standards of redistribution and therefore seems inconsistent with the constitutional and political realities of Canada. The exclusively provincial case would rule out any role of the federal government in redistributive equity, including that related to its commitment to equalization as well as that achieved by its access to redistributive taxes and transfers. It is necessary, therefore, to consider cases in which the two sharing communities coexist, with some degree of countrywide sharing coexisting with different degrees of sharing within provinces. Indeed, one might argue that this coexistence is the nature of a federation. Countrywide sharing would reflect the idea that citizenship in a country entails some expectation of comparable treatment in redistributive policies. But the federation itself is made up of separate provincial communities, some of which might have greater feelings of provincial solidarity than others, giving rise to asymmetries in redistributive policies.

The envisioned role of the federal government will be affected by what one considers to be the relative importance of the entire country versus the province as the primary sharing community. In this context, it is useful to distinguish three versions of the relevant sharing community along the spectrum of possibilities. In all cases, the fact of countrywide sharing implies that there is interprovincial redistribution. These models differ in the extent to which common interpersonal redistribution policies apply across provinces.

Predominantly Canada-wide Sharing

The *predominantly Canada-wide* version takes the country as a whole as the primary sharing community, and defines the extent of redistribution or social justice in national terms. In this version, all citizens enjoy a form of social citizenship; that is, they enjoy comparable social benefits no matter in which province they reside. As the British sociologist T.H. Marshall noted, the development of a social dimension to citizenship represented a pervasive trend across Western democracies during the twentieth century (Marshall 1950). In previous centuries, citizenship had come to embrace civil rights and political rights such as the right to vote. During the twentieth century, a social dimension was added, by creating social rights and obligations that individuals enjoyed not on the basis of their class, religion, language, or place of residence, but by virtue of their common status as citizens. Stripped to its essentials, social citizenship implies that a sick baby at one end of the country is entitled to medical care on the same terms and conditions as a sick baby at the other end of the country.

This vision of countrywide sharing implies that political representatives from across the country as a whole establish a conception of social benefits. Putting it into place requires both full fiscal redistribution between provinces, and strong, detailed countrywide standards with respect to the kinds of services and redistribution policies that should be available in all provinces. Comparable standards of vertical equity would apply, which implies that horizontal equity would apply nationwide. This version of sharing may well apply to some elements of social policy but not others. That is, there may be a consensus that Canada-wide standards should apply to some social insurance programs like health care and unemployment insurance – because equal compensation for different fortunes in one's health or employment status may be valued for citizens in all provinces – whereas different standards may be tolerated across provinces for, say, income redistribution programs such as welfare and redistributive taxation.

Predominantly Provincial Sharing

The *predominantly provincial* version of the sharing community represents the least amount of countrywide sharing among our feasible options. It leaves full scope for provincial governments to chart distinctive approaches to vertical redistribution. Countrywide sharing in this case is limited to redistributing among provinces so that all provinces have the *potential* to provide comparable overall levels of public services and redistributive equity, if they so choose. To use the terminology of the economics of fiscal federalism, inter-provincial transfers should be such that *average net fiscal benefits* are equalized across provinces.[8] At the same time, full horizontal equity would not necessarily apply – net fiscal benefits would not be equalized for each and every type of individual residing in different provinces. Some provinces might legislate higher degrees of redistribution than others. However, the system of intergovernmental transfers would ensure that each province has the potential to provide comparable net fiscal benefits to all its residents.

This version of the sharing community corresponds with the principles that underlie the current equalization system. That system involves transfers to provinces with lower revenue-raising capacities so as to enable them to raise some minimum national standard of tax revenues per capita at national average tax rates. More generally, and with health programs in mind, a system of inter-provincial equalizing transfers that redistributes among provinces in a way that fully reflects provincial differences in both revenue-raising capacity and need would satisfy this version of the sharing community.

The Dual Sharing Community

These two versions of the sharing community serve as useful bench-marks, but obviously they do not exhaust the possibilities. One might think of there being a continuum of views along the spectrum from predominantly Canada-wide to predominantly provincial sharing. It is natural to think of the latter version as being the lower limit of the spectrum because the Canadian constitution sets out as a principle the federal government's commitment to equalization, using wording that roughly corresponds with our definition of the predominantly provincial version of the sharing community. For some, however, this position on the spectrum does not leave enough room for Canadians to decide collectively to establish a common approach to social benefits that reflects a sense of social solidarity spanning the country as a whole. For others, the end of the spectrum represented by predominantly Canada-wide sharing seems to require redistribution standards resembling those one might expect in a unitary state, and to give too little scope to the regional diversities that also define Canada. Not surprisingly, much effort has been devoted to finding an intermediate position on the spectrum which balances the community of all citizens and the diversity of regional communities. One such intermediate position would involve a countrywide framework that defines some basic parameters of major social programs including health care but leaves room for provincial variation in program design and delivery mechanisms that are consistent with the framework. According to this intermediate position, which might be labelled the *dual sharing community* or a modified form of social citizenship, citizens across the country are assured of comparable, as opposed to identical, health care services.

The range of potential options is increased further by the possibility that the balance in the strength of attachment to the countrywide and provincial sharing communities might differ across the country. While much of the country might prefer the dual sharing model, for example, one region might prefer the predominantly Canada-wide sharing and another the predominantly provincial sharing model. The possibility of regional differences in the sense of attachment to community raises the possibility of asymmetrical relationships between the federal and provincial governments in a federation. To make the analysis manageable, this chapter focuses primary on the three primary conceptions of the sharing community: predominantly Canada-wide, dual, and predominantly provincial. Nevertheless, in practice, the possibility of combining different models in different parts of the same federal state is a real one.

In summary, where the federation situates itself along the spectrum will affect the role of the federal government and the design of policy instruments for effecting that role. Such choices ultimately reflect the underlying sense of community in the federation as well as the social context within which individuals feel a shared sense of obligation for each other's well-being.

Examples of Federal Sharing Communities: A Comparative View

Interestingly, most federations give substantial weight, in practice, to the idea of countrywide sharing in the area of health policy. Almost all federal states choose to engage both the central government and the provincial or state governments in health care (Banting and Corbett 2002). In this sense, multi-level governance in health care is not simply a Canadian pattern: it represents the norm among federal countries generally. However, federal countries tend to organize themselves so as to achieve significant countrywide sharing. Typically, legislation passed by the central government sets a general policy framework that defines key parameters of the health care system for the country as a whole. In many federal countries, the central government also administers important health care programs itself, dealing directly with citizens and service providers.

Moreover, where state or provincial governments manage parts of the system, they typically operate within broad parameters defined for the country as a whole, and normally rely for a substantial portion of their financing on transfers from the central government, transfers which incorporate a significant element of interregional redistribution.

Although the relative balance between levels of government does differ significantly from one federation to another, the central government in most major federations plays a much larger role than in Canada. For example:

> In Belgium and Germany, the policy parameters are defined in a highly centralized and corporatist process. The federal legislature incorporates the resulting agreements in framework legislation that specifies in detail key features of the system for the country as a whole. Program delivery then proceeds on a decentralized basis through networks of social funds.

> In Australia, the Commonwealth government plays the dominant role in two ways. First, it takes direct responsibility for major parts of the Medicare system, providing for access to doctors, pharmaceuticals, and nursing homes through programs that are administered by federal agencies operating on similar terms and conditions across the entire country. Second, it provides a special-purpose transfer to state governments to support public hospital care, and attaches highly detailed requirements concerning targets and auditing, with which states must comply. The result is a national health care system that operates on a similar basis across the country as a whole.

> In the United States, public health programs present a bipolar case. Medicare, which covers elderly and disabled Americans and represents two-thirds of total public health expenditures, is a purely federal program. Congress determines the basic policies, and a federal agency delivers the program across the country as a whole. The federal government also provides significant health services directly to military personnel and veterans. Support for poor Americans, however, demonstrates a sharp contrast. Medicaid and the State Child Health Insurance Program are federal-state programs supported by federal conditional grant programs. Federal conditions are very general, and state programs vary considerably in eligibility, service coverage, utilization limits, provider payment policies, and spending per recipient.

Overall, federal states have tended to approach a countrywide sharing community in health care, such that a sick child in one region receives heath care on comparable terms and conditions as a sick child in another region. The one partial exception among the four major federations surveyed here concerns coverage for poor American families and children. Otherwise, the primary form of territorial variation in health services in federations tends to be urban/rural differences rather regional differences, as is the case in unitary states. That is, differences between urban and rural areas within regions tend to be much greater than differences between regions.

Defining the Sharing Community in Canada

How do Canadians think of the sharing community in areas such as health care? Canadians live in a set of overlapping sharing communities that are defined by their family and personal relations, their ethnic and religious backgrounds, the languages they speak, and the local, provincial and federal arenas in which they conduct their political life. In thinking about assigning the public role in health care within the federation, we have observed that it is the relative strength of the citizens' attachments to regional and pan-Canadian political communities that is critical. Are citizens more strongly attached to their local and regional communities, and do they seek to manage public programs that matter to them at those levels? Or are they strongly committed to the pan-Canadian community, and do they wish to debate and define core public programs with fellow citizens from coast to coast to coast?

Fortunately, we have evidence on these issues.[9] Surveys of public attitudes and values confirm that Canadians have a sense of attachment or belonging to multiple communities, including both to Canada and to their province, and see no reason to choose definitively among them. Given their allegiances to both political communities, it is perhaps not surprising that Canadians want both levels of government involved in health care. Surveys regularly find that Canadians see health care as a countrywide program and overwhelmingly support the engagement of both levels of government in sustaining it. They endorse an active federal role, a preference that seems to have strengthened over the 1990s, and they expect the federal government to be involved in maintaining the system and ensuring standards. By wide margins, they want the federal and provincial governments to collaborate in the management of

the health care system, and they are uneasy about cuts in federal fiscal transfers to provinces. In addition, public attitudes toward the equalization program
suggest reasonably strong support for the idea of pan-Canadian sharing. This
commitment to a countrywide conception of health care and the engagement
of both federal and provincial levels in defining and sustaining it suggests an
underlying pan-Canadian sharing community, and is consistent with what we
have termed a dual sharing community and a modified conception of social citizenship in health care.

This vision of a dual sharing community seems also to accord with the
realities of social policy as conducted by the federal government and the
provinces up to the present time. The provinces are largely responsible for legis-
lating and delivering important public services in the areas of health, education,
and welfare. At the same time, the federal government intervenes in a number of
ways that lead to the achievement of reasonably comparable pan-Canadian standards of redistributive equity. The equalization program goes a long way toward
giving provinces the potential to provide comparable levels of these public services using comparable tax rates. The dominant role of the federal government
in the income tax system allows it to achieve reasonably uniform standards of
vertical equity in after-tax incomes. This effect is reinforced by the fairly recent
federal system of refundable tax credits, which extends national vertical equity
standards to those with low levels of income. There is an even greater degree of
national sharing for the unemployed and the elderly through the employment
insurance system and the system of public pensions. Finally, elements of a countrywide framework in health care have always existed through the broad conditions that have been attached to the original cost-shared grants and more recent
block grants for provincial health programs. Thus, there can be little doubt that
Canada-wide sharing currently exists alongside the sharing that occurs within
provinces through their redistributive programs.

In the specific case of health care, the Canada-wide framework is less
elaborate than in other federations. The federal government does not provide
health coverage directly to citizens generally; the conditions attached to intergovernmental transfers are less detailed; and the shift to block funding has largely eliminated day-to-day federal scrutiny of specific provincial decisions. In
comparative terms, the Canadian health system is clearly more decentralized,
and is best thought of as an interlocked series of provincial and territorial health
care systems. The five principles of the *Canada Health Act* and the interregional

transfers embedded in our fiscal arrangements do sustain reasonably comparable standards in key health services across the country as a whole, but interregional variation is greater than in the other federations discussed above.

There is some variation even in core hospital and physician services, which fall within the framework of the CHA. As noted earlier, the Act requires provinces to provide coverage for all medically necessary hospital and physicians' services, as well as all medically necessary surgical-dental services that require a hospital for proper delivery. However, provinces do vary at the margins in the range of services that are deemed medically necessary from one province to the next. Table 6 gives examples of services that are provided in some provinces but not others. There is also variation in the availability of doctors, nurses, and hospital beds provided across the country. It is worth noting, however, that decisions on these services reflect different provincial decisions about the delivery of health care services, rather than differences in the strength of provincial economies. Reading Tables 7 and 8 together illuminates this point. Table 7, which shows provincial per capita expenditures on health for selected years, suggests that the Maritime provinces and Quebec tend to spend less than the national average and

Table 6

UNCOVERED HEALTH SERVICES, BY PROVINCE

Uncovered Service	Province
Eye examination (ages 19-64)	PEI, NS, NB, Que, Man, Sask, Alta
Otoplasty (ear plastic-surgery)	Nfld, PEI, NB, Ont, Alta
Gastroplasty (stomach-stapling)	NB, NS
Reversal of sterilization	PEI, NS, NB, Ont, Man, Sask, Alta, BC
Psychoanalysis	Que, Man
Wart and benign skin lesion removal	NS, NB, Ont, Man, Sask, Alta, BC
In-vitro fertilization	Nfld, NS, Ont, Man
Chiropractic services	Sask
Eye refractions	Nfld, Sask

Source: Standing Senate Committee on Social Affairs, Science and Technology, *The Story So Far*. Vol. 1 of *The Health of Canadians: The Federal Role. Interim Report* (Ottawa: Queen's Printer for Canada, March 2001), table 6.1, p. 99.

Table 7

PROVINCIAL GOVERNMENTS' PER CAPITA HEALTH EXPENDITURES, 1975-2001 (dollars)

	Nfld	PEI	NS	NB	Que	Ont	Man	Sask	Alta	BC	Can
1975	358	353	323	301	400	378	368	329	384	372	376
1976	389	383	362	352	465	429	435	391	434	428	432
1977	413	419	398	391	508	462	479	435	451	465	468
1981	684	679	670	677	805	689	755	727	816	842	752
1986	1,060	1,026	1,031	1,047	1,150	1,165	1,163	1,189	1,364	1,147	1,169
1991	1,483	1,454	1,461	1,477	1,585	1,719	1,611	1,653	1,633	1,652	1,645
1996	1,650	1,563	1,413	1,637	1,590	1,681	1,694	1,605	1,469	1,848	1,652
2001[1]	2,420	2,033	2,011	2,153	1,981	2,176	2,359	2,248	2,293	2,457	2,191

[1] Data for 2001 are forecasts.
Source: Canadian Institute for Health Information (CIHI), Statistics by topic – macro-spending, table 10.

Table 8

HEALTH SERVICES IN THE PROVINCES AND TERRITORIES, 1998

	Doctors per 1,000 Population	Registered Nurses per 1,000 Population	Acute-Care Hospital Beds per 1,000 Population
Newfoundland	1.7	9.8	3.3
Prince Edward Island	1.3	9.3	3.5
Nova Scotia	1.9	9.1	3.6
New Brunswick	1.5	9.9	3.9
Quebec	2.1	7.7	3.7
Ontario	1.8	6.9	2.2
Manitoba	1.7	8.9	3.6
Saskatchewan	1.5	8.2	3.9
Alberta	1.6	7.5	2.2
British Columbia	1.9	6.9	2.2
Yukon	1.5	7.8	1.8
Northwest Territories	0.9	7.8	3.9

Source: A. Maioni. Health care in the new millenium, in H. Bakvis and G. Skogstad (eds.), *Canadian Federalism: Performance, Effectiveness, and Legitimacy,* (Oxford University Press, 2002), table 5.3, p. 97.

Table 9

PROPORTION OF THE POPULATION WITH DRUG INSURANCE COVERAGE

	Percent Covered
Newfoundland	65
Prince Edward Island	73
Nova Scotia	76
New Brunswick	67
Quebec	100
Ontario	100
Manitoba	100
Saskatchewan	100
Alberta	83
British Columbia	100
Canada	97

Source: Standing Senate Committee on Social Affairs, Science and Technology, *Issues and Options.* Vol. 4 of *The Health of Canadians - The Federal Role. Interim Report* (Ottawa: Queen's Printer for Canada, September 2001), table 1, p. 75.

the rest of the provinces more. However, differences in the cost of providing services help explain part of this pattern. Table 8 suggests that, although there is considerable variation in the numbers of doctors, registered nurses, and acute-care hospital beds across the country, the differences are not rooted primarily in provincial income levels.

Much more substantial regional differences are evident, however, in services that fall beyond the ambit of the *Canada Health Act*, such as drug therapy outside of hospitals and homecare. Drug insurance differs widely across the country. Provincial programs tend to cover low-income senior citizens and social assistance recipients in all regions, but coverage of other citizens varies considerably. Table 9 shows the proportion of the population in each province that has drug coverage from public and/or private plans. Five provinces ensure 100 percent coverage by establishing programs that provide a minimum level of coverage for all residents. For example, in 1997 the Quebec government introduced a comparatively generous public drug plan that covers everyone who does not have access to private insurance. Alberta has a comparable plan, but participation is not mandatory and a significant minority have chosen not to join and thereby avoid the provincial premium. The Atlantic provinces are at the other extreme; there are no public drug plans to cover the entire population in this part of the country, and private coverage also tends to be more restricted. In addition to such gaps in coverage, many more Canadians and their families are underinsured, in the sense that they can be placed in financial jeopardy by catastrophic drug costs.

Home care is a second area that varies greatly across the country. Although each province and territory offers some form of home care, there are major differences in eligibility, the proportion of those needing care who are covered, the range of services provided, and the level of user fees. All jurisdictions offer services such as assessment, nursing care, and home support for those they deem eligible. But only some provincial programs provide physiotherapy, speech therapy, and respiratory therapy (Standing Senate Committee 2001b, 81).

The importance of the CHA is highlighted by the greater regional differences in programs outside its scope. Nevertheless, current trends do pose important questions. When the countrywide framework was established in the postwar decades, hospital and physician services represented the core instruments in health care. Currently, however, drug therapies and home care are rapidly growing components of the sector. The fact that they also fall outside the CHA means that the pan-Canadian model of health care is more heavily modified with each passing year.

Canadians have long been committed to sharing, both within their regional communities and across the country as a whole, and they expect both levels of government to respond to important social needs such as health care. During the postwar era, Canada established its own version of a dual sharing community in health care, which took the form of reasonably comparable health services for all Canadians and represented an element of social solidarity across the country as a whole. However, it is important to recognize the limits of the Canadian approach here. In comparison with other federations, the Canadian system of health care is decentralized, and the Canadian model of sharing is more fragmented, especially outside the range of services covered by the CHA. Moreover, these limits are growing. The increasing role of health instruments that fall outside of the Act represents a quiet narrowing of social citizenship in Canada.

Every generation must judge anew the role of community sharing in the life of the country. There is no reason to assume that the postwar model should remain fixed in time. The growing importance of health instruments outside of the CHA raises questions about their possible inclusion, in some form, into a dual sharing model. In addition, critics of the Act have challenged some of the components of the original model. Some have questioned the role of the principle of public administration. Others seek to revisit the role of financial charges at the point of service. Whether or not Canadians should create more space for private delivery of health services, or introduce fees at the point of delivery, goes beyond the scope of this paper, since these questions turn fundamentally on conceptions of the ideal health care system rather than on approaches to federalism and intergovernmental relations as such. Having said that, the dual community sharing that has animated Canadian health policy over the last half-century suggests that such decisions should be made on a countrywide basis, such that Canadians continue to enjoy access to reasonably comparable health services on similar terms and conditions from coast to coast.

Efficiency in the Federation

Efficiency considerations also have implications for the federal-provincial/territorial role in health care. Two dimensions of our federal arrangements are particularly relevant here. The first is the balance between centralization and decentralization. As we shall see, efficiency concerns point in different directions on this issue. On the one hand, some efficiency concerns point in favour of decentralization, and many commentators advocate decentralization primarily on this basis. On the other hand, decentralization itself gives rise to potentially adverse efficiency effects that might justify a federal presence in certain programs, including health care. The second dimension of federal arrangements pertains to the nature of relations between the two orders of government. At any particular point on the continuum between centralization and decentralization, the nature of relations between the two levels of government can also raise questions, especially about the quality of accountability of governments to their electorates.

We begin by recounting the efficiency debates about centralization and decentralization, and then turn to the issues posed by the character of intergovernmental relations.

Centralization/Decentralization

The arguments for decentralization of the provision of public services are well developed in the literature on fiscal federalism. Some of the more prominent ones are as follows:

> *Catering to local preferences*: Lower-level governments might be better

able to tailor the design of their programs to suit the preferences of local residents. Public programs provided by the national government will tend to be uniform across the country, representing a compromise across a more diverse range of interests and preferences. Provinces, on the other hand, will be able to differentiate their programs to reflect what might be unique provincial political consensuses.

> *Information advantages*: Provincial and territorial governments are often seen as being "closer to the people," and therefore better informed about the preferences and needs of their residents. This will be especially important in the case of services delivered to individuals (including health services) that are to be targeted on the basis of need.

> *Administrative advantages*: Provinces and territories may be more efficient at administering the delivery of public services to individuals and firms, as well as targeted transfers. These kinds of programs are ultimately delivered by institutions on the ground (welfare agencies and hospitals, for example), and the management of these institutions may be more effective at the provincial rather than the federal level. There will be fewer layers of bureaucracy, and control will be facilitated by management that is closer to the point of delivery. To use the terminology of economics, there will be fewer so-called agency problems involved in controlling these delivery institutions and ensuring that the incentives of program managers are aligned with the objectives of the government rather than with their self-interest.

> *Experimentation and innovation*: To the extent that there are thirteen different provincial and territorial programs, the possibility of experimenting with program design and delivery will be enhanced. There will be more opportunities for provinces and territories to discover new ways of designing programs and to introduce completely new types of programs. This response-readiness is especially important in an area like health where new scientific and technical knowledge frequently becomes available, and public programs need to adapt to those changed circumstances. Experimentation at the provincial level also allows for trial and error that can lead to both successes and disappointments. It is more efficient to have disappointments occur on a small scale than at the national level. Successful initiatives can then be adopted across the country through provincial action or federal-provincial collaboration.

> *Intergovernmental competition*: Governments do not face the discipline of markets, which is the main engine of efficiency in the private sector. Some of the advantages of competition can be achieved through the political competition that is induced by decentralization. Governments implicitly compete with one another for mobile individuals and businesses. As well, citizens are better able to hold their governments to account if they can observe what is going on in neighbouring jurisdictions, a phenomenon that economists refer to as "yardstick competition."

In weighing these advantages of decentralized government, however, it is also important to consider a number of potentially adverse consequences of decentralization for nationwide efficiency. Addressing these negative consequences constitutes the efficiency case both for federal intervention and for a countrywide framework for policies that might be within provincial legislative jurisdiction.

There are three broad sorts of efficiency concerns that must be balanced against the advantages of decentralization. The first relates to efficiency in the "internal economic union." Decentralization can disrupt the internal economic union within a federation. It is generally agreed that economic resources should be allocated efficiently across a national economy, or what is often called the internal economic union. Efficient allocation is fostered by the free and undistorted flow of goods, services, capital, and labour across provincial borders. Unconstrained decentralized decision making can lead to distortions in these flows if provinces implement policies that favour their own residents over residents of other provinces (preferential procurement and hiring policies, fiscal measures that favour local firms or individuals, differential access to provincial public services, and discriminatory licensing policies, for example). Even if provincial policies are not intentionally discriminatory, the fact that provinces are designing their policies to suit their own needs may well give rise to distortions in the internal economic union. Provincial tax systems might differ, as may the structures of provincial public services. These problems are analogous to those that occur with respect to trade between countries, although they take on special importance in a federation that espouses the freedom of persons to take up residence and pursue a livelihood in any province.

The primary way in which the internal economic union is relevant to health care programs pertains to the mobility of individuals. The main requirement in regard to mobility is that health benefits be portable across provinces so that interprovincial movements of persons are not discouraged. There are various ways in which this concern may be addressed. In some federations, constitutional provisions do not allow provinces to distort cross-border flows or discriminate against non-residents. The Canadian constitution, however, gives relatively little guidance in this regard. A second mechanism for ensuring portability might be negotiated intergovernmental agreements. The Agreement on Internal Trade is a wide-ranging document that is intended to serve this purpose, but it has relatively weak dispute settlement provisions. The third means of tackling the issue is for the federal government to act as the guarantor of efficiency in the internal economic union. Given the structure of the Canadian constitution, the use of conditional transfers (the spending power) is the only realistic instrument that the federal government can bend to this purpose. It has been used to induce mobility provisions in provincial social programs, including the portability provisions of the *Canada Health Act*.

A second source of inefficiency in a decentralized federation arises because decisions taken in one province result in spillover benefits or costs to other provinces and their residents. These can take many forms. Changes in tax rates can induce interprovincial migration of tax bases, with the result that provinces compete by lowering tax rates and possibly also degrees of progressivity to attract high-income residents and businesses. By the same token, transfers to the less well-off and other social programs may be eroded as provinces engage in a "race to the bottom." More generally, in some cases, some of the benefits of provincial programs might accrue to residents in other provinces. This scenario constitutes the classical argument for conditional grants as a means of inducing provinces to take account of the full benefits of their programs when deciding on levels of expenditure.

The potentially adverse effects of tax competition are difficult to avoid. They are often used in the fiscal federalism literature as an argument for restricting the amount of revenue-raising responsibility assigned to provinces, especially for mobile tax bases. The fact that virtually all federations are characterized by sizable vertical fiscal gaps can be attributed to the predicted consequences of tax competition.

On the expenditure side, fiscal competition has both beneficial and detrimental effects. As we have seen, some amount of fiscal competition can be useful as a means of inducing provincial governments and their bureaucracies to be more efficient. On the down side, vigorous fiscal competition can reduce the size of programs and detract from the amount of sharing through social programs that might otherwise exist. A case can be made for using the spending power to prevent the worst effects of fiscal competition on the quality of social programs, including those in the provincial health sector, from occurring.

The third broad source of inefficiency results from "fiscally induced migration." As noted earlier, fiscal decentralization generally gives rise to differences in the ability of provinces to provide comparable levels of public services to their citizens. Provinces will have differing revenue-raising abilities, and will have different needs for public service expenditures because of the different demographic mixes of their populations. In a unitary state, the national government will typically provide common levels of public services across the nation and will finance them through a common tax structure. As a result, persons of like circumstances who are residing in like communities in different regions will have access to comparable public services and will pay comparable taxes; that is, they will receive similar net fiscal benefits (NFBs) from the national government.

This will no longer be the case in a federation in which major services are decentralized to the provincial level. Residents in provinces with high revenue-raising capacities or lower needs will typically obtain systematically higher NFBs. The consequences of systematic differences in NFBs across provinces are well known. On the one hand, they provide a purely fiscal incentive for persons and businesses to migrate to provinces with higher NFBs. This fiscally induced migration will lead to a situation in which too many resources settle in provinces with high NFBs. At the same time, to the extent that people are not mobile, otherwise identical persons living in two different provinces will obtain different NFBs from their provincial governments, leading to a violation of horizontal equity, as discussed above.

The health sector seems particularly susceptible to fiscally induced migration. Access to quality health care is a powerful motivator for people, especially those with serious illnesses. In a regionally varied health care system, people with a serious illness for which they lacked adequate coverage where they lived would have a real incentive to move to a province that provided much fuller coverage for their problem. A similar calculus would presumably also affect retirement decisions.

These efficiency problems would be avoided or muted by federal interventions that were consistent with either the predominantly Canada-wide or the predominantly provincial version of the sharing community. The former approach, which defines a common set of social benefits and obligations for citizens across the country as a whole, avoids the problem fully. In the case of the predominantly provincial sharing community the problem can be addressed by an appropriate system of intergovernmental equalization transfers. By undoing the source of NFB differentials, these transfers will enable different provinces to have the ability to provide "reasonably comparable levels of public services at reasonably comparable levels of taxation," to use the constitutional phraseology. Almost all federations (with the notable exception of the United States) have in place a system of equalization payments for this very purpose.[10]

Health programs are clearly of the sort that might give rise to NFB differentials across provinces. They are financed mainly out of provincial general revenues, and their benefits are intended to be available without distinction of income level. In the absence of intergovernmental equalizing transfers (including both equalization and the CHST), provinces with lower revenue-raising capacities would not be able to provide the same level of health services without substantially higher tax rates. Both the equalization system and the CHST serve to make it possible for all provinces to raise some minimum standard of revenues at given tax rates. At the same time, no program takes into account the differences in needs among provinces. In the case of health programs, provinces with more aged populations will have higher needs for health expenditures simply because health care costs rise with age. In principle, it is possible to incorporate needs into federal-provincial transfer systems, as can be seen in federations elsewhere (for example, Australia and South Africa).

In contrast to the predominantly Canada-wide version of the sharing community, NFB differentials will not be eliminated entirely by a system of equalizing transfers. At best, an equalization system can provide provinces with the potential for eliminating NFB differentials. If provinces have the opportunity to design their public services according to their own preferences, they may well choose programs with very different features. Such differences would pose a challenge to Canada-wide sharing, and the challenge would be exacerbated to the extent that fiscal competition itself reduces the extent of provincial sharing. But the level of interprovincial differences that would likely emerge under the predominantly provincial version of the sharing community is unlikely to pose a serious problem. The differences in NFBs that might arise from differences in provincial program structure are unlikely to be sufficient to generate substantial migration responses.

Intergovernmental Relations and Efficiency

In addition to establishing a balance between centralization and decentralization, federal states must also define the character of relationships between the two levels of government. The nature of intergovernmental relations can also have important implications for the efficiency of public policies. Observers have long argued that federal-provincial relations can generate inefficient incentive structures, constrain flexibility in program adjustment, undermine transparency and openness of governmental decision making, and weaken the accountability of governments to their electorates.

Critics tend to argue that efficient incentives, flexibility, and accountability are best preserved in a classical model of federalism, in which each level of government operates independently within its own jurisdiction, making its own policy decisions and raising its own revenues. In this arrangement, voters have a clearer view of who is responsible for government decisions, and have a better opportunity to hold governments accountable at the polls. By comparison with these relatively clean lines of accountability, stronger forms of intergovernmental collaboration and partnership in the management of public programs pose greater challenges.

Considerable attention has been devoted to the issue of whether some specific forms of federal-provincial fiscal arrangements can induce inefficient responses by provincial governments. For example, shared-cost programs might lead provinces to overspend or to skew their spending priorities. They may preclude the provinces from adopting innovative approaches to program design or financing. More generally, complex decision rules that require substantial consensus among federal and provincial governments may reduce program flexibility and impede the process of adjustment to changing conditions, a phenomenon that has been labelled the "joint decision trap" (Scharpf 1988).

In a similar fashion, the Canadian version of executive federalism, in which policy issues are resolved through negotiations between the two levels of government, is often held to weaken accountability to the electorate. Critics argue that the system accentuates the closed and secretive nature of policy making. Legislative debate plays a more limited role; participation by affected groups is more difficult; and intergovernmental secrecy can mean that public debate is less informed by the open clash of contending ideas. Moreover, given the intergovernmental parentage of important decisions, it is often difficult for citizens to understand which level of government should be held accountable on a continuing basis. Only very knowledgeable citizens can understand the complex interplay of governments that shape social programs, including health care, and even they have difficulty in deciding whom to hold accountable for policy failures.

Such tensions are not unique to Canadian federalism. The potential exists in all systems of multi-level governance. For example, considerable attention has been devoted to a "democratic deficit" in the context of the European Union as well. However, it is important not to overstate the impact. By its very nature, parliamentary democracy concentrates power, and decisions made by Canadian governments in their own jurisdiction are hardly models of open, participatory decision making.[11] Indeed, executive federalism is prominent in our system of governance because power is concentrated in the hands of cabinets and first ministers. Undoubtedly, the dynamics of intergovernmental negotiations accentuate the tendency toward secret and closed decision making in Canada. But they are not the sole reason for it.

Deciding what weight to accord these tensions when defining the role of the federal government in health care involves complex judgments in two ways. First, whatever attractions the classical model may have had in an era of smaller government, it is difficult to fully disentangle federal and provincial governments today. Second, whatever their reservations about executive federalism, Canadians still express a powerful preference for federal and provincial collaboration in the management of contemporary pressures in the health care system, as we have seen. These factors suggest that the critical challenge is not so much to disentangle governments in the health sector as to manage the interdependence of the federal and provincial governments in more open and transparent ways.

Efficiency and the Federal Role in Health Care

As in the case of the general role of the state in health care, efficiency concerns about the design of federal institutions do not point unambiguously in a single direction. As we attempt to define the balance between centralization and decentralization, we discern advantages on both sides. Decentralization promises a closer fit with local preferences, as well as informational and administrative advantages, greater scope for experimentation and innovation, and stronger intergovernmental competition. On the other hand, decentralization can disrupt the internal economic union, generate fiscal competition and spillovers, and lead to fiscally induced migration, all of which point to advantages inherent in a cross-country framework on key policy parameters. Similarly, the debate over the form of intergovernmental relations does not point unambiguously to a simple conclusion. The advantages of classical federalism in terms of incentive structures, flexibility, and accountability to the electorate need to be counterbalanced by the seeming intractability of intergovernmental interdependence in the contemporary era and the clear preference of Canadians for intergovernmental collaboration in health care.

The Federal Role in the Sharing Community: A Summary

As we have seen, the general rationale for a federal role in health care reflects both equity and efficiency concerns. Most important, the federal role depends on the conception of the sharing community that prevails in the federation. The key issue is the extent to which the sharing community is seen as the community of all citizens rather than communities defined by provincial or territorial boundaries. Further, if the pan-Canadian community is seen as an important sharing community, the role of the federal government, and the choice of instruments through which it should implement that role, will depend on whether a predominantly Canada-wide or predominantly provincial conception of that community is chosen. Is the goal to establish health care as a component of "social citizenship" such that all Canadians receive the same health services no matter where they live? Or is the goal simply to ensure that all provinces have the potential to establish comparable health services if they wish? Or is the goal to be found somewhere between these two poles, reflecting a dual sharing model that promises Canadians comparable but not identical health services across the country as a whole? Put differently, should standards of redistributive equity and social insurance be defined primarily for the country as a whole or province by province? If it is the latter, there will be no guarantee that individuals of a given type will receive comparable health services if they reside in different provinces.

Considerations of efficiency are also important in defining the federal role. As we have seen, decentralization can have a number of important efficiency advantages. However, decentralization can also generate efficiency concerns related to portability of benefits, fiscal competition among provinces, and fiscally induced migration. Similarly, concerns about the form of intergovernmental relationships do not seem strong enough to resolve issues of institutional design definitively. As a result, efficiency concerns do not point unambiguously in a single direction. Much depends, for example, on the balance one strikes among the various strengths and weaknesses of centralization and decentralization.

Redistributive equity and efficiency considerations cannot be acted on in isolation. In contemplating a federal role based primarily on values of pan-Canadian sharing, it is important that the instruments used for achieving that role not abrogate the important advantages of decentralized provision. In particular, the ability of the provinces to design and manage their own health systems, to experiment, to innovate, and to undertake new reform initiatives should not be compromised unduly by federal measures designed to achieve countrywide sharing and efficiency in the internal economic union. Put another way, the case for federal intervention is based on sharing considerations, not on the advisability of a federal role in reforming the health care system. This will be a primary consideration in our discussion of instruments in the following section, especially with respect to the use of federal instruments for a transformative role. For example, on grounds of community sharing, a stronger case can be made for the federal government using its influence to extend social citizenship to pharmacare and home care programs than to induce provinces to undertake reform of the way in which they deliver primary care.

The balances that should be struck among these various dimensions of sharing can only be determined through our democratic processes. To date, the preferences of Canadians and the federal-provincial balances that our elected leaders have crafted seem consistent with what we have called the dual sharing model. This model sees health care as a pan-Canadian enterprise, and reflects a commitment to a pan-Canadian sharing community. The model assumes that provinces are also sharing communities, and that different regions may choose to vary the mix of services and the modes of delivery in innovative ways. This blend seems consistent with current evidence on Canadian preferences. In this area, Canadians see no reason to choose between levels of government. They express a powerful preference for both the federal and provincial governments to collaborate in the maintenance and enhancement of our health services. Such collaboration does not require that health services be defined in identical fashion and delivered in identical ways across the country. But it does seem to suggest a model in which Canadians have access to quality health care services on comparable terms and conditions across the country as a whole, regardless of the province or territory in which they live.

Admittedly, the dual sharing approach to health care is more heavily weighted in favour of the provinces than in most federations, and is being narrowed steadily by changes in medical technology that enhance the importance of instruments falling beyond the CHA, such as pharmacare and home care. The current generation of Canadians will therefore have to decide anew about the range of health services that should be available to Canadians across the country on broadly comparable terms and conditions. Given the evolution of both medical technology and the demography of Canadian society, the key question for the future may be whether elderly Canadians are to have access to health services of particular relevance to them on broadly similar terms from one end of the country to the other.

An important conclusion flowing from this discussion is that it is misleading to pose the debate about the federal role in terms of an inevitable trade-off between equity and efficiency. The federal role is essentially determined by the extent to which the country as a whole rather than the province is deemed the appropriate community within which social insurance against ill health is provided, the one in which redistributive equity considerations dominate. At the same time, the manner in which the federal government fulfills this role can contribute to the efficiency of the federation rather than detract from it. The efficiency advantages of decentralization of health care can be best achieved by following the constitutional norms concerning the provinces' role in health care. Unless one adopts the exclusively countrywide sharing model, the federal government's efficiency objectives can be achieved without the need to violate provincial delivery. Predominantly provincial sharing can be achieved by a carefully designed equalization system that attends to both the revenue-raising abilities and the needs of the provinces. Such a program would enhance efficiency in the federation by undoing NFB differentials that would otherwise result from fiscal decentralization. The intermediate version of pan-Canadian sharing implicit in the dual sharing model can be achieved by setting pan-Canadian norms that can be embodied in a system of block transfers from the federal government to the provinces in support of health care. Such norms, which can be arrived at with provincial participation, need not be so intrusive as to interfere unduly with the detailed and efficient provincial delivery of health care. Moreover, the norms themselves might address efficiency issues such as the portability of health services across provincial borders. Thus, it is quite conceivable that both equity and efficiency can be enhanced by a suitably designed set of federal policies.

That is not to say that tensions between the two levels of government will dissolve. The federal government and some provinces may disagree both with the social insurance arguments for state intervention in the health sector in the first place and with the appropriate level of community sharing in the second place. To the extent that the federal government interprets the pan-Canadian consensus to be in favour of a greater degree of countrywide sharing than the provinces do, the types of standards that it will wish to see in place will appear to the provinces to be excessively intrusive. But this disagreement will be more a conflict over values than over the efficiency of federal intervention. There may also be conflicts about the processes for making decisions on these critical issues, and whether the level of financial contributions from the different levels of government are appropriate. But these issues lie more in the third dimension of choice, the instruments of federal action, to which we now turn.

THE CHOICE OF FEDERAL INSTRUMENTS

We have suggested that a comprehensive interpretation of the federal role in health care combines choices on three key dimensions: the general role of the state in health care; the particular responsibilities of the federal government in the sector; and the instruments through which the federal role is implemented. In our discussion of the first two dimensions, we have referred from time to time to the kinds of instruments that could help achieve equity and efficiency in health care. We extend the discussion of this third dimension of choice in this section.

As we have seen, the federal role in health care is sustained by considerations of both equity and efficiency. However, it is primarily equity, or more precisely social insurance considerations, that lead most OECD countries to provide health insurance through the public sector more or less universally regardless of private insurability, and to fund it largely out of general government revenues. Federal states are confronted with the additional question of whether the country or the province is the primary sharing community. In practice, sharing can coexist at both levels, and there is a spectrum along which the relevant sharing roles of the federal and provincial governments might locate.

What are the implications of this analysis for the choice of federal instruments? According to the predominantly provincial version of community sharing, which we have taken to be the end of the feasible spectrum involving the least countrywide sharing, the main role of the federal government should simply be to ensure that all provinces have the resources to provide comparable public services at comparable levels of taxation. Provinces would then be free to define the degree of sharing or redistribution within their jurisdictions as they see fit. If this view were applied to the full range of social programs, the federal redistributive effort would mainly involve transfers to provinces rather then to individuals. Of course, in financing those transfers and other federal expenditure programs, it would be necessary to take a stand on how redistributive the federal tax system should be, so some element of countrywide sharing would be inevitable. But provinces would themselves be able to choose their own tax systems to reflect their preferred degrees of redistribution.

The main policy instrument for implementing the predominantly provincial notion of community sharing would be the system of equalizing transfers to the provinces. It is important to emphasize that this currently includes not just the equalization program but also the CHST, and that these schemes focus on revenue equalization. The equalization system is designed explicitly to ensure that all provinces have the ability to raise some minimum standard level of revenues (currently the five-province standard) at national average tax rates. The CHST can be thought of as a purer, more complete, form of revenue equalization. It effectively obtains funds from a common national average tax system (federally defined) and disburses it in equal per capita terms among all provinces. It is a perfect net revenue equalization system.

At the same time, full net revenue equalization does not satisfy the predominantly provincial version of community sharing if the latter is taken to imply the literal satisfaction of the principle of equalization set out in section 36(2) of the constitution. This would require that provinces be able to provide reasonably comparable levels of public services at reasonably comparable levels of taxation. Revenue equalization only goes part way toward that objective. Provinces may also face different "needs" for public services in the sense that they differ in the composition of populations for whom the major public services are targeted. In the case of health care, there is a systematic difference in the costs of providing services to persons of different age and other characteristics. It can be argued that the predominantly provincial version of community sharing as applied to health requires that needs ought to be taken into account in allocating funds to provinces through the CHST block transfer. There are a number of examples of federations and other nations with decentralized delivery of health services that do precisely that: and provincial funding of regional health authorities is normally based on some indicator of need. The allocations could be determined using the same representative approach as is taken in the revenue equalization system. That is, needs equalization could be based on the cost of a national standard level of care for different demographic groups, in which the costs could represent some average of actual provincial costs. As with revenue equalization, the idea is to base the entitlement to needs equalization on objective measures that are outside the direct control of the recipient provinces.

The setting of norms for calculating needs-based transfers for health, although conceptually straightforward, would have complex measurement problems not unlike those found in the revenue equalization system. As well, difficult decisions would need to be made concerning the kinds of services that should be included in the standard, given that provincial health insurance coverage varies from province to province. However, they do not present an insuperable problem. Moreover, there might be ancillary advantages to basing CHST allocations on indices of need. For one, measures of need would inform the public about the magnitude of costs faced by the provinces, and might serve as a basis for informing public debates about the share that might be borne by the federal and the provincial governments. An index of need might also form the basis for allowing citizens to judge the adequacy of their own province's health care system. More generally, an index of need that was jointly agreed to by the federal government and the provinces and used as a basis for allocating federal transfers might serve to operationalize the principles set out in section 36(1) of the constitution. As we saw earlier, this section jointly commits the federal government and the provinces to "providing essential public services of reasonable quality to all Canadians" and "promoting equal opportunities for the well-being of Canadians." Both of these commitments could be interpreted as having relevance for health care.

Under the predominantly provincial form of community sharing, interprovincial equalization would be sufficient. There would be no need for pan-Canadian parameters to structure provincial programs, and each province could design its own program. Ideally, it would be a net equalization scheme, based on national average standards of revenue-raising capacity and needs. To achieve this net outcome, it may well be necessary for there to be enough of a vertical fiscal gap that the net outcome can be achieved without requiring that any provinces receive "negative" transfers. Revenue-raising capacity could be measured using a representative tax system approach as in the current equalization system, or it could be based on more aggregative measures, such as the so-called macro formulas that use a single macro measure of a province's fiscal capacity. As discussed above, needs would primarily reflect different demographic features of the provinces that are relevant for estimating the costs of providing public services to target populations. Of course, if the provinces chose quite different program and tax mixes, the design of an appropriate equalization system would become problematic. The transfers would be unconditional and would evolve as provincial fiscal programs evolved; and they would be formula-driven both in terms of their aggregate level and their interprovincial allocation.

Notions of community sharing that give more weight to countrywide sharing, including the dual sharing model, would require a wider set of instruments. A system of equalizing transfers would still be a prerequisite. But there would also be a need for mechanisms to define a common framework for health insurance across the country as a whole. Logically, there would seem to be a number of instruments available in a federal state that might be employed to this end:

> Direct federal delivery of health insurance programs;
> Direct financial transfers to citizens to support the purchase of health insurance;
> Federal fiscal transfers to provincial governments associated with a common set of policy parameters, expressed as standards or principles;
> An interprovincial compact to establish a common framework for provincial health insurance programs.

The same set of instruments is relevant in responding to the efficiency arguments for federal intervention. As we have seen, a case can be made for full equalization on grounds of efficiency as well as equity. Efficiency considerations might justify federal action to protect the functioning of the internal economic union (by avoiding barriers to economically efficient migration and inducement to migration driven purely by differential access to health services), or where fiscal competition is so strong as to jeopardize the extent of provincial sharing desired by the population. For instance, provincial sharing might be compromised by a race to the bottom in redistributive programs, tax competition that causes too little revenues to be raised to finance provincial social programs, and beggar-thy-neighbour fiscal policies.

Responding to these problems would require choosing from the same set of instruments. For instance, intergovernmental agreements might preclude provinces from engaging in discriminatory policies or destructive competition in programs. Given that social programs are involved, this would go beyond the kinds of provisions one finds in the Agreement on Internal Trade. Conditional federal transfers represent an alternative instrument, even where the relevant sharing community is the province. Conditions could be imposed on transfers to protect the portability and mobility provisions of special programs and individuals' access to them. If interprovincial competition seemed to be eroding the levels of health services desired by provincial electorates, minimal programs standards could be sustained on the basis of federal transfers.

Choices among such instruments tend to be highly sensitive to constitutional provisions and the distinctive traditions governing federal arrangements prevailing in each country. As a result, there is no single "best practice" in instrument choice. Moreover, each of these instruments permits many variations and, as in many policy domains, the real impact is determined by the implementation details. Nevertheless, each general approach does present strengths and weaknesses, and each one deserves more detailed attention.

Direct Federal Delivery

As we have seen, direct federal delivery of health insurance is a feature in many federations, including Australia and the United States; and one former provincial premier has recently suggested the transfer of direct responsibility for pharmacare to the federal level. The main feature of direct federal provision of health insurance is that it would effect full sharing countrywide, since presumably the same program would apply in all provinces. In addition, the single-payer principle would apply Canada-wide rather than at the provincial level. The case for direct federal provision thus relies on the country as a whole being the exclusive sharing community for health care (even though it is not for many other social programs).

This approach would represent a major departure in Canada. It would certainly raise interesting constitutional controversies. A federal health program such as pharmacare might survive judicial challenge if it were funded through general revenues rather than contributions or premiums. But it would certainly challenge deeply held political conventions about the division of powers in the sector and would require a significant degree of integration with existing provincial pharmacare programs.

However, this discussion does not exhaust the possibilities of direct federal action. Another option is an expansion of direct transfers to citizens through the tax transfer system.

Direct Federal Transfers to Citizens

Table 2 above demonstrated that the federal government already makes sizable implicit transfers for health care in the form of tax expenditures in the personal income tax and sales tax systems. However, these are mainly for health expenditures incurred by persons over and above what is provided in provincial health care systems. The question is whether this approach might appropriately be used as a basis for financing basic health insurance coverage.

In principle, Canada-wide sharing objectives in social programs might be achieved by a system of direct federal transfers to citizens. By being national in scope, this system would ensure that common standards of sharing would apply countrywide. Moreover, different degrees of Canada-wide versus provincial sharing could be accomplished by co-provision of transfers by both levels of government. Such an approach has proven to be successful in other areas of social policy. The federal program of refundable tax credits, for example, represents a nationally defined system of redistribution toward the poor and toward poor children, which supplements similar benefits offered through provincial social assistance programs. The question is whether this approach could be adapted to the case of health insurance.

The key feature of health insurance is the contingent nature of its assistance: payments are required only if health expenditures are incurred. Moreover, to the extent that health insurance fulfils a social insurance role, the extent of reimbursement should be independent of the recipient's means. One rather trivial way that a public health insurance program could be implemented using direct transfers to individuals is for the transfers to simply mimic payments that would otherwise be made directly to health providers; that is, health providers would bill individuals, and individuals in turn would claim the relevant amount from the government. This method might have some salutary value in terms of informing citizens of their cost of usage. But, otherwise it would simply increase administrative costs and would clearly require the cooperation of the provincial governments. Moreover, liquidity problems might be imposed on individuals if they were required to pay up-front and receive reimbursement later on.

An alternative way of achieving similar results, in theory, would be to make transfers directly to citizens and allow them to purchase their own insurance on private markets. For such a system to mimic social insurance, the transfers to each citizen would have to be differentiated according to risk so that all citizens could in fact purchase full insurance. It would obviously be very difficult to operate such a system on an ongoing basis. Moreover, by relying on the private insurance market, it would involve giving up the advantages of a single-payer system.

Programs of direct transfer to citizens might instead be viewed as ways of introducing some incentives into the use of health services by citizens. One way this might be done would be to offer only partial reimbursement of expenses incurred, which would simply be an indirect way of introducing user fees at the federal level. It might have an advantage over charging user fees directly, in that by being operated as a government program, reimbursement might be tied to ability to pay. This type of program might be a way for the federal government to actually implement a countrywide income-contingent system of user fees, given that health services are provincial programs. An alternative, more direct way might be to include some proportion of health expenses as taxable benefits for income tax purposes. A variant of this plan has recently been proposed by Aba, Goodman, and Mintz (2002). They propose that a proportion of the cost of health care services used by each individual (40 percent in their proposal) be assessed as a charge through the income tax system. However, the maximum that a family would pay would be restricted to 3 percent of income in excess of $10,000. This proposal would both exclude low-income families and ensure that the payment increases in relation to income. Since both the federal government and the provinces administer income taxes, the proposal could in principle be applied at either level of government. However, for the federal government to be involved, provinces would have to agree to set up the required administrative machinery to both bill taxpayers correctly and receive the federally collected contribution as co-payment for health costs incurred in the province. Canada-wide sharing principles would apply to the extent that the same co-payment schedule was used in all provinces. Of course, since the scheme would be intended solely as a means of addressing incentive concerns, it would have limited value as a social insurance device.

Another proposal for injecting individual incentives into health insurance that has gained some currency is the use of so-called Medical Savings Accounts (MSAs) (Ramsay 1998). The use of MSAs originated in the United States, where they are used in conjunction with private health insurance plans, typically as part of an employer-provided package. The basic idea in the American context is that the private health plan has a high deductible amount and so only covers serious or more catastrophic expenditures. Lower-cost, more routine expenditures would be covered from the MSA. The employer (or other provider) would have an amount corresponding to the size of the deductible deposited into the MSA in the individual's name. The individual would then be responsible for covering his or her own health expenses up to the deductible amount. The MSA could be used for this purpose until it is exhausted. Health expenditures above the amount of the MSA would have to be paid by the individual (though there could be some tax incentives to help defray the cost). Unused MSA funds could be carried forward for use within a specified number of future years, and eventually could accrue to the individual as part of the incentive to save on health expenditures.

The MSA could in principle be used as part of a public health insurance system. This would involve introducing a deductible provision into the system, and at the same time creating an account for each individual in the jurisdiction. This could be simply an accounting device that individuals could draw on to meet health expenditures below the deductible amount. As with private MSAs, individuals would be responsible for such expenditures once their MSA had been exhausted, and would be able to claim unspent funds as their own income.

The case for MSAs, as with the proposal of Aba, Goodman, and Mintz, is based on incentive arguments. In particular, it represents a response to concerns about moral hazard, which, as we saw, refers to the built-in incentive for individuals to overuse the health system if the costs of such use are fully paid by insurers. With a system of MSAs, individuals would implicitly bear the opportunity cost of small health expenditures. The effectiveness of the MSAs would then be judged on the basis of how much discretion individuals have in their demand for health expenditures, and how great a problem the resultant moral hazard might be. Another benefit is that they may provide a base of funds for all individuals who have no other means of financing their own health expenditure requirements. They also can be designed to retain the advantages of a single-payer system.

The disadvantage of MSAs is that they effectively undo the insurance function of the public health insurance system. Basically they require individuals to self-insure out of their own accounts, so all the pooling advantages of ordinary insurance are lost. This loss is mitigated to the extent that individuals can self-insure over time by carrying unused MSA funds forward. Nonetheless, the system remains one of self-insurance, which may be a steep price to pay to address the moral hazard issue. As well, MSAs do not fulfill the social insurance role except to the extent that the size of individual funds is somehow related to health risks. As we have mentioned, insuring against risk requires information that governments are unlikely to have.

There would be no constitutional barrier to the federal government establishing a system of MSAs. As long as benefits were financed from general government revenues, as opposed to being tied directly to contributions, such a system would represent a valid use of the spending power. From the viewpoint of federalism, however, it is not obvious that MSAs have any attraction as a federal, as opposed to a provincial, policy device. To the extent that one views the federal role as being essentially motivated by countrywide social insurance or sharing considerations, MSAs have little to recommend them as a federal policy instrument. In fact, MSAs represent an abrogation of what we have called the social insurance rationale for government intervention in health insurance.

Federal Transfers to Provincial Governments

Transfers to provincial governments have been the primary instruments in the definition of a pan-Canadian sharing community in health care. Moreover, as we have learned, the basic structure of these transfers needs to differ only incrementally between the transformative phase, when the countrywide framework is being created, and the subsequent phase, when the emphasis shifts to sustaining that framework over time. As we learned from the medicare case, a transfer with quite general conditions is sufficient to initiate a program that contains a reasonably high degree of sharing countrywide while at the same time allowing the provinces discretion to design and deliver health care systems that suit the needs and preferences of their residents and satisfy their own norms of province-wide sharing. Full traditional cost-sharing grants, such as the CAP, are not absolutely necessary. The basic structure of federal-provincial block health transfers also sustains the dual sharing conception of the federal role. A block transfer with general conditions is flexible enough to allow for the maintenance of countrywide standards, while at the same time allowing provinces the discretion to deliver their citizens' own preferred modes and levels of province sharing.

If Canadians wish to maintain some form of dual sharing communities in health care, transfers to provinces are likely to remain a central instrument. To be effective, this approach would ideally require a clear definition of relevant standards; sufficient levels and predictability of federal funding to ensure that federal policy parameters are credible and effective; and some suitable procedure for resolving disputes between the federal government and the provinces and territories. However, Canada has never fully achieved this ideal, and has fallen further from some aspects of it recently. The result has been an increasingly active debate about the future of transfer programs.

On one side are commentators who seek to reinforce the legitimacy of the federal role through a stronger, more predictable, and more visible financial commitment. For example, some have proposed a return to a global cost-sharing approach, perhaps at the level of 25 percent of aggregate provincial health expenditures. Others have suggested the reinstatement of an automatic escalator for the CHST. In this context, it is useful to distinguish between the level and the predictability of the federal transfer. The moral and political authority of the federal government to sustain a meaningful countrywide framework through the CHA is clearly correlated with the level of its financial commitment. The federal government has to be a serious financial partner to be credible. Moreover, the more exacting the federal standards, the greater the level of federal support presumably needed. It is difficult to be precise about the minimum level of federal support required. In the final analysis, the considerations are political rather than economic. What is the level of support required to preserve the legitimacy of the federal policy framework in the eyes of both provincial governments and Canadians in general? Recent challenges from provincial governments suggest that the federal government has fallen below the essential level. Whether a return to cost sharing is the best way forward, however, is less clear. Given past practice, presumably cost sharing would apply to aggregate provincial expenditures rather than to the expenditures of individual provinces. Even in the latter case, however, cost sharing would require measuring eligible provincial expenditures, and would therefore reintroduce administrative complexities and costs, and add to potential intergovernmental frictions. The advantages of this approach over a simple increase in the block transfer are unclear.

The predictability of federal support, however, remains critical. As in the case of interpersonal trust, nurturing intergovernmental trust requires transparency and predictability in relationships. Given the propensity of the federal government to make unannounced changes to the transfer system, the case for an automatic escalator that bases changes in the CHST on a formula rather than on federal discretion is strong. Various formulas for the rate of growth of such transfers are possible. Basing a formula on the rate of growth of actual provincial health expenditures would have the advantage of maintaining the federal share of funding (and therefore authority to enforce the general conditions) over time. However, it would imply the administrative and measurement costs mentioned above. At the other end of the spectrum, the escalator could be the rate of growth of GDP or GNP as was the case under the EPF. An intermediate approach that might more accurately reflect affordability would be to base the transfer on the rate of growth of federal tax bases. These latter two options have the advantage that they put the transfer on a formula basis, thereby removing discretion from the federal government. But they are based on economic aggregates that are themselves variable and unpredictable over time. The lack of predictability could be avoided to some extent by using a rolling average of the relevant economic aggregate to smoothe out changes over time. Alternatively, to avoid fluctuations altogether, one could simply adopt a constant escalator of some arbitrary percentage. This growth rate could be applied either to aggregate transfers or to per capita transfers. This formula could be a more flexible option if the percentage was periodically subject to change.

Other proposals focus primarily on making the federal contribution more visible by separating the block transfer for health from those for welfare and post-secondary education. The main argument in favour of this reform – and it is certainly a substantial one – is that a separate transfer would enhance the transparency and visibility of the federal role in health care, thereby enhancing the ability of citizens to hold governments to account. On the other side of the ledger, however, there would be difficulties in deciding on the precise allocation of transfers to such a fund. At the moment the federal government pays some lip service to the separate components of the CHST by attributing a share to each program. But until recently the attribution of share was based largely on historical data, and probably had little relationship with provincial expenditure patterns. More recently there has been an attempt to base the shares on more relevant estimates of federal support for provincial spending in health. This issue is discussed more fully in chapter 4 by Lazar, St-Hilaire, and Tremblay. Moreover, the impact of a separate transfer on provincial decisions would be marginal, since the transfers would remain fully fungible in the hands of the provinces. Finally, in the absence of increased federal commitment, a separate health transfer would necessarily be smaller than the current CHST, and would therefore dilute further the ability of the federal government to sustain federal policies.

These proposals all come from commentators committed to sustaining a pan-Canadian conception of health care. At the other extreme are proposals that would reduce the commitment to national sharing. Some have suggested converting the CHST into a straight tax point transfer to the provinces. Such a plan would result in a significant reduction in the level of national sharing in two ways. First, it would spell the end of dual community sharing in health care. It might be argued that the equivalent could be achieved by national standards negotiated among the provinces, but for reasons discussed below, that seems not to be feasible. Second, under a tax-point transfer it would be difficult to maintain even the minimal level of national sharing, which relies solely on effective equalization. Replacing CHST with tax points would make this difficult for four reasons: a) the net equalization property of the CHST would be lost, and would be unlikely to be replaced under Equalization proper; b) decentralization of more tax room would itself place much more pressure on the Equalization system and make it difficult to sustain politically; c) it would be more difficult to take account of needs, which we have argued is important for the predominantly provincial sharing model; and d) decentralizing the tax system would make it more difficult to maintain common redistributive standards through the tax-transfer system. Proponents of this option often point to the advantages of accountability. This argument, which is generally taken as self-evident, is actually quite unclear. It is not obvious how accountability for provincial health spending is compromised by the fact that some of the provinces' revenues come as fungible block grants from the federal government.

Whatever view one takes of the appropriate extent of countrywide versus provincial sharing, equalization is bound to be a key component. It is worth digressing for a moment on the principles of the design of an equalization system that would suit a decentralized federation. On the basis of both economic and constitutional principles, a strong case can be made for basing equalization in the broadest sense on both revenue-raising ability and needs. In the current fiscal arrangements, the Equalization system is specifically designed to equalize the ability of the have-not provinces to raise revenues comparable to the five standard provinces using national average tax rates. There is no doubt that the revenue-equalization system could be fine-tuned and improved in various ways, many of which are documented in the 2002 Report on Equalization by the Standing Senate Committee on National Finance. At the same time, the CHST system can partly be interpreted as a very crude needs-based equalization system, where the measurement of need is based on equal per capita spending requirements. To incorporate needs more carefully into the fiscal arrangements system, the per capita transfer of the CHST could be adjusted by adopting the same representative provincial method as is used to equalize for tax capacity. The procedure would work in the case of health as follows. A national average cost of providing medical and hospital services to identifiable groups of persons could be calculated. These groups could include age groups, genders, geographical descriptors such as urban or rural, and perhaps ethnic groups in the population whose health care needs vary substantially from others, such as Aboriginal peoples. For each group, a national average per capita cost of providing a standard package of medical and hospital services would be calculated. For each province, these could be aggregated up to determine the average per capita cost of providing medical and hospital services to the population as a whole. Each province's per capita health transfer could then be adjusted to account for differences in needs across provinces.

Such a scheme would have a number of features. First, the needs-based equalization could be carried out as part of the CHST transfer system, and, unlike with the Equalization system, it could be a net scheme (provided the size of the CHST were large enough). Second, the needs adjustment would be appropriate for all points along the relevant community-sharing spectrum. It would be compatible with varying sizes of vertical transfers. Third, because the system would be based on countrywide average per capita costs, there would be no incentive for provinces to vary their own spending patterns. Moreover, the incentive to attract more desirable demographic types to the province would be blunted. Fourth, there would be considerable discretion to decide how finely to divide the population into different segments. That would be partially driven by the extent to which different identifiable groups incur different health costs. Finally, as with the Equalization system, there would be unavoidable measurement and design problems, the more so, the more the fiscal system was decentralized. Since different provinces choose different definitions of insurable services, some compromise would be required in choosing the national average standard of services on which to base the needs calculation. In fact, incorporating needs into equalization systems is quite feasible, as examples from other federations have shown. Even a new multi-level government like that of South Africa has a reasonably sophisticated system of needs equalization along the lines described above.

The preceding discussion focused primarily on the sustaining role of the federal government. Advocates of a more transformative federal role, one that provides greater leadership in responding to new challenges in health care, probably must look to other instruments. Take, for example, pharmacare and home care. It would be difficult to incorporate these increasingly important areas into the dual sharing model by simply increasing transfers flowing through the CHST. Rather, transformative action would require repeating the precedent established for hospital and medical services. At the outset, this would involve new transfer programs, with a stronger shared-cost component. When established, these programs might then be incorporated into the general block fund transfer mechanism.

Two particular observations about the use of federal-provincial transfers for transformative purposes are in order. First, in the case of pharmacare and home care, the transformation to fully public programs would not be starting from scratch. Unlike in the earlier cases of hospital and medical insurance, a substantial proportion of the population of most provinces is already covered by either public or private health insurance programs. Turning these into fully funded public insurance schemes would not be anywhere near as financially ambitious as instituting such programs where none previously existed (although the actual transformation might be no less contentious). Logically, this might suggest that the extent of federal support needed to engineer the transition would be correspondingly lower. However, the political reality is that provinces are under considerable pressure from cost increases in the traditional core health services, and encouraging them to extend coverage in newer areas might well require a greater federal contribution.

Second, as mentioned earlier, the main rationale for federal involvement turns on the social insurance argument, and especially the notion that the umbrella for social insurance should cover Canada as a whole. The case for federal involvement in the actual design and reform of health services has not been made. On the contrary, the presumption is that the provinces are better suited to legislate and deliver health programs, a presumption that is also reflected in the constitution. The implication is that a case has not been made for using federal grants as a medium for the reform of health care. Thus, one does not contemplate the transformative role as including the use of federal transfers to induce the provinces into, say, adopting a particular model for primary health care or affecting the balance of in-patient and outpatient services. The reason that pharmacare might be viewed as a suitable candidate for the transformative role rests on the argument that it is an element of social insurance, not on the idea of encouraging the use of pharmaceuticals per se.

Interprovincial Compact on Health Services

During the 1990s the weakening of traditional instruments of federal influence triggered a search for alternative mechanisms for sustaining a Canada-wide approach to social programs. In that context, some analysts argued that programs do not have to be federal to be national, and that a compact negotiated by provincial governments among themselves could sustain a common approach to programs such as health care.[12] In the most extreme version of this approach, the CHST would be replaced by a transfer of tax points, and provincial governments would take up the burden of national leadership by developing a compact on core principles of social policy.

As critics of such suggestions have emphasized, this approach faces significant problems in regard to collective action (Kennett 1998). Provincial governments are elected by provincial electorates to respond to provincial concerns and interests. The key question is: why would provincial governments voluntarily agree to constrain their policy-making autonomy in the area of health policy? In the current context, provincial governments do so in return for federal financial support. Absent such support, they have limited incentive to plan their programs with the interests or preferences of residents of other jurisdictions in mind. To the extent that there is a countrywide consensus about the kind of sharing that ought to be reflected in provincial health programs, it might be argued that provinces ought to be able to negotiate an agreement on a set of pan-Canadian principles to govern their own programs. But consensus would not guarantee that an effective interprovincial response would actually emerge. The problems of achieving collective agreements when all participants must agree are well known: each participant has enormous bargaining power when unanimity is required. Moreover, given the mobility of individuals – including medical professionals – and businesses, there would be incentives for some government to "free-ride" or to engage in social dumping despite such an agreement. In the absence of a decision rule enabling a majority of provinces to impose a collective outcome on dissenting provinces and an effective binding dispute settlement mechanism, outcomes would be governed by consensus decision making. As a result, there would be strong pressure to reach a lowest-common-denominator outcome. It seems highly unlikely that a strong Canada-wide policy framework could emerge from such a system. The example of the relatively toothless Agreement on Internal Trade, which in principle should lead to collective gains for all provinces, is instructive in this regard.

These difficulties on the policy side reappear on the financial side. The fullest version of the interprovincial approach, which replaces the CHST with a transfer of tax points, would lead to all of the problems of sustaining a strong system of interregional transfers discussed above. It seems unlikely that an effective system of interregional sharing could be negotiated among provincial governments. The current Equalization program is a federal program, financed through federal tax revenues and established by federal legislation. Although provincial premiers often articulate views about the program, their assent is not formally required. An interprovincial sharing mechanism would require wealthier provinces to agree to a sharing formula and send cheques to some pooling mechanism. The probability that this process would generate as strong a system of interprovincial transfers as the current system seems low. At a minimum, it would be a high-risk strategy for have-not provinces.

In the words of one commentator, the strategy of relying on an interprovincial compact to sustain a Canada-wide sharing community rests on "heroic" assumptions about the role of provincial governments (Kennett 1998). While it is true that programs do not have to be exclusively federal to be national, there seems to be no escape from the world of federal-provincial collaboration.

Asymmetrical Approaches

Other commentators have suggested that it would be possible to develop an asymmetrical approach to health care, one that would allow individual provinces greater flexibility in the definition of health care services. This proposal is most often advanced in relation to the province of Quebec.

Such proposals are usually premised on the distinctive nature of political identity and community in Quebec compared to other provinces. The essential proposition is that Quebec represents a distinct society within Canada, and that a different conception of the relative importance of the Canadian and provincial sharing communities prevails there. Surveys of public attitudes do suggest that political identities and the sense of attachment to Canada are qualitatively different in Quebec than other provinces.

The precedent of the Canada and Quebec Pension Plans points to possible ways in which such an asymmetrical relation could be established in practice. The difficulty with this approach, however, is its acceptability to other provinces. In the decades since the establishment of the Canada and Quebec Pension Plans, much greater emphasis has been placed on the norm of the equality of the provinces, especially in western Canada. It is not at all clear that the asymmetrical arrangements that were negotiated in the mid-1960s could be established today, even in the case of contributory pensions. In the case of health care, other provinces would probably also insist on any additional flexibility that was made available to Quebec, and the distinction between an asymmetrical model and a simple decentralization would narrow substantially. As a result, it would be difficult to preserve a pan-Canadian approach to health care even in Canada outside of Quebec. In theory, asymmetrical federalism seems like an attractive mechanism for accommodating the distinctive role of Quebec in Canada. In practice, however, it seems likely to trigger a wider set of provincial opt-outs that would erode the broader proposition that Canadians value a shared vision of their social future.

In summary, the federal government has a limited set of instruments available to pursue its transformative and sustaining roles in the Canadian health care system: direct delivery, direct transfers to citizens, and transfers to provinces. In addition, an interprovincial compact remains an instrument with some potential for limited purposes. Adapting the mix of instruments to changing realities remains a continuing challenge in federal states.

The combination of constitutional provisions and traditional federal-provincial practice places most of the burden on one instrument, transfers to the provinces. Hence an important dilemma remains. The basic legitimacy of the primary instrument available to sustain a countrywide sharing community in health care has increasingly been challenged within the processes of federal-provincial relations in Canada. Yet no other instrument seems capable of filling the void. A key question, therefore, is whether it is possible to reinforce the legitimacy of the federal spending power. This would seem to require re-establishing a consensus on appropriate fiscal shares, federal-provincial decision processes, and dispute resolution. These issues are taken up in more detail in the following chapters.

SUMMARY

A comprehensive interpretation of the federal role in health care incorporates judgments on three separate dimensions of choice: the general role of the state in health care; the particular role of the federal government in health care; and the instruments through which the federal government carries out its role. These dimensions of choice are distinctive, in that each raises a different range of considerations, but they are also cumulative. For those who oppose a general role for the state in health care, the second and third dimensions are not relevant. For those who support a role for the state in health care but oppose federal intervention in the sector, the choice of federal instruments is moot.

We have argued that the general role of the state in health care is sustained by considerations of both equity and efficiency. The primary rationale for the extent of government intervention common in most OECD countries is to be found in considerations of equity and social insurance. The central proposition is that, in a humane society, persons ought to be compensated for differences in their risk of ill health over which they have no control. Some people are unlucky, often from birth, in having a systematically higher risk of illness than others. We cannot know for sure about these differences in health status and illness insurability in advance, but they are real. Governments have therefore established social insurance programs to offset such differences in luck and insurability by, in effect, creating a universal pooling insurance scheme. This equity case for public health insurance is reinforced by efficiency considerations, since single-payer systems can have important advantages in reducing administrative costs, balancing the collective organizations representing health care professionals, and strengthening cost controls, all of which are important. Public action is also critical in overcoming externalities in the field of public health. Yet, when all is said and done, the core of the case for the comprehensive role that governments have assumed in health care is rooted in the logic of social insurance. It represents a form of sharing and redistribution that depends in the final analysis on a collective sense of responsibility among individuals for other members of their community.

Federal states such as Canada confront a second dimension of choice as they decide on the boundaries of the community within which this sharing takes place. Are our commitments to each other bounded by the pan-Canadian community of all citizens, the community of people living in our own province, or a mix of both? Or to pose the questions in other words: Is the goal to establish health care as an element of "social citizenship" such that all citizens receive health services on the same terms and conditions irrespective of where they live? Is the goal simply to ensure that all regions have the potential to establish the same level of health services if they wish? Or is the goal somewhere between these poles, reflecting a dual sharing community approach that promises comparable but not identical health insurance programs across the country as a whole?

The preferences of Canadians as revealed in public opinion surveys, and the federal-provincial balances that their elected governments have established in the past are consistent with this intermediate model, which we have called the dual sharing community model. This model sees health care as a pan-Canadian enterprise and reflects a commitment to a pan-Canadian sharing community. The model also assumes that provinces are sharing communities as well, and that different regions may choose to vary many important features of health services and the modes of their delivery in innovative ways. Health services, as a result, will not be, and need not be, identical across the country. But a broad pan-Canadian framework remains important in this model. It holds that Canadians should have access to quality health care services on comparable terms and conditions across the country as a whole. The bedrock of this approach is the conviction that that a sick baby in British Columbia should be entitled to health services on broadly comparable terms as a sick baby in Atlantic Canada.

Although the role of the federal government is rooted primarily in a commitment to a pan-Canadian definition of the sharing community, efficiency considerations are also important in defining the balance between federal and provincial governments. Decentralization has undoubted advantages that point to the desirability of local delivery of complex programs such as health services. However, decentralization can also generate important efficiency problems regarding the portability of benefits, fiscal competition among provinces, and fiscally induced migration. In addition to basic equity concerns, it is simply inefficient to have people with serious illnesses moving from one part of the country to another to qualify for adequate health coverage. Thus the debate about the federal role in health care does not simply pit equity against efficiency considerations. Capturing the benefits of both involves a judicious balancing in the federal-provincial division of labour.

The third dimension of choice, the selection of federal instruments, is also dependent on which conception of the pan-Canadian sharing community is selected. The predominantly provincial conception points primarily to equalization of the fiscal capacity of provincial governments through instruments such as the formal Equalization program – perhaps augmented to reflect different needs for provincial health expenditures – and the CHST. Conceptions of the sharing community that put more weight on Canada as the relevant community, including the dual sharing community model, require a broad policy framework for the country as a whole, and therefore point to a wider range of instruments. In the

Canadian case, the primary instrument remains federal transfers to provinces that are conditional on provincial acceptance of common principles or standards. Ideally, such an instrument would be sustained by a broad federal-provincial consensus on the ways in which the common policy framework would be determined, the appropriate financial responsibilities of the two levels of government, and a mechanism for resolving particular disputes, issues that will be addressed in the following chapters.

NOTES

1   In the case of unemployment insurance, the transfer was complete; in the case of contributory pensions, the constitutional amendments retained provincial paramountcy, such that provinces can choose to establish contributory pension schemes if they wish. Only Quebec has exercised this option.

2   This usage of the POGG power has been criticized by Hogg (2000, 17.3b), who holds that the legislation is better seen as criminal law. It is worth noting as well that section 91(11) gives the federal government responsibility for "Quarantine and the Establishment and Maintenance of Marine Hospitals."

3   The mechanism of coverage of the poor and hard-to-insure varied among these governments. Alberta offered public subsidies to the poor and hard-to-insure with which to purchase private coverage; British Columbia and Ontario created government agencies to insure those who could not obtain private coverage (Taylor 1987, 338-41).

4   See Alberta 1995. The differential size of the sector can be seen in the monthly penalties calculated by the federal government: Alberta $422,000; Newfoundland $11,000; Manitoba $68,000; and Nova Scotia $4,500.

5   The actual role of the state in implementing these interpersonal transfers-cum-insurance could vary. The state could simply make the transfers and rely on the private market to provide insurance. Or, the government itself could provide the insurance. In a world with full information available both to the government and the insurance industry, the two would be equivalent.

6   Nonetheless, some observers have advocated funding the non-catastrophic part of health expenditures through assessments based on users' taxable income (Aba, Goodman, and Mintz 2002).

7   As we stress below, identical treatment of like persons will have to be tempered even in a unitary nation if there are different costs associated with providing services to different persons. For example, it may well be the case that the level of services available in rural areas is different from that in urban areas. This reflects a standard equity/efficiency trade-off. Our concern is really with differences across provinces with respect to services provided to given types of persons in comparable circumstances.

8   Net fiscal benefits refer to the difference between the value of public services that an individual enjoys and their tax payments. For a discussion of the concept and its application in fiscal federalism see Boadway (2000).

9   The next two paragraphs draw on the survey of data on public attitudes in Mendelsohn (2001).

10 Equalization systems fulfill at the same time another efficiency purpose. They provide a sort of regional insurance to provinces against idiosyncratic fiscal shocks that they might be faced with. Thus, equalization-receiving provinces that suffer an unexpected decline in their tax bases will be sheltered from the full effects of that decline by an increase in equalization payments. In a unitary state, this kind of insurance is implicit in the nationally defined system of taxation and public services. In the absence of equalization, part of that regional insurance would be lost.

11 A long-standing critique of decision making within the federal government as concentrated, closed, and secretive can be traced from Smith (1977) to Savoie (1999).

12 This case was developed most fully by Courchene (1996). For a variety of assessments of this proposal, see Cameron (1997).

CHAPTER 2

COOPERATION AND DISPUTE RESOLUTION IN CANADIAN HEALTH CARE

DAVID CAMERON AND JENNIFER MCCREA-LOGIE

C ooperation and conflict, consensus and dissonance, collaboration and competition – these are features of all federations, as they are of most if not all forms of human association.[1] In Canada, as in other federal systems, the political forces of conflict and cooperation are mediated through the particular institutions and processes of the federation. Our interest in this study lies in exploring these forces as they are expressed in intergovernmental relations, particularly in the health care field; specifically, we plan to look at the origins and nature of intergovernmental cooperation and conflict, and the arrangements that have been employed, or might be employed, to foster beneficial cooperation and resolve destructive conflict.

Before we proceed to the theoretical and comparative discussion of dispute resolution mechanisms, an overview of the intergovernmental disputes in the health care field will be helpful. Ottawa has used its spending power to uphold national standards in health care in areas of provincial jurisdiction that it could not directly regulate, given constitutional requirements. The provinces protest that Ottawa does not transfer sufficient resources to them to give it the moral and political authority it needs to encourage them to uphold the principles of the *Canada Health Act* (CHA) over the long term. Thus, they resent the hierarchy and paternalism implicit in the unilateral federal control over health care funding, and over enforcement of the conditions of the CHA, as Ottawa disregards the constitutional, financial, policy, and administrative dominance of the provinces in the field itself. Health disputes intensify periodically when Ottawa intervenes to prevent the provinces from contravening the principles of the CHA, an example being the case of Alberta's and other provinces' approval of private clinics charging user fees. We make the case that reforms to institutionalize joint federal-provincial decision making through the establishment of a formal dispute resolution mechanism could ease tensions in the health and fiscal systems.

CONCEPTS AND ISSUES

Dispute Resolution Mechanisms

While acknowledging the dynamism and fluidity of the processes of cooperation and conflict in federations, it is nevertheless possible to identify several different approaches to conflict management in such states as these.[2]

Dispute Avoidance

One approach entails undertaking policies or initiatives designed to avoid the dispute in the first place; an example of this might be the transfer of tax points from Ottawa to the provinces so as to reduce or eliminate the conflicts that are sure to flare up about the level of ongoing federal transfers. It should be recognized that some initiatives can have the unintended effect of simply shifting the location of the conflict elsewhere. In this case, for example, the transfer of tax points would place extra weight on the equalization system and raise questions about whether the federal government had done enough in its horizontal redistribution programs to ensure that weaker provinces were compensated for the differential impact of a more decentralized taxation system. Integrating institutions, such as the party system or the second chamber, serve both to avoid or minimize conflict in federal systems, and to offer useful channels for its resolution when it breaks out. Dispute avoidance is most likely to be an attractive option when the parties involved have shared policy goals and are engaged in a relationship where there is a high level of trust and ongoing dialogue and negotiation.

Formal Dispute Resolution

Another approach is to tackle the resolution of disputes formally, by establishing official institutions and mechanisms, often based on constitutional provisions. These dispute mechanisms may seek to create the incentives for the parties directly concerned to sort things out among themselves. For example, the South African Constitution explicitly states that it is the responsibility of govern-

ments to avoid third-party, or judicial intervention. Consider section 41(1)(h) of
the South African Constitution:

> All spheres of government and all organs of the state within
> each sphere must:
> (h) co-operate with one another in mutual trust and good
>   faith by –
>   (i)   fostering friendly relations;
>   (ii) assisting and supporting one another;
>   (iii) informing one another of, and consulting one another
>   on, matters of common interest;
>   (iv) co-ordinating their actions and legislation with one
>   another;
>   (v)   adhering to agreed procedures; and
>   (vi) avoiding legal proceedings against one another.

This is a constitutional code of conduct, imposing a legal obligation on the participants to approach intergovernmental relations in a spirit of partnership rather
than opposition. Since the provision is only six years old, it is perhaps too soon
to say how compelling this constitutional injunction will prove to be.

The German Constitutional Court has elaborated the principle of "federal comity," which enjoins the Bund and Länder governments to behave in a fashion that is "friendly to the idea of federation." This principle is credited by some
with limiting the growth of German federal legislative power. The Canadian
Supreme Court's identification of "federalism" as a basic principle of the constitutional order not only helped to clarify the proper character of any secession process
in the country, but has also imposed a clearer obligation on the federal actors to
conduct themselves in a manner consistent with this fundamental reality.[3]

Dispute settlement mechanisms may invoke third parties to become
involved in fact-finding, mediation, arbitration, or formal resolution by a court
or tribunal.[4] In a federation the judiciary has as one of its central functions the
authoritative settlement of jurisdictional and other disputes among the con-
stituent members. Beyond the normal judicial processes, such as were followed
in the dispute concerning the cap on the Canada Assistance Plan (CAP) in 1990,
the ability of the actors in the Canadian constitutional system to make a reference
to the courts to test the constitutionality of their own initiatives or the initiatives
of another federal actor is a fairly definitive legal procedure for seeking to settle
entrenched disagreements.

Informal Dispute Resolution

Informal dispute resolution approaches are quite diverse. Meetings of officials, ministers, and first ministers, are the classic devices in Canada's system of executive federalism for settling conflict and reaching agreement on matters involving both orders of government. Recently, as we have seen, Canada has taken a leaf out of the book of international trade dispute settlement practices, applying, with modest success, a broadly similar approach to the domestic Agreement on Internal Trade (AIT).[5] The Social Union Framework Agreement (SUFA) contemplates the elaboration of an explicit dispute settlement process to cope with conflict in the social policy field, and, in fact, in response to considerable provincial pressure, the federal health minister, Anne McLellan, has recently addressed this matter (Cotter 2002; Mahoney and Laghi 2002). We will take a look at her proposal toward the end of this chapter.

Cooperation and Conflict

It would be a mistake to assume that cooperation is always good and conflict bad; both, as we have said, are inevitably facts of life in federal systems, and their respective consequences can be noxious or beneficial depending on the circumstances.[6] This being so, a capacity to challenge non-beneficial cooperation, to accommodate useful conflict, and to resolve disputes that impede the effective functioning of the system is an indicator of a mature form of government.

Drawing on our reading of the work of Peter Kellett and Diana Dalton (2001), we would suggest that useful intergovernmental conflict normally occurs in the following circumstances: when there is an authoritative voice whose pronouncements are definitive and legitimate; when the dispute management process generates energy and motivation; when substantive policy concerns take precedence over considerations of turf, status, credit-claiming, and blame avoidance; when the short-term outcome is a resolution of the matter under dispute, possibly with a new modus operandi. Alternatively, the short-term outcome could be non-confrontation, involving avoidance behaviour,[7] where the disputing parties redirect their attention from the contentious matter to cooperative initiatives as new issues arise on the policy agenda. The long-term outcome of constructive conflict is the commitment of governments to participate in ongoing dialogue and negotiation.

In contrast, destructive intergovernmental conflict is typically characterized: by the absence of an authoritative voice whose pronouncements are definitive and legitimate; by a dispute management process that follows rigid, predictable patterns; by quibbles over turf that overshadow substantive policy concerns; by the creation of a worse situation in the short term where there is a failure to deal with the hard issues, gravitation to lowest-common-denominator solutions, a blurring of issues, and a freezing-out of the public in decision making;[8] and by a long-term tendency for intergovernmental relations to deteriorate into stonewalling and escalating tensions, and a unilateral decision by one of the disputing parties to resort to silence and withdrawal.

Horizontal and Vertical Relationships

In a multi-governance system, such as that of the Canadian federation, patterns of cooperation and conflict express themselves in a complex variety of ways; horizontally, which is to say, between and among provinces; and vertically, between the provinces and the federal government. Joanne Bay Brzinski notes: "In the process of representing interests, elected leaders in a federal system have to decide which interests and which set of constituents (regional or federal) they will serve. Citizens seeking representation must likewise select the government (regional or federal) to which to appeal for response" (1999, 46). Consequently, the policies that arise in a federal system represent the diverse national and local needs of citizens and privilege some interests over others. Inevitably, policy differences arise but they do not necessarily imply conflict; nor does intergovernmental harmony necessarily require "harmonization" of all policies.

Sometimes cooperation between governments becomes a resource to assist in pursuing a conflict with another government or governments. In the early 1980s, the Government of Ontario, under Premier Bill Davis, cooperated with and supported Ottawa on two highly controversial policies – the National Energy Program (NEP) and constitutional patriation – both of which precipitated a bitter dispute between Ottawa and several other provinces. In the late 1990s, the provinces and territories, minus Quebec, leagued together in opposition to the Government of Canada's fiscal transfer and social policies.

In the health care field, the most important lines of tension flow vertically between Ottawa and the provinces rather than among the provinces themselves. While there are interprovincial difficulties that arise from time to time (for example, the dispute between Ontario and Quebec about Gatineau residents seeking medical services in Ottawa hospitals), by far the most problematic intergovernmental relationship in the health care field is federal-provincial. That is the focus of this chapter.

Institutions and Events

One can draw a useful analytical distinction between an ongoing process and a particular episode, or between a system and the events that occur within the system. Do the institutional arrangements in a political system tend to foster productive cooperation and minimize destructive conflict, or do they do the reverse? That is a system question, clearly distinguishable from a question about specific occurrences within the system. Are governments in conflict over a particular matter, and, if so, how is it being resolved? That, in contrast, is a question about a specific dispute, not a question about the system within which it occurs.

Having made the analytical distinction, one needs at once to qualify it, by recognizing that, in practical and operational reality, it can be blurred. What is a system, after all, but an almost infinite series of individual events? Forces of conflict and cooperation play themselves out over time. It is rarely the case, for example, that there is an isolated dispute whose resolution will have no longer-term implications for the parties to the conflict. A disagreement is embedded in an ongoing political process, and its resolution will in turn shape the subsequent evolution of the political relationships of which it is a part. Working together and working against one another – these elemental forces both shape the political culture and institutions of the particular society in which they are set and are in turn shaped by their specific context.

Having said that, however, an examination of the political landscape from either an institutional or an episodic perspective raises different issues and points to a distinct set of concerns. If one looks at the Canadian federation from an institutional or systems point of view, several structural elements present themselves to the eye of someone interested in forms of cooperation and conflict:

> The first-past-the-post electoral system plus parliamentary government makes for very powerful executives at both the national and the sub-national levels, and creates a pattern of executive-driven intergovernmental relations. The role of the legislatures and Parliament in the functioning of the federation is minimal to non-existent.

> The fragmented nature of the political-party system in Canada, together with the reality of very weak political parties, means that party processes cannot perform as integrating institutions in the federation.

> The absence of a constitutionally rooted intergovernmental body, like the *Bundesrat* in the Federal Republic of Germany, deprives the Canadian federal system of another potentially significant institution for

linking governments and jurisdictions together.

> The absence in Canada of an integrated public service supporting both federal and provincial governments, together with the relatively low level of mobility between federal and provincial bureaucracies, sharply limits the integrating potential of Canada's public administration.

> The way in which crown authority and responsible government are structured in Canada means that governments cannot contractually bind each other. This constitutional reality contributes to the unenforceability of intergovernmental agreements and accords.

These structural characteristics of Canadian federalism mean that the country is weakly endowed with the multi-dimensional institutional glue that helps to hold many other federations together. Executive relations between federal and provincial governments must carry the lion's share of the burden of integration and perform the central role in reconciling the federal and provincial business of the country. The Supreme Court of Canada, itself an Ottawa-appointed rather than a "federal" institution, stands as the ultimate backstop in regulating intergovernmental relationships that have become dysfunctional, but, by their nature, the courts are institutions to be resorted to only in extremis.

This means that, barring the courts, there is no effective monitor of the vertical intergovernmental relationship.[9] While Ottawa is able, at least to some extent, to perform as the monitor of horizontal relationships and disputes among the provinces,[10] there is no equivalent institution that can perform this function with respect to the vertical relationship between Ottawa itself and the provincial governments. Federal relations are shaped decisively by the actions and behaviour of federal and provincial executives, but, when these relations fall into disrepair, or when there is acute conflict, there is no agency other than the actors themselves that is capable of intervening to set things aright.

What Canada has, then, is this: a system in which the critical relations among the federal units are narrow and focused, rather than multiple and dispersed; these relations rely almost exclusively on governments, not on political parties, on legislatures, or on an effective federal upper chamber. It is a system in which intergovernmental relations are weakly institutionalized, with intermittent meetings of first ministers awaiting the call of the Prime Minister – no decision-making rules, and no settled processes for tackling the resolution of disputes. The European Union, an association of sovereign states which is not yet a federation, is by comparison vastly better equipped than Canada in this respect, with a set of powerful common institutions to conduct, oversee, and regulate the public business of Europe.

In these circumstances, the chief instrument that Canada employs to shape the common business of the federation is Ottawa's autonomous capacity to define its own role in the federation, which is normally expressed in fiscal terms. We will discuss this in a moment. When specific disputes arise in this context, they are typically resolved via a political process in which the federal government is ultimately both the prosecutor and the judge.[11] There is effectively no non-judicial third-party capacity to oversee the federal-provincial relationship, as there is in some other federations (for example, Australia with the Commonwealth Grants Commission and South Africa with the Financial and Fiscal Commission). It seems plausible to contend that the absence of a dispute settlement process, in which both or all parties to the dispute can have confidence, has pushed the Canadian intergovernmental system toward the negative rather than the productive side of the conflictual ledger.

It is possible that the double-barrelled prosecutor-and-judge role of the federal government with respect to vertical competition may not simply be a problem in itself but may compromise Ottawa's capacity to exercise its horizontal monitoring functions as well. The most significant field for the expression of intergovernmental vertical competition is unquestionably the fiscal transfer system, particularly insofar as it is focused on the provision of federal support for provincial programs rather than (as in the case of equalization) on fiscal redistribution among the provinces.[12] Federal transfers in support of health, education, and social assistance have been in existence long enough to be understood as a structural feature of the federation, yet the system lies entirely within the hands of the federal government.[13] The provincial search during the Charlottetown negotiations for a mechanism to make intergovernmental agreements binding was an attempt to correct what many regarded as a design flaw in our system of intergovernmental relations. The Government of Canada's prosecutor-and-judge function with respect to monitoring its own actions vis-à-vis the provinces means that it is not acceptable to the provinces as an impartial monitor of interprovincial competition; provincial suspicion of federal intentions in the regulation of securities seems to be an indication of this (Coleman 2002).

Canada would benefit from an effective dispute settlement process in the health care field that would respect federal principles (that is, the two levels of government would agree to a political process for resolving conflicts). Ideally, a third party, whose pronouncements were definitive and legitimate, would oversee the federal-provincial relationship, offering recommendations to address the destructive intergovernmental conflicts that sometimes impede the proper functioning of the health care system. It would be guided by clear rules, be perceived as transparent and impartial, be accessible to all those who have a legitimate interest in the outcomes, and facilitate clear, efficacious, and timely settlement of disputes.

THE CANADIAN EXPERIENCE

I t would be a mistake to assume that the Canadian federal system is mostly about conflict simply because it is the disagreements and the federal-provincial battles that receive the greatest public attention. By far the largest proportion of intergovernmental relations in Canada is marked by informal, effective, sustained cooperative relations between and among Canada's governments. The country could not function on any other basis. Federal and provincial public servants work productively together, out of the limelight, year in and year out, sharing information, solving problems, and reconciling programs and administrative responsibilities. In the line departments, where most of the day-to-day business of government is carried on, officials from both orders of government work in an atmosphere of mutual respect, sharing values, recognizing one another's specialized expertise, and acknowledging shared codes of professional conduct.

The conflict that attracts public notice is, almost by definition, political in character. If it is sufficiently persistent and acute, this type of conflict, which characteristically marks public and political debates, can penetrate the ranks of the bureaucracy; in these circumstances the ongoing business of the federation risks being compromised by division and destructive conflict. This state of affairs has existed at several points in our postwar political experience and has exacerbated regional tensions. Intergovernmental conflicts have developed quite often between Ottawa and sovereigntist governments in Quebec; between Alberta and Ottawa during the NEP period (Milne 1986, 87-95); among several governments during the constitutional patriation exercise; and between Queen's Park and Ottawa during the Harris years. Yet these cases are in the minority compared to the vast range of common endeavours on which federal and provincial officials cooperate.[14]

Intergovernmental Relations since the Second World War

The roots of our present system for the provision of health care to Canadians go back to the early postwar years. The federal government's spending power was the critical Canadian instrument fostering the expansion and consolidation of the system, but a singular focus on the federal role tells only a part of the story. One might locate the origins of public health care in Canada in a dialectical relationship that prevailed between the provincial governments and Ottawa. A Canada-wide public health insurance scheme was first seriously proposed by the federal government at a Dominion-Provincial First Ministers' Conference at the end of the Second World War, but was dropped for lack of support (Cohn 1996, 169). Public hospital care was actually introduced first in Saskatchewan in 1947, with British Columbia and Alberta[15] following suit in 1948 and 1950 respectively – all of this before the federal government became directly in involved in 1957. The federal government's role was to pick up on an important social-policy initiative begun by several provinces, and, through moral suasion and money, convince the other provinces to come on board. Saskatchewan again was the first jurisdiction to initiate public support for medicare in 1962, followed in due course by Ottawa, which in 1966 fostered the establishment of a Canada-wide medicare program. The acknowledged dominance of federal fiscal transfers in shaping and supporting provincial provision of health services has obscured the significant role of the provinces as incubators of social reform and managers of social policy, a feature of the Canadian system that has continued in various ways to this day.

The Canadian health care system is the most impressive product of a complex set of cooperative and conflictual relations between governments over an extended period of time, each side endowed with significant political resources, and neither side finally capable of dominating the other. In looking back, one can see that a good deal of the friction in the system has served a beneficial purpose.

The first chapter in this volume speaks of the constitutional foundations upon which government roles in health care rest, describes the nature and use of the federal spending power, and briefly charts the evolution of intergovernmental relations in respect of health care. Chapter 3 provides a general account of the history of federal and provincial public finance since the end of the Second World War, while chapter 4 depicts the evolution of the federal transfer system in respect of health and other social programs.

From 1945 to the early 1970s there was a dramatic increase in the size of the public sector, especially at the provincial level, as central elements of the Canadian welfare state were introduced. The creation of major new programs, for example, in the areas of health, social assistance, and post-secondary education, and the provision of federal transfers and some taxation room to the provinces were key elements in this story. Between the early 1970s and the beginning of the 1990s, social programs were consolidated, as both federal and provincial governments sought greater fiscal predictability and policy autonomy. In the service of these objectives, there was a move away from federal-provincial shared-cost programs to block-funded fiscal transfers.[16] The shift suited Ottawa, because it did not wish to see its expenditure patterns in the area determined by the provinces' spending on health care and education; it suited the provinces, because they did not wish to have their priorities distorted by the existence of "50-cent dollars" and because they found the accounting requirements that cost sharing required burdensome. Less satisfactorily from the point of view of Ottawa, the federal government lost its leverage over provincial social programs, which it sought to recover through the passage in 1984 of the *Canada Health Act* (to be discussed below).

In the early 1990s governments across the country made fighting the deficit their top priority, and sought to contain or reduce their financial commitments to the major social programs. During this period (1992-96) the rate of growth in per capita health expenditures in Canada flattened out before beginning to rise again in 1997. In the late 1990s most Canadian governments entered a new era of budgetary health, with Alberta and Ottawa in particular experiencing significant surpluses, but health care continued to be without question the biggest item driving up provincial costs, as it is today.

Students of federalism have used a number of terms to describe the style and operation of the federal process in these various phases of Canada's historical development.[17] Some of the phrases that have been used are: "cooperative federalism,"[18] "administrative federalism,"[19] "executive federalism,"[20] "summit federalism,"[21] "competitive federalism,"[22] and "collaborative federalism."[23] These are not scientific terms. While both the periodization and the characterization of the several styles of federalism and intergovernmental relations vary from author to author, the important thing to realize from the point of view of our story, is that – whatever the periodization and characterization – a central element of the account has to do with the balance and the relationship between cooperative and conflictual practices.

Program-specific relations among relatively decentralized governments and bureaucracies, for example, distinguished cooperative federalism in the 1950s and 1960s. Ottawa was widely acknowledged to be the senior government (the major exception to this view being Quebec); practical arrangements were typically worked out among officials in line departments, and the level of tension was low.

What some authors have called competitive federalism emerged in the late 1960s and existed throughout the 1970s and early 1980s, marked by a higher level of intergovernmental tension. Central agencies took over files and linked them together to fashion corporate intergovernmental strategies; first ministers became more directly involved; the status of politicians and their governments became more directly implicated in the conduct of the business of the federation; and issues were increasingly framed in zero-sum terms, making them awkward candidates for artful compromise.

Some writers have argued that a discernibly different form of intergovernmental relations, dubbed collaborative federalism, emerged in the course of the 1990s. In part a response to federal fiscal retreat, collaborative federalism refers to the growing practice of provinces and territories, working together, to initiate serious discussion of national policy questions. Sometimes Ottawa is involved; sometimes not. Perhaps the distinguishing features of this style of intergovernmental relations are an assumption of equality among all participating governments and a belief that provinces and territories, acting on their own, are capable of fashioning programs and initiatives in the national interest. One example of a product of collaborative federalism is the Ottawa-led negotiation of the Agreement on Internal Trade, signed in 1994 and implemented in 1995. Another, this time initiated and carried forward by the provinces and territories, is the Social Union Framework Agreement, agreed to by all governments except Quebec in February 1999.

A review of Canada's postwar experience with federalism permits some observations about the sources and levels of conflict in federal-provincial relations (Cameron and Simeon 2000, 71-73). They will be greater:

> *When differing ideologies exist.* If there is tacit agreement among governments and citizens about the nature of politics, the role of government, the central problem confronting the public sector, the extent to which radical change is necessary, and so forth, this will reduce the likelihood that intergovernmental relations will be poisonous. In the case of health

care, if the provinces and federal government are in agreement about the value of national health insurance, the principles of the *Canada Health Act*, and the role of the private sector, the likelihood of conflict over the federal government's enforcement of the Act is diminished.

> *When the status, recognition, and identity of regions, communities, and governments are seen to be at stake in intergovernmental negotiations.* Using shared perspectives and expertise to solve practical problems encourages compromise; challenging a player's status or identity is almost certain to create conflict. Symbolic issues are much more difficult to resolve than practical problems. Increasingly, from the 1960s, intergovernmental relations came to embody "identity politics." The "facility fee" confrontation is an example of a highly charged symbolic issue. Premier Ralph Klein has allowed user fees for private clinics to proliferate in Alberta since the 1990s as part of his drive to broaden the role of the private sector in the health care system and to uphold the province's autonomy, even though his critics have argued that these fees contravene the *Canada Health Act* (Boase 2001).

> *When issues play out differentially along regional or linguistic lines.* The NEP set the west, particularly Alberta, against central Canada. Phrases such as "Let the Eastern bastards freeze in the dark" and the "blue-eyed sheiks" are coarse reminders of the interregional animosity that existed at that time. The CF-18 incident envenomed French-English relations and was one of the chief regional grievances behind the formation of the Reform Party. The federal cap on CAP drove a wedge between the wealthy provinces (Alberta, British Columbia, and Ontario) and all the others; it was the impulse behind the push for constitutionally binding intergovernmental agreements during the Charlottetown negotiations.

> *When neither government is prepared to defer to the other.* In the immediate postwar period, there was considerable agreement among both citizens and governments that Ottawa was the "senior" partner – equipped with political and financial strength and a self-confident bureaucracy. By the 1970s Quebec had come to see itself as the primary political expression of the Quebec people, and western provinces had come to see themselves as defenders of a regional interest that was not represented in Ottawa, with its weak senate and its governing parties that had to pay attention to the more populous Central Canada. Neither their politi-

cians nor their increasingly professional bureaucracies were prepared to defer to Ottawa.

> *When the primary concerns of governments become blame avoidance, the winning of credit, and the enhancement of their own political status relative to other governments.* While these are obviously virtually universal phenomena, the factors listed above affect whether such concerns are in the foreground or background during intergovernmental negotiations. The framework for cooperation and conflict is shaped by a number of practical factors: the nature of the issue involved (high politics, involving symbolically freighted issues or specific program-based matters); the site at which the issue is being addressed (at the level of first ministers, for example, as distinct from the level of senior officials, or line department civil servants); and the substantive content of the issue (money, for example, as opposed to jurisdiction).

Let us turn now to several examples of the way in which conflict has been dealt with in the Canadian federal system outside the field of health care. We will reserve our discussion of the *Canada Health Act* and the Social Union Framework Agreement to the final section of this report, where we examine various models of dispute resolution in the health care field.

Dealing with Conflict in the Canadian Federation: Some Examples

In our examination of Canadian experience, we will pay particular attention to several characteristics of dispute settlement mechanisms: their authoritativeness, compatibility with federal principles, formality, scope, accessibility, transparency, frequency of use, and enforceability. The authoritativeness of dispute mechanisms is bolstered when a third party whose pronouncements are definitive and legitimate offers recommendations to the conflicting parties for resolving their disputes. The authoritativeness of decisions and rulings is based on the legitimacy of the process in the eyes of the parties to the conflict. Is the process open and fair? Is the decision-making authority impartial and balanced in its judgments? A mechanism could be considered compatible with federal values if it recognizes that both levels of government are on an equal footing and have their own competences and policy-making capacities. Both levels of government agree to participate in the design of the dispute mechanism, choose representatives to be a part of the body, and follow its procedures to bring an end to destructive conflicts. The formality of dispute mechanisms turns chiefly on whether they have a constitutional or legal foundation. Some dispute resolution mechanisms contain provisions that encourage the conflicting parties to engage in dispute avoidance and informal dispute resolution processes such as mediation before resorting to more formal ones such as resolution by a court or tribunal. Dispute mechanisms range in scope from narrow (focusing exclusively on CHA interpretation, for example) to broad (including for instance, CHA interpretation, fiscal transfers, mobility, and future joint initiatives, as envisioned in the Social Union Framework Agreement). Accessibility depends on the number of people who are party to the agreement and can use the mechanism. Is the mechanism only open to government actors or are interest groups and private citizens also potential participants in the dispute resolution process? Transparency refers to the ease with which the public can access the process, including viewing the documents that are submitted by the conflicting parties and the reports that are produced by the dispute settlement body. The frequency of use depends on the cost, length of deliberations, and the accessibility of the mechanism. The frequency with which a mechanism is resorted to is also related to the perceived likelihood of its leading to a settled resolution of the conflict, which will allow the parties to move on. Enforceability of the dispute mechanism has to do with the binding or non-binding nature of the recommendations, the existence of an appeals process, and the severity of the penalties for non-compliance.

The Charlottetown Accord

The Charlottetown Accord (1992) aimed at addressing some of the enduring problems of federal-provincial power sharing by clarifying the roles and responsibilities of the two levels of government in several different policy sectors. It represented the Mulroney government's second attempt to bring about constitutional reform acceptable to Quebecers, and included changes in Aboriginal self-government and senate reform. What is relevant for our purposes is that it made provisions for conferring legal status on intergovernmental agreements and for creating dispute mechanisms to resolve issues concerning the common market and self-government, although the details were very sketchy. Had the Charlottetown Accord been enacted, the first ministers would have been responsible for determining the role, mandate, and composition of the common market dispute mechanism. The mechanism for resolving self-government disputes would have involved mediation and arbitration and would have been set out in a political accord.

In 1992 Canadians rejected the Charlottetown Accord in a referendum. Thus, a wide-ranging constitutional package did not prove to be a useful vehicle for introducing a dispute settlement mechanism. Incremental agreements between the provinces and territories and the federal government are more promising vehicles for creating dispute mechanisms. They can more easily be implemented than constitutional reforms because they do not require as many individuals to give them their stamp of approval and the issues under consideration can more easily be disaggregated.

Environmental Policy: 1987-1990

In the environmental policy field, as in health care, there have been vigorous debates over the appropriate role of the national government in a federal system since there is some overlap of jurisdictional responsibility in both areas. We will examine federal-provincial relations in environmental policy during two time periods: 1987 to 1990, and 1991 to the present. The former period illustrates an informal federal leadership approach to dispute resolution where harmonious intergovernmental relations were put to the test, whereas the latter illustrates a more collaborative approach. The environmental example will show that collaboration between federal and provincial governments does not necessarily produce better policy outcomes than when the federal government takes a leadership role.

During the late 1980s the federal government sought to renew its regulatory activity in the area of environmental assessment through the *Canadian Environmental Protection Act* (1988) even though the provincial governments, particularly Quebec and Alberta, strongly objected to its "interference" in provincial resource-management decisions.[24] In a sense, the federal government had its leadership role thrust upon it. It was motivated to take a stronger leadership role than it had traditionally claimed by a federal court decision in 1989, which ruled that the government "had to adhere to the terms of its own Environmental Assessment and Review Process (EARP) and conduct environmental assessments on two dams on the Rafferty and Alameda rivers" (Conrad 1999, 40). Pressure from environmentalists and the court's verdict made it impossible for the federal government to "restore intergovernmental harmony simply by retreating from the field,"[25] as it had tried to do in the past.

A number of different mechanisms were in use between 1986 and 1990, including informal (for example, meetings between provincial and federal officials at advisory meetings) and formal dispute mechanisms such as the federal court. The authoritativeness of the federal government's unilateral initiatives (including the 1988 *Canadian Environmental Protection Act*, the *Canadian Environmental Assessment Act*, and the 1990 Green Plan) was bolstered by the court decision and public opinion, which has "consistently supported a stronger federal role in the protection of the environment" (Winfield 2002, 124). Federal relations were strained during this time period, but there is little evidence that the governments' adherence to the principle of federalism suffered. One of the advantages of competitive federalism was that there was very little overlap and duplication between the federal and provincial programs (Winfield 2002, 127). The scope of federal environmental policy expanded because there was an increase in international pressures on Ottawa to enact more sustainable policies, and citizens became more determined that the environmental ramifications of economic development should be considered (see Skogstad and Kopas 1992). Accessibility grew as environmental groups learned to use the courts to encourage government to take a more proactive stance in enforcing regulatory standards. Governments needed to at least appear to be more responsive to the public. They invited industry representatives and environmental groups to comment on regulatory changes in key forums such as the Canadian Council of Ministers of the Environment. Meetings of provincial and federal officials became more frequent. Policy innovation and enforcement of environmental regulations became a priority.

In the 1990s the federal government shifted from using a leadership model to a more traditional cooperative one. Mark Winfield attributes the shift to "national unity concerns and neo-liberal ideas" and regrets that they "have intruded into and overridden environmental protection goals" (2002, 124).

Environmental Policy: 1991 to the Present

Part of the impetus behind the harmonization initiative in the 1990s was to illustrate the federal government's flexibility and the potential for non-constitutional policy reform with respect to one of the leading irritants in intergovernmental relations (Winfield 2002, 127). A collaborative approach in the area of environmental policy is clearly illustrated by the Canada-wide Accord on Environmental Harmonization (1998) and its three sub-agreements on inspections, national standard setting, and environmental assessment. The Accord was signed by all provinces that were represented in the Canadian Council of

Ministers of the Environment, except Quebec. Conrad (1999) notes that in sign-ing the Accord the federal and provincial governments "agreed to move toward a radical reallocation of environmental responsibility, shifting away from the bilat-eral arrangements or less formal multilateral arrangements, to ... multilateral coordination and joint action" (43). The governments agreed to cooperate in conducting a single environmental assessment and review process for cross-juris-dictional issues. This cooperation was intended to make it easier for them to share information and expertise on environmental problems.

The government that is "best situated," using criteria such as physical proximity and capacity to address client and local needs, which appear to favour the provinces in most cases, is to deliver the services under the "one-window" mechanism (Winfield 2002, 129). The Accord and the sub-agreements can be altered only with the unanimous consent of the signatories, although a government can withdraw from the arrangements on six months' notice. If there is an intergov-ernmental disagreement within the inspections sub-agreement, six months of con-sultations are required, after which, if the concerned government is still not satisfied, it has the option of withdrawing from the sub-agreement after the six-month notice period. Disagreements with respect to the implementation of nation-al standards call for an effort on the part of the concerned governments to develop an "alternative plan," but there is no provision for the dissatisfied level of govern-ment to act where it judges the other government has failed to acquit its obligations satisfactorily (Winfield 2002, 129-30).

Winfield argues that the collaborative approach to environmental issues has greatly reduced the level of intergovernmental tensions in the field, but notes that, with the race to the bottom among the provinces continuing, it is apparent that good intergovernmental relations do not necessarily equal good substantive policy outcomes. He argues that the earlier, conflictual era of competitive feder-alism "seemed to produce far better results for the protection of the environment" (2002, 131-32). The federal government will be hard pressed to regain the lead-ership authority it needs to respond to domestic and international developments related to environmental matters.

Canada's Agreement on Internal Trade

The Agreement on Internal Trade,[26] signed in 1994 by all Canadian governments, provides an example of a quasi-formal dispute settlement mech-anism in a collaborative setting. It is not as formal as a legal document, since it is a political accord, and is not justiciable. Nevertheless, the creation by all governments of the Internal Trade Secretariat in Winnipeg indicated a determination to institutionalize the arrangements, and the Agreement certainly requires governments to engage in a greater level of consultation or "process" when introducing measures affecting internal trade than was the case before it was enacted (Certified General Accountants 2001, 5). The Agreement is aimed at reducing barriers to the free movement of goods, services, investments, and members of the workforce across Canada. As in the health care case, harmonization was a contentious concept in the negotiation of the AIT, with the federal government wanting to assert national standards and the provinces resisting them (Doern and MacDonald 1999, 136).

The dispute settlement mechanism, described in chapter 17 of the Agreement on Internal Trade, is designed to facilitate the resolution of disputes between governments, and between governments and businesses. If disputes are not settled through cooperation (consultation, mediation, and conciliation) they can be referred to a panel for arbitration. Individuals, companies, and governments can use the mechanism. An individual or a business can access the process in one of two ways:

> An individual or a business may request that their government pursue the government-to-government dispute resolution process. This process may lead to a request for the assistance of the Committee on Internal Trade and a dispute resolution panel of experts.

> If the government chooses not to step in, an individual or business may proceed under the private party-to-government dispute resolution process and request consultations. At this stage the complaint will be assessed by an independent screener who will determine the merit of the request. If a complaint has merit, a panel is formed (see MacDonald 2002, 146).

The transparency provisions of the AIT are limited. Consultations are confidential. Although all proceedings before a panel are public, all documents filed are accessible only to the parties (see Doern and MacDonald 1999, 139).

The panel process is time-consuming (there is a 545-day wait for the submission and implementation of a panel report, and a further 365 days for meetings to discuss non-compliance). The panel can make its findings public and offer recommendations (Alberta 1997). The two government-to-government disputes that have been subject to the panel process have both led to provincial compliance with the panel findings (MacDonald 2002, 146). The decision from the first person-to-government dispute resolution panel under the Agreement on Internal Trade was made public in December 2001, sixty days after its issuance, to put pressure on the party complained against (Ontario) to comply with the recommendations in the panel report (Internal Trade Secretariat 2001).

Critics point out that "aspects of the mechanism make the AIT more complex and cumbersome than it should be (for example, limited private-party access, lack of a right to appeal, and dubious enforceability measures, not to mention multiple procedures for different industries)" (Clendenning 1997, 47). Its detractors regret that the scope of the institution is somewhat limited since, if Ottawa is unhappy with the functioning of the AIT, it has the option of bypassing the mechanism entirely and introducing legislation to remove barriers, using its constitutional trade and commerce powers (Howse 1996, 13-14). For example, Bryan Schwartz argues:

> Given its limited scope of application and many exceptions, the AIT is a smallish and rather mild-mannered tiger. When it becomes clear that the terms of the agreement are offended, the guilty party is expected, as a matter of honour, to mend its ways. If it does not do so, the agreement may be cited to bring public attention to the offender's shameful conduct. If the offender is still unrepentant, the agreement can provide no further relief except that the victimized party is authorized to retaliate. (1995, 212-13)

Defenders of the AIT dispute mechanism, however, praise it as "a first step" in a longer process of improving intergovernmental trade relations. Furthermore, they argue that in circumstances such as those in Canada, in which the probability of repeated trade is very high, the incentive on the part of the actors to play by the rules of the game may be very high, making a political process, rather than a binding legal one, effective. Indeed, as time passes, and the AIT becomes more deeply institutionalized, "the politically based dispute resolution mechanism may be all that is necessary to maintain the AIT" (MacDonald 2002, 147).

A number of lessons can be drawn from the AIT example which may have relevance for the health care case, such as the importance of including incentives for conflicting parties to settle their disputes through blame avoidance, and the need to use informal dispute resolution processes before using formal ones. The AIT experience also suggests that a dispute mechanism does not need to be legally binding to be effective, but that there must be sufficient political and economic incentives to encourage individuals, companies, and governments to use it.

Labour Market Policy

The labour market has also been the topic of sustained discussions among academics and policymakers over the appropriate role of the national government. The Charlottetown Accord envisioned making labour policy the exclusive jurisdiction of the provinces in order to relieve some of the intergovernmental tension relating to this matter. That proposed change, along with the introduction of a dispute mechanism for the common market and the other provisions in the Charlottetown Accord, was rejected in 1992. The bilateral Labour Market Development Agreements, signed in 1996 and 1997 by Ottawa and eleven of the twelve provinces and territories, are of interest because they embody an attempt by the Government of Canada to reach concord in a controversial intergovernmental file by a process of differential decentralization. In 1996 Ottawa offered to transfer all of its labour market programs plus the associated funding and staff to the provinces, provided certain basic conditions were met. The Labour Market Development Agreements that were signed between the federal government and the provinces and territories have been classified into several types: the "co-management model" (Newfoundland and Labrador, British Columbia, Prince Edward Island, and Yukon Territory); "full-transfer agreements" (New Brunswick, Quebec, Manitoba, Saskatchewan, Alberta, Northwest Territories, and Nunavut); and a "strategic partnership" (Nova Scotia). Only Ontario has yet to sign an agreement. Thomas Klassen observes that:

> Under the co-management model, there is no transfer of resources (either dollars or staff) to the provinces, but a joint management of program design and implementation ... The full-transfer model, on the other hand, involves provinces assuming responsibility for labour market policy and program delivery within the federal funding and client eligibility constraints. The federal government retains responsibility for the delivery of EI benefits and pan-Canadian initiatives such as national labour market information and exchange, as well as responding to economic emergencies ...
> The only requirement of the [strategic partnership] agreement is that a joint-management committee be established to examine the areas of joint cooperation and collaboration. (2000, 177)

The advantage of this new regime is that it allowed the provinces to "negotiate and tailor their particular agreements to meet their specific needs and wishes" (Hanson 1999, 132-33). However, the Agreements offer few opportunities for citizen engagement, have weak accountability mechanisms, and do not as yet include Ontario. Moreover, as Klassen comments, the danger of the new regime for the provinces is that "they provide services but ultimately the federal government, along with macroeconomic conditions, determine the size of the caseload" (2000, 194).

What has been the effect of this initiative? Herman Bakvis (2000) contends that it was an intergovernmental success, in the sense that it effectively resolved some long-standing issues in the intergovernmental arena. On the other hand, he acknowledges that, at the federal political level, there is some disenchantment with the loss of visibility and the minimal credit Ottawa has won for its initiative; that, in Quebec, checkerboard federalism – asymmetry for all – does not directly address that community's desire for distinct recognition; and that, in terms of good public policy, devolution inevitably undermines the country's capacity to formulate national labour market strategies (215-16). The labour market case illustrates that the federal and the provincial and territorial governments can design innovative and workable asymmetrical solutions to long-standing intergovernmental problems, but that these may imply increasing inequities across the nation.

SOME RELEVANT COMPARABLE EXPERIENCE

Here we examine a number of approaches to conflict management that have been employed elsewhere in the world. We begin by reporting on arrangements (ranging from most advanced to least advanced) designed to resolve disputes among international actors. In the second section we explore relevant experience in other countries that are in some ways similar to the Canadian federation. Here, as in our discussion of the Canadian experience, the criteria for comparing the dispute mechanisms include: their authoritativeness, compatibility with federal principles, formality, scope, accessibility, transparency, frequency of use, and enforceability record. It is important to examine their design closely because provisions of existing national and international dispute mechanisms that have proven to be effective can be borrowed for the creation of new mechanisms in other sectors and countries.

International Organizations

The European Union has been described as more advanced than the other examples of international mechanisms that follow. Clendenning, for example, considers the European Union to be the most highly developed on several counts:

> It provides direct access for both private and public parties through national courts and the European Court of Justice. In addition, it provides for the direct effect of secondary legislation and allows Commission directives to supersede national legislation in the establishment of the economic union. Indeed, the EU has made continuing strides in expanding the scope of the economic union through amendments to the Treaty of Rome, the adoption of Commission directives and compliance precedents established by Court of Justice rulings. (1997, 45)

We will describe the dispute mechanisms of the European Union in more detail before examining two other international mechanisms, the World Trade Organization and the North American Free Trade Agreement; and national mechanisms in two federal countries, Belgium and Australia.

The European Union

The European Union (EU) has a highly rules-based, confederal structure that some observers have suggested has relevance for dispute resolution in the Canadian social union (Biggs 1996, 22). In order to participate in the EU, governments must consent to share a measure of their sovereignty with a network of supranational institutions. Informal processes (for example, meetings in advance of official conciliations) smooth the interaction between institutions responsible for the adoption of European Union legislation (Garman and Hilditch 1998, 283), including the European Commission, the Council, the Parliament and the Court of Justice (ECJ). The Union is supported by a group of officials dedicated to making the whole system work.

The commissioners have the authority to oversee and implement treaties between member states without being directly accountable to their own governments. The Council of Ministers is the main legislative body with the mandate to define the EU's general policy guidelines. Regarding the matter of transparency, Steven McGiffen critically observes that: "In common with the other major decision-making bodies of the European Union – with the exception of the European Parliament – the European Council shrouds itself in a Kremlin-like secrecy which seems to many quite out of keeping with what might be expected from a community of democratic nations" (2001, 15). The Parliament, which derives its authority directly from the voters of the member states, considers the Commission's proposals and shares budgetary powers with the Council. Depending on the type of policy instrument emanating from the Council of Ministers, enforceability varies. Regulations are automatically binding in member states without any action on the part of their government; directives give each member state the opportunity to decide how to achieve the objective prescribed by the European Union; decisions target a particular member state, company, or individual; and recommendations are completely non-binding.

The Court of Justice is the most formal body for conflict resolution. The ECJ mechanism is used frequently and its scope is very broad, encompassing all of the legal issues that arise in the member states. The Court's decisions are highly credible since "the Commission, its member states, business firms and individuals can all take action directly to enforce EU provisions with the certainty that Union law will supersede any national law" (Clendenning 1997, 6).

Critics have suggested that the European Union suffers from a "democratic deficit" because the supranational institutions like the Council of Ministers and the European Court of Justice meet in secret and are not directly elected, yet they have the power to direct national legislatures. Other observers, like Moravcsik (1993, 515), contend that the " 'democratic deficit' may be a fundamental source of its success" (Biggs 1996, 23). Governments can bargain and reach consensus with relatively little constraint from citizens and interest groups on issues related to all sectors and types of barriers. At the same time, business firms and individuals do have access to the EU dispute settlement mechanisms, which is one of the reasons that they have been used frequently. The EU example shows the importance of informal processes for resolving disputes even when a highly formal structure like the ECJ is in place.

The World Trade Organization

The World Trade Organization (WTO), which came into being in 1994 after the Uruguay Round of trade negotiations, is based on the principle of formal equality among actors. The dispute mechanism of the World Trade Organization is highly developed, especially compared with that of its precursor, the General Agreement on Tarriffs and Trade (GATT). It was set up in order to prevent the competitive raising of trade barriers and to ensure that major players did not shirk their GATT responsibilities at the expense of poorer countries.

The World Trade Organization is a forum for resolving disputes among countries through consultation or, failing that, a procedure that includes the possibility of a panel and an appeal. Any interested member states can participate in the process as "third parties." The panel may consult experts, upon agreement from the disputing members, in order to determine whether or not a member has violated its WTO obligations.

Decisions of WTO panels may be appealed to the standing WTO Appellate Body, where seven members with experience in law and international trade re-examine the case. The WTO's Appellate Body has the authority to reject the expert panel's interpretation of the agreements and overturn its ruling. The final step in the WTO's dispute mechanism process is as follows: the decision of the panel or Appellate Body is "presented to all WTO Members for adoption at a meeting of the Dispute Settlement Body (DSB). Panel and Appellate Body decisions are adopted by so-called 'negative consensus': they are adopted unless there is a consensus of all DSB Members not to do so. Once adopted by the Members, the report becomes a 'WTO ruling'" (Department of Foreign Affairs and International Trade 2001).

The dispute mechanism is available only for contracting parties to the Agreement; hence its frequency of use is limited. If individuals or firms have grievances that they want resolved through this mechanism, they have to persuade their own governments to take up their cause (Clendenning 1997, 9), in which case panels composed of three members seek a resolution. The decisions and rulings that are made by the panel are highly credible, since measures are taken to prevent the panel from becoming vulnerable to political influence. For example, the members on the panel do not come from countries that are party to the dispute. Although the deliberations and written submissions of the panels are confidential, the disputing parties have the option, which Canada uses, of disclosing their own positions to the public. Parties have some incentive to comply with the recommendations, since compensation is theoretically "available in the event that the recommendations and rulings of a panel of the Appellate Body are not implemented within a reasonable period of time" (Epps 2001, 71). However, enforcement of compensation is difficult. The primary remedy is to bring the offending measures into conformity with the relevant agreement.

Critics contend that the WTO does not provide adequate protection for smaller countries that are not economically able to retaliate effectively against stronger economies (Zekos 1999; Bhagwati 2001). As well, William Davey (2000, 167-70) suggests that the WTO dispute settlement system is weakened by the absence of permanent panellists and sufficient staff support. Nevertheless, the WTO has attracted positive commentary for its success in opening markets, increasing predictability in trade relations among states, and improving on the impressive dispute settlement record that existed under GATT (Grané 2001). Whereas 300 disputes were dealt with through GATT between 1947 and 1994, 167 cases were dealt with by the WTO between 1995 and March 1999 (WTO 1999, 5). The number of cases indicates the members' confidence in the WTO dispute resolution process. Observers have also stressed the importance of the Appellate Body as an innovative feature that bolsters the WTO's "impartiality, integrity and independence" (Clendenning 1997, 54) and could be incorporated into other dispute resolution mechanisms.

The North American Free Trade Agreement

The North American Free Trade Agreement (NAFTA) is the successor to the Canada-US Free Trade Agreement (FTA) (Rosa 1993, 255) and is designed to eliminate barriers to trade in goods and services between Canada, the United States, and Mexico. Like the FTA, it has formal dispute mechanisms that involve consultation, arbitration, and mediation (although mediation is used infrequently).[27] Chapter 20 provisions of NAFTA (under chapter 18 of the FTA) involve government-to-government proceedings. Chapter 19 provisions govern the settlement of anti-dumping and countervailing duty cases and allow individuals and companies to bring cases against governments even without the consent of their home government (Appleton 1999, 94). NAFTA created a binational panel process to review trade determinations by domestic agencies and apply the law of the importing country (Hoberg and Howe 1999, 4). Parties are required to resolve the dispute by agreement in accordance with an arbitral panel's findings within thirty days of the release of the report (Crommelin 2001, 142).

Canadian critics argue that the credibility of NAFTA decisions may be compromised for several reasons: (1) The proceedings lack transparency. All panel hearings and submissions are treated as confidential, and only the final report is released fifteen days after it is submitted to the Commission; (2) There is no opportunity for non-parties such as interested members of the public to participate, although expert testimony may be permitted if both parties approve; (3) There is an inherent bias favouring the nation with the majority of panellists; (4) The arbitrators "may not have any familiarity with Canadian law or health policy objectives and little real sense of Canadian values"; (5) "Arbitral panels are not required to follow the decisions of previous panels. This means that there is uncertainty whenever a dispute comes before such a panel"; (6) "There is no right of appeal or judicial review from the decision of an arbitral panel" (Epps 2001, 103-4). An expert challenge panel can address allegations of gross misconduct but, unlike the WTO's Appellate Body, it cannot confront the issue of interpretation.

The strengths of the FTA and NAFTA dispute settlement mechanisms are that they provide: "(1) a specific forum in the Commission for consultation and mediation; (2) a defined timetable set for stages of dispute-settlement procedure; (3) an option to retaliate with 'equivalent effects' if either party is not satisfied by the Commission decision; (4) a more rapid process than that of the GATT; and (5) the development of a body of 'jurisprudence' on Canadian-US [and Mexican in the case of NAFTA] trade within the Commission" (Campbell and Pal 1991, 220).

In general, the FTA and NAFTA dispute settlement mechanisms have created a more predictable trading environment, but observers have made compelling recommendations to strengthen them. Some of the lessons that could be drawn for the health care case are that the credibility of a dispute mechanism can be improved by making it more transparent, allowing interested members of the public to participate, requiring panels to follow earlier decisions, and making provisions for an appellate body with panellists appointed for specific terms to review rulings.

Dispute Resolution Bodies in Other Countries

Belgium's Conseil d'État

Belgium's Conseil d'État (supreme administrative court) and Comité de Concertation are of interest because they are authoritative institutions in a complex, decentralized environment, and their pronouncements for resolving intergovernmental disputes are widely viewed as legitimate (Commission on Fiscal Imbalance 2001b, 33). Subnational governments in Belgium (as in Canada) play a significant role in central decision making, just as member states do at the supranational level in the EU. The Conseil d'État is an example of a formal dispute mechanism with a broad mandate. It reviews draft legislation prior to implementation, including all constitutional amendments, to ensure that each order of government does not overstep its jurisdiction. In some cases, its assistance in reviewing legislation is compulsory; in other instances it is optional. Its decisions are credible since it is composed of experts in various fields who have a reputation for providing uniform, consistent interpretations of legislation. Its decisions are enforceable. It can annul administrative acts and regulations that are incompatible with existing legal opinions, or suspend their execution. The Conseil d'État has the power to refer draft legislation to the Comité de concertation if the legislation risks sparking jurisdictional conflict. The committee, which is composed of representatives of all governments, then reaches a consensus on the contentious matter. If legislation is developed that may exceed the competence of the level of government, governmental actors or interested individuals can refer the matter to the Court of Arbitrage, which acts as an independent arbitrator among the federal state, the communities, and the regions, and protects the rights of citizens. The Court has the authority to cancel the offending legislation within six months of its publication and to rule on preliminary questions.

These dispute resolution mechanisms allow intergovernmental issues to be treated in technical and legal ways and minimize the political considerations that would otherwise surround disputes.

Australia's Council of Australian Governments

The Council of Australian Governments (COAG), which was established in 1992, is a collaborative forum where disputes between the federal, state, and territorial governments can be resolved through negotiation.[28] It evolved out of traditional premiers conferences as a way of making Australian intergovernmental relations more cooperative and productive. Margaret Biggs identifies the features that distinguish COAG from premiers conferences: "What distinguishes COAG from the Ministerial Council system is that it addresses areas of national significance and has a central agency, 'whole of government' perspective. COAG is a forum for spearheading reform, challenging existing processes and thinking, and making the cross-sectoral linkages and trade-offs that are often essential to a 'national' solution" (1996, 26).

The scope of COAG is very broad. Within this intergovernmental body, political actors tackle such difficult issues as competition, Aboriginal policy, and taxation policy. Representatives of the two levels of government have used the forum to initiate "major policy reforms across a wide range of sectors, in relatively short periods of time" (Biggs 1996, 28). There is a lot of pressure on parties to reach an agreement in the latter stages of the negotiation because COAG operates under a unanimity rule. If a consensus is not reached, the parties have few options for settlement other than handing over outstanding issues to other intergovernmental bodies. COAG decisions are not enforceable and its existence is tenuous. Since it was created by agreement, it could simply be dissolved if the parties no longer supported it.

The credibility of COAG is diminished by the fact that the public is not privy to the negotiations but is only informed of the results through communiqués at the end of the meetings. Some critics are concerned that COAG has the potential to undermine parliamentary accountability (Painter 1996). Nevertheless, the forum attracts a lot of popular support and praise from policy experts for creating more cooperative intergovernmental relations by facilitating the development of shared language and relationships (Painter 2001).

COPING WITH CONFLICT AND DISPUTES IN THE HEALTH CARE FIELD

After setting out some of the factors that will frame our analysis of dispute resolution approaches, we will examine the *Canada Health Act* (CHA), both because it is central to the Canadian health care system and because it offers a useful base-case scenario for considering alternative ways of tackling the resolution of conflict in the health care field in the Canadian federation. This analysis will lead to a framework for understanding the nature of conflict in the health field, which we will then use as the foundation for an evaluation of a number of alternative approaches to the resolution of conflicts between the federal and provincial governments in the field of health. Our focus, as we have said, is on disputes among governments, not on conflicts in the private sector or conflicts between citizens and the state. We do not include any discussion of possibilities that would require constitutional change, as these lie beyond the range of practical politics.

In a federal state, the pattern of conflict is established to a substantial degree by the distribution of jurisdictional authority between and among the federated governments. These conflicts may be rooted in the aspirations and convictions of the populations in the various parts of the country, or they may be more restricted to the political ambitions of political leaders and other actors.

Some conflicts are so deeply rooted in the cleavages and fault lines of the country that they are better regarded as eternal facts of political life than as disagreements that may, in principle, be resolved. For example, the nationalist conflict concerning Quebec's status within or outside of Canada is of this character. Efforts at conflict resolution have involved the entire Canadian state, its political parties, its legislative and judicial institutions, and its people. This is not the sort of conflict we are speaking of in this paper, although it is eminently capable of spawning the second- and third-order conflicts that *are* the subject of our study. Indeed, Quebec's constitutional views and its position on health care jurisdiction set it decidedly apart from all the other provinces – so much so that much of the discussion of alternatives in this paper, which presupposes normal participation of the government actors in the system, does not really apply at all to Quebec, whose involvement in national health care discussions is greatly limited and deeply ambivalent.

While a conflict will almost always be framed in the vocabulary of justice and fairness, a dispute may have its origins in one or more of a fairly wide range of differences: ideological or policy disagreements; a quarrel over money and resources; the drive for status or reputation; the desire for political credit or public reputation; the ambition to control and direct; and differences of view about programs and program implementation. For the purposes of our discussion here, we will focus chiefly on money and policy authority as the two main matters around which disputes tend to form in the health care field. This is not to say that the quest for political credit, political ideology, and jockeying for reputation and position have no role to play, but simply to say that such factors tend to be implicit or unacknowledged in the dispute and are mediated through the formal, public discourse, which normally focuses on money and policy authority. The federal-provincial fiscal transfer system and the provisions of the *Canada Health Act* are emblematic of this twofold reality.

Given the realities of politics, the needs of politicians and the differing orientations of widely dispersed communities in the Canadian federation, recurrent conflict should be taken as a given. The point is not to get rid of it, but to try to ensure that there are productive channels for its expression and for its resolution when the time is right. Conflict can arise at the level of officials, ministers, or first ministers. As we said earlier, the record of collaboration and quiet, effective conflict management is very good in Canada at the level of officials and line departments; the great majority of the public business of Canada is carried on efficiently beyond the hurly-burly of political debate. It is when intergovernmental conflict breaks out at the political level of ministers – and, especially, first ministers – that the concern for dispute resolution processes arises. This is the level at which our investigation proceeds.

The Canada Health Act

The main instruments for regulating governmental behaviour in the health field are the *Canada Health Act* and the ten provincial health acts. The *Canada Health Act* is a case of one of the actors, heavily implicated in a complex system, announcing rules for the conduct of the other actors, and determining for itself whether the rules have been flouted, and whether a penalty should be imposed.[29]

Because of its central importance to the Canadian health care system, we will examine how the *Canada Health Act* has operated over time. What is of particular interest is the role that formal sanctions have played in shaping behaviour and in exacerbating or diminishing conflict between Ottawa and the provincial governments. Underlying the CHA are several assumptions: that there is a national interest in maintaining a public health insurance system in the country; that Canadians, wherever they live, are entitled to broadly comparable services; and that the federal government has a responsibility to enforce provincial compliance with respect to key elements of the health insurance system.

What has been the impact of the CHA on federal-provincial cooperation and conflict? What are the options for using the Act as a dispute mechanism in the future? These are the questions that are central to our discussion. In order to set the context, let us review the terms of the Act, the processes and arrangements for enforcing compliance, the cases in which a penalty was imposed or was contemplated but was not imposed, and the strengths and weaknesses of the current system.

The *Canada Health Act*, which was enacted in 1984, re-established the four principles that have been in place since medicare was introduced, and added the principle of accessibility. The five criteria with which provincial health insurance plans must comply before they qualify for a cash contribution from the federal government are public administration, comprehensiveness, universality, portability, and accessibility.[30] The Act also bans extra-billing and user charges. If provinces contravene these two conditions, there is an automatic dollar-for-dollar penalty. As the *Canada Health Act Overview* explains, an automatic penalty means that "if it has been determined that a province has allowed $500,000 in extra-billing by physicians, the federal transfer payment to that province would be reduced by that amount" (Health Canada 2002). Through orders-in-council, financial penalties can legally be imposed for not complying with the five criteria and two conditions of the Act. However, no discretionary penalties have ever been applied for contravening the conditions of universality, comprehensiveness, and accessibility. The *Canada Health Act Overview* indicates that if the penalty is discretionary, "the amount of any deduction is based on the gravity of the default." The Canada Health Act Division, part of the Intergovernmental Affairs Directorate, Health Policy and Communications Branch, Health Canada, is responsible for administering the CHA. It advises the Minister of Health on whether to make deductions. The Minister then communicates the amount of any deductions to Finance officials after informing the province of the problem, obtaining its explanations, drafting a report on its concerns, and sometimes holding a meeting with the province to discuss the issue.[31]

Federal government enforcement of the Act has been sporadic, a fact that reflects the deeply politicized nature of the process. The federal government imposed around $245 million in cash penalties against seven provinces for extra-billing in the first three years after the Act was introduced. After the violations ended, the money was reimbursed. The *Canada Health Act Overview* notes that "the second period of deductions related to extra-billing in British Columbia during the period 1992-1995" (Health Canada 2002). British Columbia lost $2,025,000 in Established Program Financing (EPF) transfer payments because some doctors extra-billed. Then, in the second half of the 1990s, $6 million was withheld from the provinces, specifically Newfoundland and Labrador, Nova Scotia, Manitoba, and Alberta, where patients had been charged a facility fee for medically necessary services at private clinics. Since 1999 Nova Scotia has lost $57,360 in transfer payments for contravening the Act concerning the federal policy on private clinics.[32]

There have been many instances in which a penalty was contemplated but was not imposed. For instance, the provincial governments have contravened the spirit of the CHA by providing uneven access to abortion services (there are no services in Prince Edward Island, and only in 1996 did Alberta shift from no coverage to full coverage at clinics) and by denying medical services to British Columbians if they did not pay fees to be enrolled in health insurance. In fact, the discretionary penalty provisions of the Act have never been applied.[33]

The Auditor General has been critical of the federal government because it has never required the provinces to give the detailed information required in section 23 of the Act (the provinces are expected to indicate the degree of their compliance with the Act in general and the extent to which they have satisfied the five criteria and two conditions); nor has Health Canada provided this information to Parliament.[34] The federal government's lack of political will to systematically enforce the CHA may be traced to its reluctance to get involved in an intergovernmental dispute in an area of provincial jurisdiction unless it is obviously in the short-term interest of the federal political leadership.[35] Enforcement is not subject to the initiative of non-governmental actors: citizens and non-governmental organizations do not currently enjoy the right of launching actions under the CHA – only the Government of Canada can do that.[36] So, although the CHA is highly popular with Canadians, citizens have been effectively locked out of its processes.

It is important to consider the effect of the CHA on federal-provincial cooperation and conflict, since the only formal dispute resolution mechanism associated with an intergovernmental impasse in the federal-provincial/territorial health conference system pertains to the principles and conditions identified in the Act (O'Reilly 2001, 119). The federal government's style of enforcement of the CHA contributes to federal-provincial cooperation only insofar as some of the provincial leaders may secretly be relieved that national principles like the portability of services exist. But it has been argued that Ottawa's approach to enforcement does much more to exacerbate intergovernmental tension than to relieve it. As Joan Boase has observed, the intergovernmental negotiations to resolve conflict relating to CHA interpretation and enforcement have tended to be "highly politicized, confrontational, and competitive. This has resulted in residual feelings of intergovernmental resentment, suspicion, and frustration well beyond the health arena" (Boase 2001, 194). At the same time, Health Canada (2002) implies that it is important not to overstate the degree of conflict in this area. It emphasizes that almost all CHA-related disputes have been resolved through informal consultation with the offending governments without resorting to penalties. It is undeniable that the existence of this federal legislation has helped to preserve the basic architecture

of the Canadian health care system, at least insofar as it rests on the five principles specified in the statute. While we cannot know for certain how health
care in Canada would have evolved in the absence of the CHA, it seems clear
that, without it, respect for the basic principles that have shaped its operation
would have been attenuated over time.

All these factors make the *Canada Health Act* a very interesting case in
point in the dispute resolution field. It is federal legislation, passed by the
Parliament of Canada alone. Using federal fiscal transfers as leverage, it provides for the imposition of fiscal penalties on provinces that do not comply
with its five principles and two conditions. The principles are vague and unde-
fined. The administration of the Act is highly political, in that the federal government chooses not to apply its provisions impartially and systematically, but
circumstantially and politically. The regulatory process is not accepted as legitimate by the provinces. Yet it seems certain that its existence has had a good
deal to do with the preservation of the basic national architecture of the health
care system in this country. Altogether, it leads to a surprising conclusion: that
a highly political, selectively applied, unilaterally interpreted federal Act, intervening in a field of undoubted provincial jurisdiction, can have beneficial public policy results.

Having said that, we must recognize that the capacity of the Government
of Canada to influence provincial behaviour in the health care field has not relied
solely on a piece of legislation, but on the fact that the legislation is paired with a
significant federal fiscal presence in the system. As Tom Kent (1997) and others
have pointed out, this fiscal presence has been allowed to fade in recent years, leading perilously close to a situation in which Ottawa claims a voice without substantive participation. Beyond the instability that this introduces into the system, the
disjunction between voice and presence risks, over time, depriving the federal government of the public legitimacy that has buttressed its role vis-à-vis the provinces
in the past.

The Anatomy of Conflict in the Canadian Health Care Field

Federal-provincial conflict in the field of health is the product of two
structural forces: one has to do with policy, and the other with money.

With respect to policy, the provincial health care programs are embedded in a broadly accepted national policy framework expressed by the five prin-

ciples of accessibility, portability, public administration, universality, and comprehensiveness.[37] Extra-billing by doctors and user fees for medical services are widely viewed as being incompatible with the public insurance philosophy that underlies the Canadian health system. The *Canada Health Act*, and the more recent Social Union Framework Agreement (SUFA), offer the authoritative enunciation of the policy framework within which Canadian health services are to be provided. As an intergovernmental agreement, SUFA confirms the general acknowledgment on the part of Canada's governments that the five principles are structural features of the Canadian system. While the Government of Quebec refused to sign SUFA, it was not on grounds of disagreement with the principles.

As for the question of money, fiscal transfers from the federal government have supported provincial health programs for even longer than the policy framework described above has been in existence. Almost half a century's continuous experience with federal fiscal transfers to the provinces in support of health entitles the impartial observer to conclude that this too is a structural feature of Canada's health care system.

It is, then, not surprisingly, chiefly with respect to money and policy that intergovernmental disputes arise. When they do, an intergovernmental imbalance appears in the processes by which conflicts are addressed.

While there is a good deal of intergovernmental discussion about the nature and level of federal transfers in support of provincial health programs, the technical instrument employed to effect transfers is parliamentary legislation. In other words, with respect to this crucial element of the federal-provincial relationship, it is ultimately Ottawa, and Ottawa alone, that makes the final determination as to the nature, level, growth, and duration of the fiscal transfer. Ottawa's sovereignty in this matter has been confirmed in the courts. There is no formal or informal dispute resolution mechanism relating to this structural feature of the Canadian intergovernmental health support system. There is federal-provincial discussion, negotiation, and contestation, but at the end of the day the Government of Canada unilaterally decides on the terms and conditions of the transfers and submits legislation to Parliament to that effect.

As for the policy side of the intergovernmental relationship, the determining instrument is again a piece of federal legislation, the *Canada Health Act*, which provides for the imposition of financial penalties on provincial governments that fail to abide by its terms – terms, be it noted, that relate to matters falling clearly within provincial jurisdiction. While there is a process of exchange and discussion with the given province prior to federal action, the decision whether to impose a penalty and, if so, how much, rests with the Government of Canada alone. Again, then, disputes are ultimately resolved by the federal government acting on its own.

We spoke above of several features of dispute settlement mechanisms: their formality, scope, frequency of use, enforceability, and credibility. Canada's mechanisms for dealing with intergovernmental conflict in the health field are informal or non-existent, narrow in scope, and intermittent and unpredictable in their application. They are, broadly speaking, enforceable – that is to say, the federal government's decisions, once made, are usually complied with: in the fiscal domain, the provinces have no choice; in the policy field, the financial penalty, or perhaps public opprobrium, is normally enough to bring provincial governments into line. However, the process and the decisions arising from the process are not typically regarded as legitimate by the provinces, although they would normally be positively viewed among much of the population in English-speaking Canada.

In reflecting on existing arrangements for dispute resolution in this field, there are two dimensions to which we must pay particular attention. The first is the character of the mechanism itself: is there a mechanism, and, if so, what does it provide? In particular, does it meet what one might call the "authority test"? An authoritative voice is critical to an enduring dispute settlement process. When one is dealing with autonomous, democratically elected actors in a federal system, a voice of authority implies two things: that its pronouncements are definitive, and that they are legitimate. Are decisions reached via the given dispute settlement mechanism definitive? – that is, do they authoritatively resolve the conflict? And are they legitimate – that is, do they derive from a procedure that both sides acknowledge as fair and impartial? The second dimension is the scope of the mechanism: to what issues does the mechanism apply? How broad is its sweep? Does it apply to the main elements in the relationship or to only a portion of them?

When approaching it from this perspective, what one discovers in Canada is a system tilted radically in favour of the federal government. To the extent that a dispute settlement mechanism exists, it applies only to the policy dimension of the relationship, not to the fiscal aspect. Within the policy dimension, disputes under CHA are ultimately decided by the federal government – one of the parties to the dispute. With respect to the fiscal transfer system, there is effectively no mechanism at all, and disagreements are simply left unresolved, with Ottawa finally determining what it is and is not prepared to do. Provincial governments in both domains are subject to the will of the Government of Canada.

This one-sidedness seems dysfunctional, given that the paternalistic position of the central government at the time of Confederation has long since been superseded in most areas by the operating principle of federal-provincial equality; and anomalous, given that health is an area of provincial jurisdiction. Health is the largest expenditure item modern governments face. Current arrangements for coping with intergovernmental relations in the health field suggest a costly institutional immaturity in the Canadian federation that is unlikely to serve the interests and needs of citizens very well. They foster a recurrent and, in some respects, intentionally obfuscatory debate between governments, in which it is impossible to agree even on the most basic numbers. How much does Ottawa really contribute to the provinces in support of health care? Governments cannot agree, and it is almost as if they have been complicit in designing a system in which it is not possible to agree, and in which each side can therefore evade responsibility by shifting blame to the other. This avoidance does not build confidence among Canadian citizens that their welfare is at the centre of the debate.

The actor for whom the current system works best is the federal government. As we have seen, it holds most of the cards; it is viewed by many citizens in English-speaking Canada as the monitor of provincial health care behaviour; and it chooses, with a fairly high degree of autonomy, when and how it will involve itself in the policy field. The grinding, day-to-day management of the system is left to the provincial governments, for whom the often mercurial participation of the federal government is yet another element of uncertainty. Claude Forget has employed an arresting image to describe the conduct of the Government of Canada vis-à-vis the provincial health care systems. He says that the federal government invests in provincial health care like a bondholder but wishes to behave like an equity shareholder; it seeks voice without risk and influence without responsibility. Forget argues that the provinces assume a wide range of risks in performing their health care responsibilities – medical, financial, management, and demographic. In the federal government, they confront not a partner who is prepared to share the risks and burdens of the enterprise, but a creditor who maintains an arm's-length relationship from the provinces and seeks to exercise control from a distance.[38]

Using the framework of analysis outlined above, we will block out several alternative dispute settlement models, using the CHA and the existing fiscal transfer regime as the base-case example. In each case, we pay particular attention to the character and scope of the mechanism and relate the model to one of the three notions of the sharing community elaborated by Keith Banting and Robin Boadway in chapter 1.

DISPUTE SETTLEMENT MODELS

The Three Notions of the Sharing Community

The idea of the "sharing community" that Banting and Boadway develop refers to the breadth of the community over which health insurance programs are designed to apply. It does not refer to the decision-making process (which is our focus here), but to the extent of the community in Canada over which redistribution, common policy structures, and assumptions of mutual citizen obligation are understood to prevail.[39] The authors describe, but set aside, two extreme versions: exclusive Canada-wide sharing (as in a unitary state), whereby all citizens of a given category receive identical treatment no matter where in the country they reside; and the exclusive provincial sharing community, which effectively assumes no country-wide sharing whatsoever.

Between these extremes, Banting and Boadway identify and discuss three relevant or imaginable alternative conceptions of the sharing community:

> *The predominantly Canada-wide sharing community*: This conception would have strong, detailed national standards and strong interregional transfers. It might have a considerable direct federal delivery role.

> *The dual sharing community*: This conception would have a full equalization system as well as broad, common program principles applying to health care, as in the current regime. It might be supported by fiscal transfers from the central government to the regional governments.

> *The predominantly provincial sharing community*: With this conception, sharing would occur primarily via an un-earmarked equalization transfer, possibly via federal income taxation with selected programs, like

pensions and unemployment insurance, delivered by Ottawa. There would be no conditions associated with an instrument like the CHST, and no equivalent to the *Canada Health Act*.

Since these are alternative conceptions of sharing not decision-making models, it would theoretically be possible to have, let us say, a predominantly Canada-wide sharing community, supported, not by an active federal government exercising oversight and control, but by a powerful intergovernmental compact laying out obligations and responsibilities for all public-sector actors. In reality, however, a predominantly Canada-wide sharing community would likely assign a significant role to the federal government; a predominantly provincial sharing community would likely assign a relatively minor role to the federal government and a correspondingly large role to the provinces; and a dual sharing community would likely assign a balanced role to each order of government.

The relationship between the different conceptions of the sharing community and potential forms of dispute resolution is complex and relies on a number of factors that need to be specified. As a starting proposition, one might argue that the more intense and mutually dependent the relationship among governments is, the greater will be the need for a well-developed dispute settlement arrangement; if there is little or no connection among governments, there will be few disputes and minimal need for conflict resolution processes. The nature of the dispute settlement process may vary, not only by virtue of the relationship's intensity but also by virtue of the nature of the actors that are in relationship with one another. The nature of disputes and the consequent character of the settlement mechanism are likely to differ according to whether it is a question of the federal government playing a preponderant role or a group of provinces working within the framework of a powerful intergovernmental compact.

But there is more to it. One needs to make a distinction between logic and need, on the one hand, and the practical reality of the situation, derived from politics and circumstance, on the other. It may be that the long-standing structural relationship that exists between Ottawa and the provinces in the health care field logically calls for a well-developed dispute settlement mechanism, but the reality is rather different, as we have seen. Why is Canada so weakly endowed with institutions and processes in this area? There appear to be two chief reasons.

The first is the jurisdictional reality of the Canadian federation. Health care is a primary provincial responsibility; Ottawa chooses to contribute to its support, but, in principle, it might not. This discretionary role creates very different circumstantial pressures and unequal leverage of one actor over the other; while Ottawa, at least at the level of theory, has the option of withdrawing from the intergovernmental relationship and terminating its commitment to the support of health care, there is no way in which the provinces could exercise an option to cease to involve themselves in health care provision and simply vacate the field. Thus there is a power imbalance; Ottawa has the upper hand.

The second reason why Canada's dispute settlement system is not what one might theoretically expect it to be is what might be called the "pay for say" principle. The federal government has substantial freedom of action to determine the conditions under which it will offer financial support to provincial governments. It can therefore structure the framework of the intergovernmental relationship within which it is prepared to participate. It has never wanted an impartial, equitable dispute settlement mechanism to govern its relationship with the provinces, and it has had the power to avoid it.

Considerations of power and circumstance, then, should be very much borne in mind as one reflects on hypothetical alternative dispute settlement regimes. The models we outline below are organized from the least to the most highly developed. This structure makes analytical sense, but the question of how any one of these relates to any given practical reality is a matter for detailed consideration in the circumstances that exist, not a matter of mechanical application.

Alternative Models
Model 1. Federal Withdrawal

A designation of intergovernmental roles and relationships consistent with the notion of predominantly provincial sharing communities might involve the following type of arrangements. Ottawa might transfer tax points to the provinces to allow them to fulfill their health care responsibilities as they see fit, and reduce the cash transfers to little or nothing. It might place greater emphasis on the equalization system to redistribute resources in a way that would permit the fiscally weaker provinces to acquit their health care responsibilities to their residents, but the amount to be spent on health care and the way in which it is to be spent would be left to provincial governments. Ottawa would abrogate the *Canada Health Act*, and leave it to the provinces to manage the health care system in a fashion that meets the aspirations of their regional communities.

Governments might agree that the principle of interprovincial mobility would be respected, or, as Lazar, St-Hilaire and Tremblay suggest in Chapter 4, Ottawa might retain sufficient cash leverage to enforce that principle. Ottawa would effectively withdraw from the field, perhaps restricting itself to specific, limited activities, such as public health promotion and the regulation of pharmaceuticals, where the logic of a Canada-wide approach is self-evident. This is the model closest to the preferences of Quebec.

This model, involving substantial federal withdrawal, would address the problem of federal-provincial disputes by diminishing the degree to which the two orders of government are in relationship with one another. The absence of an explicit federal-provincial dispute settlement mechanism would not be felt as a significant institutional lack in such circumstances. The regulation of any common national standards would be maintained by the provinces, through an interprovincial dispute settlement mechanism.

Given the politics of health and the contemporary Canadian system, this model would clearly be a radical change of approach. Nevertheless, one has only to look at the way in which Canadians manage their education systems to see how an arrangement that is in fact very similar works in practice. With the significant exception of federal support for research, Canada's provincial governments run their systems of primary, secondary, and higher education in virtually complete autonomy, with what is effectively no national intervention, not even with respect to mobility; yet it is probably fair to say that these provincial educational regimes, collectively, operate according to shared principles and display common characteristics to the same extent that provincial health care systems do. There is no "Canada Education Act" to parallel the CHA, and the provincial governments have successfully fended off Ottawa's intermittent desire to intervene in this field, but the schools and universities of the country resemble one another to a remarkable degree, and the constraints on interprovincial educational mobility are, all in all, quite limited in their scope. This reality reminds us that public policy and government action are not the only means by which communities preserve themselves and the values they cherish; the notion of "established programs," as in the Established Programs Financing Arrangements legislation of 1977 may in fact refer implicitly to the degree to which certain public programs and policies are embedded in the preferences and expectations of the citizens themselves. A country is more than its public-administration architecture.

Model 2. The Base-Case Model

This system, with which Canadians are familiar, provides for no explicit conflict resolution regime that applies to both the fiscal and policy dimensions of the intergovernmental relationship. Thus the scope is narrow. The federal government sees itself as the dominant player in the field, despite the management and administrative primacy of the provinces, and has structured its central policy instruments to reflect that view. This is apparent in both the fiscal and the policy authority dimensions of the health care field.

Federal fiscal arrangements, despite their considerable structural variety over the years, have always been grounded in federal statute and subject to amendment by the Parliament of Canada. Provinces have been invited to express their views and they have sought to influence federal decisions about the kind and levels of support on offer, but there has never been any question that the final word in the matter rests with Ottawa. There is no authoritative procedure by which provinces can hold the Government of Canada to account for the fulfillment of its fiscal commitments to the provinces. The federal government is free to do what it wishes with respect to the level of transfers it promises and can change its undertakings at any time as circumstances dictate.[40]

At times, the Government of Canada designed the fiscal transfer system itself to achieve certain policy goals. Examples of this strategy can be found in the era of conditional grants, and in the provisions of the Canada Assistance Plan until its disappearance, announced in the 1995 federal budget (Cohn 1996). But even in the era of block grants under the Established Programs Financing arrangements, the federal government felt entitled to assert its policy oversight of Canadian health care. The passage of the CHA in 1984 introduced policy and program compliance requirements for the provinces that laid out the federal government's conditions for giving the block transfer, and discouraged certain forms of provincial behaviour.

The procedures under the CHA for determining provincial non-compliance and consequent penalties described earlier in the paper are perfectly consistent with the assumption of a federal oversight and control function. *Prima facie* cases of non-compliance are identified and investigated by the federal government. Provinces have an opportunity to submit whatever evidence they wish, to counter Ottawa's concern, but a finding of non-compliance is made by the federal government on its own, as is the imposition of any penalty. Should the province contest the finding and the penalty, there is no appeal process, except

the political one of going back to the same federal authority that made the determination in the first place.

The processes under the CHA, which apply to the policy side, clearly
favour the federal government. Ottawa designed the procedures, passed the legislation, decides when to trigger the process, and determines whether penalties
will be imposed and what they will be. By most standards of conflict resolution,
this design would be judged deficient on several grounds: the relationship
between the actors is paternalistic rather than egalitarian; only one party has
recourse to the instrument; one of the parties acts both as prosecutor and judge;
as a consequence, the process and the decisions, while they may be effective, are
not regarded as legitimate by all of the government participants.

Model 3. The Social Union Framework Agreement

The Social Union Framework Agreement (SUFA) emerged in the late
1990s as the provinces and territories struggled to cope with the sharp reduction
in federal support for social programs. They were looking for ways to express and
protect the common interest in provincial social programs in the absence of a vigorous federal-government presence, to put pressure on Ottawa to re-engage in
the field, and to fashion a more productive, less unilateral style of intergovernmental relations.

SUFA can be understood in part as an attempt to address the absence of
an autonomous monitor to manage competition and conflict between the
provinces and the federal government. This absence should not be understood
simply as the lack of a dispute settlement mechanism to regulate particular conflicts between Ottawa and a province or provinces relating to a specific matter,
although that was clearly part of the provincial and territorial concern. The
design of the framework as a whole reflects an effort to establish a system in
which the various relationships between the federal and provincial governments
in the social policy field are rendered more stable, more predictable, and more
balanced as between the two orders of government.

While a number of observers associate this initiative with the emergence
in recent years of a model of collaborative federalism, it should not for that reason be assumed that SUFA contemplates nothing but collaboration among
Canada's federal partners. As William Forward, then Assistant Deputy Minister of
Ontario's Ministry of Intergovernmental Affairs, observed, SUFA is an example of
"governments' agreeing on a workplan for co-operation and a rulebook for com-

petition" (Bakvis and Skogstad 2002, 11). It assumes that both are an ongoing, inevitable reality in intergovernmental relations, and seeks to place conflictual and cooperative behaviour in an orderly frame of reference, and to expose both forms of conduct to the fuller scrutiny of the public.

Perhaps the major innovation, from the point of view of our story, is the effort to redefine the federal-provincial interface on a broader and more synthetic basis, as "the social union," and to subject that complex set of relations and joint activities to the disciplines of collaborative federalism. Thus, section 6 of the Agreement, "Dispute Avoidance and Resolution," is clearly intended to apply to the broad range of intergovernmental social policy matters, and not just to a particular program. Indeed, SUFA makes this breadth explicit by stating that "dispute avoidance and resolution will apply to commitments on mobility, intergovernmental transfers, interpretation of the *Canada Health Act* principles, and, as appropriate, on any new joint initiative." The scope is considerably broadened and explicitly includes federal fiscal transfers. In this way it seeks to deal with one of the deficiencies in the current arrangements.

With respect to the other deficiency, namely, federal dominance of the dispute settlement mechanism itself, it is silent. The provisions are at a very general level, referring to dispute avoidance, fact-finding, mediation, third-party involvement, and public reporting, but the Agreement does not develop any of the ideas in detail. Clearly, that was as far as the federal-provincial negotiations were capable of going at that stage, and, as we will see below, the federal government is not yet prepared to abdicate its privileged position in the intergovernmental process.

Were the federal government prepared to do so, however, the Social Union Framework Agreement might be creatively used as the basis for developing a more balanced and impartial dispute resolution regime. In its present form, the Agreement has clearly broadened the scope or ambit of any such regime; consistent with its central philosophy, it could be employed to construct a dispute settlement process of fuller legitimacy. This might be done even with the continued existence of the CHA, if the Government of Canada declared that it was prepared to have the fiscal transfer arrangements subjected to the provisions of the regime, and if it and the provincial and territorial governments indicated that they would be bound by the determinations made by a dispute settlement process to which they had all agreed. Presumably, the provisions of the CHA would need to be clarified through federal-provincial negotiation, so that conduct in compliance or in contravention could be specified with greater certainty. This approach would be perfectly consistent with the collaborative, partnership philosophy that informs the document as a whole.

Model 4. The McLellan Dispute Settlement Process

The Social Union Framework Agreement was in part a provincial attempt to balance the forces between the two orders of government in the social policy field. On the money and resources front, there is an attempt to broaden the scope and impose a kind of code of conduct on the federal government's use of the spending power, with notice provisions and the like. As we have seen, the last section of the Agreement asserts the need to develop a formal federal-provincial dispute settlement mechanism that would offer all participants a more settled and orderly process for addressing both fiscal and policy disputes. This provision is of particular importance to the provinces, and, until recently, had been strongly resisted by the federal government. The idea is to subject the federal government to disciplines and accountabilities parallel to those Ottawa has sought to impose, with some success, on the provinces.

In a letter dated 2 April 2002 to her counterpart in Alberta, Federal Minister of Health Anne McLellan proposed a dispute settlement process that appears to respond to the concerns of at least some of the provinces, although it does not fundamentally alter the play of intergovernmental forces and is restricted in its ambit to the CHA, not applying to mobility, intergovernmental transfers, or any other joint initiative, as is contemplated by SUFA.

The letter begins with a discussion of dispute avoidance, arguing that governments need to continue to participate actively in the ad hoc federal/provincial-territorial committees on CHA issues and to exchange information on issues as they arise. The Minister commits Health Canada to providing advance assessments of specific issues upon request to any province or territory.

If dispute avoidance fails, either the federal or the provincial minister of health could initiate the dispute resolution process by following required procedures that would apparently look something like this. A disputes panel would have to be struck and report before any steps were taken by the federal government to enforce the provisions of the CHA. Governments in conflict over the meaning and applicability of the CHA to a particular case would have to agree to collect and share relevant information, prepare a fact-finding report, and make an honest effort to negotiate an end to the dispute. If the issue remained unresolved, either minister of health could initiate the dispute panel process by writing to his or her coun-terpart. Within thirty days a panel would be set up, composed of a federal appointee, a provincial appointee, and a third-party chairperson agreeable to both sides. The panel would have sixty days to hand down a report, based on its assessment of the issue in dispute in the light of the provisions of the CHA. The report would be made public.

The federal minister could accept or ignore the report; McLellan's letter states that "the Minister of Health for Canada has the final authority to interpret and enforce the *Canada Health Act.*" As the *Globe and Mail* says, it is "a new, non-binding dispute-settlement mechanism that would give the provinces the right to a hearing before they face fines for breaching the *Canada Health Act.*" The federal minister is quoted as saying: "I take that [the panel report] into consideration in deciding, which is my right and my right alone, whether I will enforce the *Canada Health Act*" (Mahoney and Laghi, 2002). This is a step away from unadorned unilateral federal action, since it provides for a federal-provincial process of fact-finding and reporting, but the ultimate authority to determine the outcome remains unequivocally in federal hands. In that sense, then, the Government of Canada remains both prosecutor and judge, although the other actors in a system of federal dominance possess limited tools to challenge federal action that were not available to them before. The procedure remains definitive, and its legitimacy has been increased, although it is still compromised by the dominant role of Ottawa. Furthermore, it is not a procedure that applies to federal fiscal transfers.

Model 5. Interlocking Legislation

If there were an intergovernmental will to introduce a substantial degree of formality and certainty into the relationship between Ottawa and the provinces in the health care field, an approach mooted by Richard Zuker is the notion of interlocking legislation; that is to say, interrelated legislation that would be passed through Parliament and the legislatures of the provinces establishing a pattern of reciprocal obligations in the area of health care. Once established, these arrangements would endow the system with significant stability and predictability, because of the mutual obligations created. We will quote directly from the discussion paper Zuker presented at a recent Manitoba conference:[41]

> The parties would agree to a funding formula for a period of time
> with required review provisions ... The federal legislation would

include a provision that the funding formula could not be changed without the approval of a certain number of provinces (and territories?) representing a certain percentage of the population. (For the CPP, it's 7 provinces and 50% of the population.)

In exchange, all provincial and territorial governments would pass the equivalent of the *Canada Health Act*, with the provision that the legislation could not be amended without federal government approval. The federal government legislation would state that some or all of the funding to a provincial or territorial government that amended its CHA-equivalent legislation without federal government approval could be suspended, perhaps with a schedule of fines. In turn, the provincial and territorial government legislation would automatically become null and void, if the federal government modified the funding arrangement without the requisite provincial and territorial government approvals. It is high stakes poker, but that is the general idea.

This approach effectively ties together the policy and fiscal components of the intergovernmental health care regime and imposes equivalent obligations on all the actors in the system. Clearly, to introduce an initiative of this kind would call on a degree of cooperative behaviour and intergovernmental concord that the country has not witnessed for some time. Equally clearly, since both orders of government would be subjecting themselves to an interlocking set of obligations, it would reflect the underlying philosophy of dual sharing communities in which governmental representatives of both communities find the means to work together on the basis of equality.

Model 6. Bringing the Public In

Canadian governments have been decidedly reluctant to open up their intergovernmental decision-making processes to the active participation of the public, yet giving the public a voice in the proceedings is a potentially powerful tool for aiding the resolution of disputes in a manner that advances the public interest and not simply the interests of the participating governments.

Model 6, developed by Richard Simeon after reading a draft of this chapter, develops one possible approach and is grounded in a recognition of the following realities:

> Ottawa is not going to transfer to a provincially dominated body its

right to make its own fiscal decisions, nor is it likely to forgo its ultimate capacity to determine contraventions of the principles of the *Canada Health Act*.

> Provinces are not going to agree to any mechanism which provides for significant unilateral federal intervention in the operation of their provincial health care systems, nor will they assent to a mechanism that entrenches the hierarchical federal position Ottawa has long enjoyed.

Hence, there is unlikely to be agreement on any purely intergovernmental mechanism that embodies these constraints.

In these circumstances, a promising way to get beyond the impasse and establish a new mechanism is to inject third parties and the public into the process. As governments, understandably, will not cede authoritative decision-making power on finance or policy to any such third party, it should be seen as an advisory and facilitative body. Contrary to the views of many, such a role would not necessarily make a body of this kind powerless; indeed, to the extent that it was open, transparent, demonstrably fair, and solely committed to the central values guiding health care in Canada, the recommendations of this body could have considerable legitimacy and persuasive power.

The governments of Canada, then, might agree to create a jointly appointed and funded "Canadian Health Care Commission." No significant federal action with respect to funding or enforcement under the CHA could go into effect until the commission had considered the matter and issued its recommendations. Thus, if the Government of Canada believed that a province had violated the Act, it could not withhold funds before the commission had examined the issue. Similarly, no provincial health care legislation *with significant implications for other provinces or for the national system as a whole* (a very important qualification) could go into effect before it had been assessed by the commission.

The commission would report to the governments and legislatures of all provincial jurisdictions. It would be mandated to hold public hearings where appropriate, and its deliberations and recommendations would be open to public scrutiny. Governments, provider groups, and concerned citizens could seek standing before the commission. One of its initial tasks would be to draw up a specification and codification of the principles of the *Canada Health Act*.[42] It would attempt to spell out how these principles would be operationalized, and what they mean, in the current health care context. While the CHA would remain in place as a piece of national legislation, a more fleshed out and mod-

ernized statement of principles, accepted by governments, would make it clear
that the Canadian health care system is a concern and responsibility of all
Canadian governments and their citizens. This document, once developed, could
be submitted to governments and then ratified by them in a new intergovernmental accord.

An initiative of this kind could bring the public much more fully into
the health care debate and give citizens a voice in the major decisions their governments are confronting, but it would do so while preserving the autonomy of
both orders of government. On the evidence, it is not an undertaking that
Canada's governments would find easy to accept; the role assigned to the public
in SUFA, for example, is quite carefully confined, and the governments themselves determine the processes of public involvement. The Canada Health Care
Commission, once established, would almost certainly be difficult for governments to control – which, after all, is just the point; the voices of the citizens
would be freely expressed, and heard. Governments would not be obliged to
accede to those views, but they would have a powerful moral incentive to explain
their decisions in reference to them, thereby elevating the quality and expanding
the scope of public debate. Such an arrangement might prove to be an instrument for focusing more attention on what citizens need in their health care systems, and less on what governments seek to protect in their intergovernmental
relations.

TOWARD A MATURE PARTNERSHIP

We will conclude this chapter with a series of points that summarize our
main findings in our exploration of potential avenues to resolve conflict
and foster cooperation in the Canadian federal system, particularly in the
health care arena.

> Before there can be a concern with conflict – or with cooperation for
> that matter – there first needs to be a significant relationship. A close
> relationship means that more connections, patterns of exchange, points
> of concord and friction exist than would be the case with a shallow or
> superficial relationship. The actors are more engaged in the relation-
> ship, it matters more, and it is, inevitably, composed of elements of dis-
> agreement as well as consensus and agreement.

> The idea of the sharing community speaks to conceptions of collective identity and redistribution, not, as such, to the agencies and instruments that give effect to that sharing. Thus, one could in theory have a predominantly Canada-wide sharing community in which there was no role for the federal government; the principles reflecting collective identity and redistribution would be operationalized by interprovincial compact; and disputes (which would in this scenario be among the provinces) would be addressed by interprovincial processes to which all provinces have agreed. A given conception of the sharing community may receive expression through a variety of institutional arrangements.

> The federal and provincial governments have been jointly involved in the provision of health care to Canadians for generations. The relationship between the two orders of government is structural, both with respect to fiscal support of the system and with respect to its policy design.

> History, constitutional law, and the preferences of Canadians have combined to produce a rough equality among federal and provincial governments and a dual notion of sharing communities in the health domain.

> The dispute settlement arrangements currently in place do not reflect this. To the extent that they exist, they are clearly biased in favour of one of the parties to the relationship. This can be understood as a kind of institutional immaturity that has negative effects on political responsibility and public debate.

> An appropriate relationship needs to be established between the conception of the sharing community and the institutional arrangements designed to support it. In the Canadian federal system, the more the emphasis is placed on the notion of the Canada-wide sharing community, the more intense the relations among governments become. The more intense they become, the more disputes there will be, and the more necessary a mature system for managing conflict becomes. It is difficult to imagine that provinces would agree to stronger versions of Canada-wide sharing in the health care field in the absence of muscular, balanced, and impartial procedures for managing the inevitable conflicts between and among federal, provincial, and territorial governments.

Our findings imply a major shift in the federal government's conception of its role. It currently views its role chiefly as an external monitor of provincial behaviour and as a beneficent donor of federal largesse, rather than as an actor deeply implicated in the workings of a highly complex system and deeply responsible for its success or failure. The question is whether Ottawa is prepared to transform that role, become a partner with the provinces in supporting the health care system in Canada and accept the disciplines, burdens, sharing of responsibilities, and satisfactions that go along with working in a partnership.

A more mature system also implies a shift in the way in which the provinces conceive their relationship with the federal government. If Ottawa wants maximum political credit for maintaining the Canadian health care system with minimum involvement, the provinces for their part appear to want more federal money for health care, but with no strings attached. Provincial governments have often found it expedient to exploit the existence of an irresponsible external actor in the health field, attacking the arbitrary reduction by the federal government of its fiscal contributions, rather than acknowledging their own management problems; if Ottawa contributed what it should, all would be well. Clearly, a shift to a notion of federal-provincial partnership would require the cessation of this blame-avoidance behaviour, and the assumption, with the federal government, of joint responsibility for the functioning of the system.

Finally, a bolder and more sweeping commitment to genuine public participation in making the nation's health care choices could assist in greatly altering the way in which Canada's single most important social program is shaped. Governments are currently mutually complicit in keeping the public at arm's length, and in limiting the role of the country's legislators. The timidity of one affects the behaviour of all; no premier or health minister is prepared to risk the disapprobation of colleagues by pushing the issue too hard. Yet giving back a measure of political power to citizens – allowing them to be actors, rather than simply reactors – would be a potent means of suppressing the dysfunctional elements of intergovernmental relations in Canada today, and of increasing the likelihood that the health care decisions taken on behalf of Canadians will actually serve them well.

NOTES

1   Kellett and Dalton (2001, 9) review some
of the literature on the positive and constructive aspects of conflict. Heisey (1991)
explains that humankind is both individu-
alistic and communal, we are similar and
different, and the tension between these
complementary but opposing forces
results in conflict. Further, Rapoport
(1992) illustrates that conflict and cooperation are essential to each other's existence. They are complementary as a
"union of opposites" (87). Each, Rapoport
argues, is a "cardinal principle of life"
(81). They stimulate each other, and at the
same time, justify themselves by the existence of the other (81). Conflict can be,
therefore, both natural and beneficial.
The key, according to Arnett (1986), is to
allow these natural oppositions to exist in
creative tension such that they generate
ideas and new possibilities. Thus, conflict
should not necessarily be viewed as a
negative or dysfunctional form of communication (Cahn 1997).

2   See Michael Crommelin (2001), whose discussion was helpful here.

3   Crommelin (2001, 139-40), cites these
examples.

4   Deutsch (1991, 49-50) describes the types
of skills that third parties need to help
conflicting parties constructively resolve
their conflicts.

5   The Agreement on Internal Trade provisions include dispute avoidance and formal and informal dispute resolution
processes. See Doern and MacDonald
(1999, 137-39).

6   Walton (1987) identifies three possible
general benefits of conflict. First, conflict
can generate a certain level of energy
and motivation. Second, in bringing out
varying viewpoints, conflict can increase
levels of creativity and innovation. Third,
people can gain a deeper understanding
of their situation and themselves from
engaging in conflicts.

7   For a discussion of deliberate "gaps of
unsettlement" in the Canadian
Constitution, see Thomas (1993).

8   Scharpf distinguishes between three
types of arrangements (networks,
regimes and joint decision systems) that
evolve to facilitate multi-level joint action
between both state and non-state actors.
"Networks facilitate trust and information
sharing, reducing transaction costs and
creating opportunity structures for problem solving ... Regimes are characterised
by ongoing rule structures that may be
imposed from above, or be mutually
agreed on, imposing obligations and
increasing the costs of certain kinds of
damaging unilateral action. Joint decision
systems, finally, are 'constellations in
which parties are either physically or
legally unable to reach their purposes
through unilateral action and in which
joint action depends on the nearly unanimous agreement of all parties involved'"
(Scharpf 1997, 143). Scharpf argues that
federations that place too much emphasis
on securing intergovernmental agreement can suffer from delay, deadlock, and
other drawbacks associated with the
"joint decision trap." Similarly, Breton
(1985) defends the virtues of competitive
over collaborative federalism.

9   Albert Breton uses this notion in his
Supplementary Statement to the Royal
Commission on Canada's Economic
Development Prospects. He suggests that
the role of the Supreme Court "is likely to
be considerably larger than it should be
unless the Senate is reformed in a way
that introduces an effective provincial
dimension in the federal Parliament"
(1985, 520).

10   As an example of horizontal monitoring,
the equalization program is based on federal legislation and is managed by the
federal government. While there are federal-provincial discussions prior to any
significant change in the system, the ultimate shot is called by Ottawa. Breton
mentions the old Borden line for energy

distribution, as well as federal regional economic-development policies as other examples of this horizontal monitoring function. The Agreement on Internal Trade, which is meant to reduce economic barriers among provinces, is another example of horizontal monitoring; it was initiated by the federal government, as was the attempt to insert a strong economic union provision into the Charlottetown Accord. The federal government has, however, been incapable of performing its horizontal monitoring function in relation to the "nationalization" of provincial responsibilities for securities regulation, which seems a classic case in which provincial jurisdictional jealousies block a reform that is almost universally regarded as a long-overdue adjustment to the framework of the Canadian economy.

11   It is important to note, as Watts does, however, that the federal government imposes fewer conditions on its federal transfers than any other federation. In the United States, 100 percent of federal grants to the states are conditional; less than 5 percent are conditional in Canada, if the FPF and CHST transfers are treated as unconditional (1999b, 49).

12   It is ironic that horizontal redistribution, which after all involves the transfer of funds from wealthier to poorer parts of the country, should be far less controversial than vertical fiscal transfers.

13   This point was made perfectly clear by the court case launched by British Columbia, and, as government intervenors, the Attorney Generals for Ontario, Manitoba, Alberta, and Saskatchewan, which contested the federal government's decision to impose a cap on the growth of the Canada Assistance Plan transfers for Ontario, Alberta, and British Columbia. <http://www.lexum.umontreal.ca/csc_scc/en/pub/1991/vol2/html/1991scr2_0525.htm >

14   The Canadian Intergovernmental Conference Secretariat lists twenty-five high-level intergovernmental conferences between January and April 2002. <http://www.scics.gc.ca/confer02_e.html> (3 June 2002).

15   Alberta's scheme covered only a part of the provincial population.

16   The Canada Assistance Program, which covered 50 percent of provincial expenditures for social assistance, continued essentially unchanged until 1990, when the Mulroney government capped the transfers going to Ontario, Alberta, and British Columbia. It disappeared entirely with the creation of the CHST in 1995.

17   David Milne (1986, 12–13) uses the terms "quasi-federalism," "classical federalism," "emergency federalism," "cooperative federalism," and "double-image federalism" to classify the evolution of Canadian federalism.

18   Kenneth Kernaghan and David Siegel observe: "It is difficult to pinpoint the precise date when *cooperative federalism* emerged, but Donald Smiley noted in the early 1960s that the development of Canadian federalism since 1945 had been 'a process of continuous and piecemeal adjustment between the two levels of government', and that these adjustments had overwhelmingly been through 'interaction between federal and provincial executives' rather than through formal constitutional amendment of judicial interpretation" (1995, 453).

19   Administrative federalism, also referred to as bureaucratic federalism, implies that bureaucratic executives are at least as dominant as political executives in the practice of Canadian federalism (Van Loon and Whittington 1987, 522–4).

20   Jackson et al. note that "*executive federalism,* represents an attenuation of federal power [over cooperative federalism]. The clearest sign of the change from cooperative to executive federalism was the movement of intergovernmental talks from among public servants behind closed doors to among politicians in the full glare of publicity" (Jackson, Jackson, and Baxter-Moore 1986, 222).

21   Summit federalism refers to the tendency for intergovernmental relations in Canada to be carried out in committees, usually at the level of first ministers.

22   Albert Breton (1985, 498) argues that competitive federalism is superior to cooperative federalism on the grounds that a system that makes greater use of checks and balances for impeding the passage of legislation stimulates discussion and is more efficient in the long run.

23   Judith Maxwell describes collaborative federalism as a model that "involves joint management and joint decision-making." For a more detailed description of collaborative federalism, see Simeon and Cameron (2002, 279–81).

24   Johns 2001. For an explanation of the federal government's unilateral approach in this field from 1987-1990, see Conrad (1999, 40).

25   Kathryn Harrison (1996, 116) made this observation.

26   For analyses of the Agreement on Internal Trade, see Certified General Accountants (2001) and Leeson (2000).

27   Steven K. Andersen (2000) identifies the barriers to mediation that currently exist with the participating NAFTA countries as: "cultural differences, language barriers, and legal traditions."

28   For a discussion of public health reforms initiated by the Council of Australian Governments, see Lin and King (2000, 251).

29   Choudhry (1996, 476) emphasizes that the current political reality where the CHA "is commonly described as imposing obligations on provincial governments who wish to receive federal monies for Medicare" is quite distinct from the legal situation. He says "Federal statutes in areas of provincial jurisdiction (such as health insurance) cannot, by themselves, impose legal obligations on provincial governments. As a matter of law, the CHA imposes obligations on the federal government. It defines the conditions that must be met by the provinces for federal payments to be legal. If a provincial plan falls short of these conditions, the federal government is obliged to take certain enforcement measures, which, in the extreme, can include withholding all contributions to the offending province."

30   For a copy of the CHA text, history, and annual reports, see the Government of Canada Web site <http://www.hc-sc.gc.ca/medicare/home.htm> (20 May 2002).

31   See Auditor General of Canada (1999, 29-12). See also Madore (2000).

32   For a list of the deductions by province or territory since the passage of the CHA, see Health Canada (2001, 14-15).

33   For a list of non-compliance issues that the Auditor General considered unresolved in 1999, see Auditor General of Canada (1999, 29-15 and 29-16). The Auditor General attributes the federal government's approach of not speedily resolving compliance issues to national unity concerns.

34   Auditor General of Canada (1999, 29-17).

35   For example, see Canadian Press Newswire 14 November 2000. Klein shoots back at Chrétien over threats of fines for private clinics.

36   Choudhry (1996, 501) identifies three cases in which the CHA argument was unsuccessfully raised: Lexogest, B.C. Civil Liberties, and Morgentaler v. P.E.I. Substantial legal hurdles would discourage most potential claimants from launching a suit that examined the compliance of a provincial plan with the CHA criteria. For example, an applicant would need to demonstrate that the agreement was legally enforceable. However, the case law on intergovernmental agreements to date does not point in this direction. "A claimant must obtain third-party standing to challenge this agreement; however, this issue is unresolved under existing case law." *The Medical Post* describes a recent case where a lawsuit arguing that a provincial plan was in conflict with the *Canada Health Act* failed to

receive certification. In June 2001 a B.C. doctor tried unsuccessfully to launch a class action against the provincial Medical Services Plan, which he alleged to have "violated federal law by failing to reimburse doctors who provided medical services to patients not insured under the plan." The B.C. judge, Justice Baker, refused to certify the class action on the grounds that his "*Canada Health Act* argument was 'bound to fail,' given that previous court cases have ruled the statute is principally a funding mechanism, and doesn't create a right for all residents generally to obtain health-care services" (Fitz-James 2001).

37   Quebec accepts the validity of the principles, but not the federal government's role in defining and enforcing them.

38   Claude Forget, at a meeting to discuss drafts of these chapters, Montreal, 19 April 2002.

39   Raymond Breton once remarked that a country is a territory over which redistribution occurs.

40   The court case on the selective imposition of a cap on the Canada Assistance Plan confirmed the legality of this reality.

41   Zuker (2002).

42   A body such as this might assume responsibility for the panels on medical services suggested by Richard Zuker in his discussion paper: "Perhaps, we could have a national body – national, not federal – that would be charged with establishing guidelines for what services should be insured. The outcomes need not be black or white only – there could be 'gray' services, too, that would be recommended for partial coverage. There would likely need to be several panels for various areas of medical services. These panels could have members drawn from doctors, nurses, other health professionals, user groups, etc. Perhaps, these panels could go even further and recommend services levels, such a waiting times, and perhaps even procedures, based on up-to-date research findings. Regardless of the extent of the mandate, provincial governments would still be free to make their own choices. This type of body could increase the probability ... for babies in Victoria, St John's and rural Saskatchewan to obtain similar services. Moreover it could provide a firmer basis for Canadians to assess their health care systems, both absolutely and comparatively" (2002).

CHAPTER 3

VERTICAL FISCAL IMBALANCE:
MYTH OR REALITY?

HARVEY LAZAR, FRANCE ST-HILAIRE,
AND JEAN-FRANÇOIS TREMBLAY

The issue of vertical fiscal imbalance has been a principal irritant in Canadian intergovernmental relations since the mid-1990s. Indeed, the political controversy surrounding that issue permeates much of the ongoing debate on the funding and policy role of the federal government in determining the future of public health care.

Federal and provincial/territorial governments share the cost of financing health care. How the burden is and should be shared, however, has become a matter of dispute between the orders of government, particularly as program costs continue to escalate and the provinces and territories find that their slice of health care spending continues to grow. The provinces and territories argue that they are saddled with an unfair structural situation whereby the amount of revenue they raise is insufficient relative to their expenditure responsibilities, whereas the federal government collects more revenue than it needs relative to its spending obligations. They point to Ottawa's large budgetary surpluses since 1997 as evidence of this. According to the provinces, there is a fiscal imbalance (VFI) between the federal and provincial/territorial governments, and this imbalance needs to be corrected. They have therefore called for a redesign of federal fiscal arrangements – including the division of revenues – in order for them to have the resources and management flexibility required to cope with their rapidly rising costs. The federal government, for its part, disputes the idea that there is a vertical fiscal imbalance, particularly since the provinces have no formal constraint on their ability to raise revenue. It further argues that considerable increases in its cash transfers to the provinces in recent years do not seem to have significantly improved the health care system.

This sort of controversy over the question of fiscal imbalance is not unprecedented in Canada. Similar disputes have taken place in different forms at different times in the past. For instance in the early 1980s, it was the federal government that was claiming the existence of a fiscal imbalance favouring the provinces. However, after the introduction of the Canada Health and Social Transfer (CHST) in 1996, the provinces argued that they were the ones that were disadvantaged by a vertical fiscal imbalance since, in their view, they had unfairly been made major, involuntary contributors to the balancing of the federal government's budget. Given the difficulty in explaining this rather obscure concept to the public, the provinces intertwined it with the health care issue in their bid to obtain increased and stable funding from the federal government over the long term.

Observers are divided over whether a vertical fiscal imbalance exists and, if it does, whether it should be interpreted as an enduring feature of the division of taxing and spending powers in the Canadian federation or whether it reflects a policy choice (Norrie 2002, 23-4). In the second section of this chapter we describe some of the events and arguments at play in the ongoing federal-provincial dispute over the VFI issue. In the third we examine the concept of vertical fiscal imbalance (and the related concept of vertical fiscal gap) and outline the difficulties involved in applying this concept in a Canadian context. After analysing and comparing three recent Canadian studies that present estimates of vertical fiscal imbalance, we examine the relative state of public finances of each order of government since the postwar years and the changes in federal-provincial fiscal relations that have taken place over time, in an effort to bring some historical context to the current VFI debate. The conclusions and options on federal health care funding that we offer in the last two chapters of this volume are not ultimately predicated on the existence or extent of vertical fiscal imbalance. Nonetheless, we believe that this question needs to be analysed, so that the reader understands the important issues it raises and the way it factors into the debate on health care financing in Canada.

THE DEBATE ON FISCAL IMBALANCE AND
FEDERAL HEALTH CARE FUNDING

The Origins of the Current VFI Debate

The current federal-provincial dispute on vertical fiscal imbalance was triggered by the 1995 federal budget, which was the centrepiece of Ottawa's strategy for restoring federal public finances. At that time, the federal minister of finance announced that two of the largest federal transfers to provinces – Established Programs Financing (EPF) and the Canada Assistance Plan (CAP) – would be rolled into a single federal block transfer, the CHST. The transfer would be conditional on provinces' upholding the principles of the *Canada Health Act* and continuing to provide social assistance without minimum residency requirements. As initially presented in the 1995 budget, the cash component of the CHST was to be reduced from approximately $17 billion in 1994/95 to $12.8 billion in 1996/97 and to $10.3 billion in 1997/98.[1] The federal finance minister, in his House of Commons budget speech, observed that the cash portion of major transfers represented 21 percent of Ottawa's total program spending and therefore could not remain untouched, given the broad goals of the budget. He presented the reductions, however, as cuts from a base that included both tax points and cash, and thus did not lay out explicitly the magnitude of the cash reductions (Department of Finance 1995a, 17-19).

The fiscal measures announced in the 1995 federal budget contributed significantly to the large and swift improvements in federal public finances that have since occurred.[2] What is in dispute, however, is whether the measures adopted to improve federal finances were harder on provincial governments than on other federal programs. Did the federal government cut transfers to the provinces more significantly than it cut its own expenditures? Provinces have argued this position vigorously, and their point of view is part and parcel of the fiscal imbalance debate. As for the federal government, it has denied this charge. In essence, since 1995 both orders of government have been arguing the fairness of the federal government's fiscal stance and the related the issue of vertical fiscal imbalance.

Let's begin with a summary of how Ottawa defended its position. It argued that provinces were still enjoying the full benefits of the tax room that had been transferred to them in 1977 when it moved from cost-sharing grants for health and post-secondary education to block funding under EPF. In addition, Equalization payments had not been reduced in either the 1994 or 1995 federal budgets. Taken together, the major fiscal transfers to the provinces – made up of EPF, CAP, and Equalization, and including EPF tax points whose value increases in line with income tax revenues – had not been cut in percentage terms more than other federal programs. The 1995 budget documents thus declared that cuts in transfers for major social programs "are less than cuts to other federal program spending."[3] In the budget speech itself, Minister Martin declared: "As a matter of fairness and balance, we believe that the provinces should not be expected to bear more of the fiscal burden than we are prepared to impose on ourselves. This budget meets that test" (Department of Finance 1995a, 18).

At the regularly scheduled Annual Premiers' Conference (APC) in August 1995 in St John's, premiers expressed their anger in somewhat muted terms. They observed: "It is unacceptable for the federal government to, on the one hand reduce federal transfers to provinces and territories, and on the other prescribe the structure and standards of provincial and territorial social programs."[4] The premiers agreed to establish the Provincial/Territorial (P/T) Ministerial Council on Social Policy Reform and Renewal "to consult on federal reform initiatives and discuss common policy positions."[5] In the following year, at the APC of August 1996, the premiers (except the premier of Quebec) directed their finance ministers to "work with their federal counterparts to ensure that an agenda for the redesign of financial arrangements proceeds and is coordinated with social policy renewal." In so doing, they began to take a series of steps to support their view that the federal position on the financing of national social programs was politically untenable.

In 1997, P/T finance ministers submitted a background paper to premiers that has served as a fundamental underpinning of their position on the issue of fiscal imbalance. Among other things, the paper declared the following:

> The tax points that were transferred from Ottawa to the provinces twenty years earlier are "not an ongoing federal transfer to provinces, any more than the provincial tax room shifted under the Wartime Tax Agreements constitutes an ongoing provincial transfer to the federal government."[6]

> The federal cuts in cash transfers to the provinces in respect of health, post-secondary education, and social assistance and services between 1994/95 and 1998/99 were 33 percent, whereas reductions for other (i.e., direct) federal programs were only one percent.[7]

> "There is a fiscal imbalance between the federal government and the provinces, even after the federal transfer system is taken into account," and

this imbalance is "likely to widen."

> "Finding the right distribution of fiscal resources between the federal gov-
ernment and the provinces means dealing with both the existing imbalance and the need for new financial arrangements to reflect any coming
rebalancing of federal-provincial roles."[8]

The report also sets out three options for addressing the fiscal imbalance, including enhanced cash transfers, a reallocation of equalized tax points, and realignment of tax fields.

These conclusions were endorsed publicly by the APC in August
1997 at St. Andrews-by-the-Sea. The premiers also declared: "Coordinating
the redesign of financial arrangements with social policy renewal will require
addressing provincial/territorial differences in the ability to raise revenues and
ensure that individuals are treated as fairly as possible no matter where they
reside in Canada."[9] In effect, they were affirming that the need to correct the
vertical fiscal imbalance was not inconsistent with ongoing efforts to reduce
horizontal fiscal imbalances.

By this time, provinces and territories were following a three-pronged
approach in their efforts to undo the damage associated with the CHST transfer
cuts. First, they were attempting to persuade the federal government to enter into
a new framework agreement on the development and management of social policy in Canada. Their objectives in pursuing this initiative were to secure some
limits on the use of the federal spending power and to obtain formal procedures
for dispute resolution. Second, they were undertaking detailed studies on vertical fiscal imbalance that they hoped would enable them to persuade the federal
government (and the public) of the validity of their financial claims. Third, they
were also developing proposals to improve Equalization.

At the December 1997 First Ministers' Meeting, all first ministers, with
the exception of the premier of Quebec, agreed to initiate talks on a new framework for Canada's social union. The joint communiqué from the meetings set out
objectives for the negotiations that were to ensue. There was no reference, however, to fiscal imbalance as an item of discussion.[10] The premiers wanted to have
these issues addressed as a package, but Ottawa apparently preferred to have
them handled independently of one another.

Over the following year negotiations took place on what would eventually become the Social Union Framework Agreement (SUFA). While these negotiations were proceeding, P/T leaders continued to demand that the cuts to CHST

cash transfers be restored. Their strategy, however, had undergone a significant change. By this time, public concern about the future of Canada's health care system had grown considerably, and provinces were also concerned that Ottawa, with its recent and anticipated budgetary surpluses, might attempt to launch a new Canada-wide shared-cost health program such as pharmacare or home care. Thus, the news release emanating from the 1998 Saskatoon meeting of the APC declared: "As their first priority for new federal spending, Premiers emphasized that the federal government must restore its funding to health care through the existing CHST arrangements. Premiers also agreed that funding for core health services, once restored, must be stable and adequate, before new health care programs are established."[11]

While in substantive terms, the P/T position had not changed, the focus on health, rather than more broadly on CHST-related social programs (i.e., health, post-secondary education, and social services) marked a departure in their public communications strategy. Health care was by then at the top of the public agenda. Therefore provinces judged that it might be easier for them to secure incremental funds from the federal government if they committed to spend any additional transfers on health care only.

The federal and provincial/territorial governments signed the Social Union Framework Agreement in February 1999 in the run-up to the federal budget. By this time the federal government's fiscal position had improved quite significantly. Thus, a deal on SUFA with terms that Ottawa could accept turned out to be the *quid pro quo* for an improvement in the federal government's CHST cash payment.

Even as the provinces were mounting their critique of the CHST and beginning their campaign on fiscal imbalance, the federal government had already begun to improve the cash component of the CHST. In its 1996 budget Ottawa had announced a five-year arrangement that included a new cash floor provision of $11 billion to limit the impact of reductions announced in 1995. In the 1998 federal budget, the cash floor was raised to $12.5 billion. The 1999 federal budget went much further, however, with a one-time CHST supplement for health care of $3.5 billion and a $2.5-billion increase in the CHST cash base to $15 billion for a three-year period. The 2000 federal budget provided an additional one-time CHST health supplement of $2.5 billion.

At the Winnipeg APC in August 2000, premiers drew attention to the fact that the federal government's surpluses were projected to rise quickly as a result of greater than expected growth in revenues and reduced expenditure commitments. In contrast, the provinces and territories would "be hard pressed to keep their budgets in balance over this same period."[12] To lend substance to their views, premiers released a report entitled *Understanding Canada's Health Care Costs*, which documented in detail the growing cost pressures on provincial health care systems. The premiers again called for the "immediate and full restoration of the CHST to 1994/95 levels, together with an escalator," claiming that these measures would still leave Ottawa with "substantial surpluses."

Meanwhile, the provincial and federal governments were in the process of negotiating a new agreement on health. The federal government was willing to further increase it cash commitment to CHST if and only if it was part of a substantial, commonly agreed upon commitment to health care reform by all governments. In September 2000 first ministers met in Ottawa and released a detailed and broad-ranging "Communiqué on Health," setting out a vision and set of principles for the future of health care and an action plan for health system renewal (First Ministers 2000a). In conjunction with this Health Accord, the federal government announced a further investment of $23.4 billion over five years. Of this, $21.1 billion would be expended through the CHST (with $18.9 billion earmarked for health care and $2.2 billion for early childhood development), thus providing the provinces and territories with "stable, predictable, and growing funding through to 2005/06."[13]

He Said/She Said: The VFI Debate Following the 2000 Health Accord

Despite the large increases in CHST announced prior to and as part of the 2000 Health Accord, provincial and territorial governments continued to maintain that the federal cash contribution for health, education, and social assistance and services is not adequate or equitable. They insist that there is still a large and growing fiscal imbalance between the two orders of government, that the cash associated with the CHST is too limited, given ongoing cost pressures, and that other aspects of the CHST are inappropriate. They point in particular to the lack of a solid federal commitment to provincial social programs beyond the CHST cash floor and the absence of formal provisions for growth (escalator). In addition to producing their own series of reports on VFI, the provinces have also commissioned independent studies to support the validity of their case against the federal government. Each public statement on the issue by the provinces has, of course, been met with equally vigorous federal counter-arguments.

In essence, the provinces argue that the federal government has revenue-raising abilities that considerably exceed the cost of fulfilling its program responsibilities, while they lack the revenue-raising capacity to meet their constitutional obligations, especially in the areas of health, education, and social services, which are recognized as key public priorities. They further argue that the costs of delivering these large and important programs are rising more rapidly than federal program costs, while their revenues are growing at a significantly slower pace than federal revenues.[14] The following excerpts from the 2001 and 2002 reports of the provincial and territorial finance ministers on fiscal imbalance capture the provinces' position:

> To accomplish their crucial programming goals, provinces and territories must have access to adequate funding, both from their own-source revenues and from federal government transfers. This adequacy has not been achieved with respect to federal transfers.

> Past cuts to federal support for provincial social programs, especially those that accompanied the CHST have widened the fiscal imbalance. Between 1994/95 and 1998/99, annual federal transfers under the CHST were cut by one-third – $6.2 billion. Despite a partial restoration in 2000/01, federal CHST payments were still $3.2 billion lower than in 1994/95. In contrast, annual provincial and territorial spending on health care, education, and social services was an estimated $18.8 billion higher than in 1994/95.

> Even with the increased payments announced at the September 2000 First Ministers' Meeting, future CHST growth … will be less than that of the cost of the main programs it helps fund. As a result, the federal contribution, expressed as a percentage of provincial and territorial social program expenditures, will once again decline.

> It is clear that the changes to the CHST announced by the federal government in September 2000 represent neither an adequate nor a durable solution to the problems of fiscal imbalance and funding of major social programs.[15]

The P/T documents also quote extensively from the work of Professor G.C. Ruggeri, which indicates that the federal surplus is likely to continue to grow over the next two decades, while the provinces' fiscal situation is deemed "precarious." We examine Professor Ruggeri's research in the next section.

The issue of vertical fiscal imbalance has received considerable attention in Quebec in particular. In 2001 the Government of Quebec appointed the

Commission on Fiscal Imbalance headed by Yves Séguin. Its report, entitled *A New Division of Canada's Financial Resources*, was released in March 2002. It also concludes that there is a structural imbalance in revenues and spending between Ottawa and the Quebec government. Moreover, the Commission considers the system of intergovernmental transfers to be inadequate and points to the federal spending power as part of the problem. The report states:

> > The CHST "is the most problematic transfer program" because it "applies to fields of jurisdiction attributed to the provinces, and its attendant conditions, as well as its defining terms, clearly limit the provinces' decision-making and budgetary autonomy in these fields of jurisdiction." Federal budgetary cuts compound these difficulties. As for Equalization, it "fails to eliminate major differences in the fiscal capacities of the provinces" due to several deficiencies in program design.

> > The federal spending power exacerbates these difficulties. The use of this power distorts provincial budgetary choices, from one perspective, and has a destabilizing impact, from another (when Ottawa withdraws from joint programs or reduces transfers). It is only because of the fiscal imbalance that Ottawa has the money to use the spending power. Doing away with the imbalance would thus improve autonomy and reduce distortions.

The Commission's main recommendation to restore fiscal balance was to abolish the CHST and have the federal government transfer the GST as an own-revenue source to the provinces.[16] With the release of its report, the Commission also made public a study undertaken on its behalf by the Conference Board of Canada (2002a) on the long-term fiscal outlook for the federal and Quebec governments supporting its conclusions.

While the provinces and territories were building their case for improved intergovernmental fiscal arrangements, the federal government responded in two ways. It implicitly acknowledged that there was some validity in the provincial/territorial position to the extent that it did increase (quite substantially) the size of the CHST transfer in the late 1990s and early 2000s. At the same time, it has been steadfast in contesting the existence of a vertical fiscal imbalance.

In an effort to counter provincial claims, the federal government also produced a number of reports laying out its arguments.[17] In particular, it points out that both orders have access to the same major revenue bases and are able to set their own rates. Moreover, provincial revenues (including federal transfers) have exceeded federal revenues for more than two decades, and provinces have exclusive access to certain revenue bases such as royalties, which are growing rapidly. On the expenditure side, Ottawa argues that provincial health spending has been rising sharply, but not if it is measured as a share of the economy. It also points to its own spending pressures in areas such as elderly benefits, Aboriginals, skills and learning, and national security.

The 2002 document produced by the Department of Finance lays out further arguments:

> As a result of the $100 billion five-year tax reduction plan announced in 2000 and the recent economic slowdown, federal revenues are expected to grow by an average annual rate of only 1.9 percent between 2000/01 and 2005/06.

> In contrast, federal cash transfers to the provinces are expected to grow at an average annual rate of 6.1 percent over the same period (more than three times faster than revenues).

> Federal surpluses are recent and "quite small compared with the large deficits that preceded them." Provinces' deficits have been much smaller. The federal debt burden is twice that of the provinces (federal debt charges totalled $42 billion in 2001/02 relative to $22 billion for the provinces). This reduces the federal government's fiscal room to manoeuvre and makes it more vulnerable to volatility in global interest rates.

> The fact that virtually all provinces have chosen to reduce taxes in recent years implies that they believe that they have sufficient revenues to manage their spending pressures. Indeed, provincial tax cuts enacted since 1995 will reduce revenues by about $20 billion this year.[18]

Thus, while the Commission on the Future of Health Care in Canada deliberated about ways of improving the sustainability of public health insurance in Canada, federal and provincial governments were engaged in a "he said, she said" debate about whether or not there is an imbalance in Canada's fiscal arrangements. Provinces clearly believe that there is an imbalance, while Ottawa insists that "the 'fiscal imbalance' is a myth."[19] Provinces also argue that not enough is being done by Ottawa to deal with horizontal fiscal imbalances. The federal government displays various charts and graphs that suggest the opposite. Central to this dispute is a disagreement on the adequacy of federal funding for provincial health care programs.

VERTICAL FISCAL GAP AND VERTICAL FISCAL IMBALANCE: WORKING CONCEPTS AND LINKAGES

The key issue in the debate over vertical fiscal imbalance is the relative capacity of each order of government to raise its own revenues to fund its own expenditures. In the economics literature, unfortunately, the term "vertical fiscal gap" is sometimes used interchangeably with the term "fiscal imbalance." These concepts, however, convey different ideas, and the distinction between them is quite important in the context of the present analysis.

In many federal systems, the constitution assigns greater revenue-raising authority to the central government than is required to meet its expenditure responsibilities, while state or provincial governments are assigned significant expenditure responsibilities but with less than corresponding taxing powers. This "mismatch" in the allocation of revenues and spending obligations can provide important benefits. Having more taxation take place via the central government fosters greater tax harmonization and reduces economic distortions and administrative costs. The "excess revenue" also enables the central government to pursue certain economic efficiency and equity objectives at a national level by transferring revenues to state or provincial governments in variety of ways. At the same time, having people-related public expenditures take place through regional or subnational governments allows them to better respond to local needs and preferences. The main drawback to this revenue/expenditure mismatch is that it makes it more difficult for citizens to determine which order of government is responsible for what. It may also result in less accountability and less local autonomy than would be the case if the government that spent was also the one that taxed (according to the principle of fiscal responsibility).

Although the extent of the mismatch differs widely among federations, the central government typically transfers a share of its revenues to the regional order of government to fill the gap. These intergovernmental transfers provide a measure of the "vertical fiscal gap." Generally speaking, the size of the vertical fiscal gap (VFG) is a function of the degree to which (a) public spending is decentralized and (b) revenue raising is centralized. Together, these two factors determine the extent to which subnational governments must rely on the central government to supplement their own-source revenues.

From that perspective, the concept of vertical fiscal gap is nothing more than an accounting identity. The size of the fiscal gap between orders of government is defined by the magnitude of the cash transfers that flow from one order of government to another. Based on this definition, the vertical fiscal gap between the federal and provincial governments in Canada decreased steadily over the two decades that ended in the late 1990s. During that period, the size of federal government transfers to the provinces, as a share of provincial revenues, was declining. Stated differently, provincial reliance on own-source revenue was on the rise. To the extent that CHST transfers have increased over the last few years, however, the vertical fiscal gap has again begun to rise. This perspective on the actual VFG, it will be clear, provides no criteria for determining whether it is too large, too small, or about right.

One way to assess whether the actual VFG is adequate would be to compare it to the desired or optimal vertical fiscal gap between the two orders of government. To the extent that there is a difference between the *actual* and *optimal* level, this may be a way to identify and measure any fiscal imbalance that might exist. For instance, in an ideal model – one that assumes the existence of an optimal allocation of expenditure and taxation between orders of government – the size of the intergovernmental transfers would be such as to enable each level of government to meet its expenditure obligations and achieve budget balance. Unfortunately, there is no ideal model from which to determine the optimal size of vertical fiscal gap. Indeed such an exercise is very much of a normative nature. For instance, the way one views the nature of the federation would very much affect the way one weighs the benefits of centralized revenue collection and nation-wide programming against the benefits of decentralization (spending adapted to local needs and preferences) and fiscal responsibility. As for the balance between state and market, the larger (or smaller) the state's role the more (or less) concerns about the efficient allocation of tax powers and expenditure functions are likely to matter. Each of these considerations has different implications for the design and amount of intergovernmental transfers. In short, the range of views on the optimal vertical fiscal gap is likely to correspond to the range of views about the nature of the federation and the role of the government in the economy.

In chapter 1, Keith Banting and Robin Boadway describe three alternative views of the role of the federal government in health care. In effect, they provide three quite different visions of the Canadian sharing community and hence of the Canadian federation. In their model of a *predominantly Canada-wide sharing community,* they envisage the whole of Canada as the primary sharing community. While this model can apply in the context of either a large or a small role for the state, for our purposes it is useful to think of it initially in the context of a larger role. What might be the VFG implications in such a setting? For one thing, the federal government would want to *ensure* that important social programs were available in all provinces and territories on fairly comparable terms. Since key social services, including health care, are generally designed and delivered by provinces, Ottawa would almost certainly use conditional transfers to provinces to persuade them to design and deliver these programs on terms that are consistent with the idea of a country-wide sharing community. The federal authorities would also want to make sure that the size of the transfers was large enough that provinces would be reluctant to challenge the conditions. (This is not to say that there could not, and should not, be extensive federal-provincial dialogue before such a decision is taken.) The consequence of such an action, of course, would be to increase federal transfers to the provinces and territories and thus enlarge the vertical fiscal gap.

Under this same model, there might be other reasons for the gap to rise. For example, the five-province standard for Equalization could be improved to better ensure that less wealthy provinces are in a position to provide services consistent with pan-Canadian norms, leading to larger federal transfers to recipient provinces.[20] It is also consistent with this vision of the federation for the federal government to occupy the dominant role in the personal income tax field because this is the only large progressive tax base that allows Ottawa to effectively fulfill its redistributive role. In short, it would be consistent with the predominantly Canada-wide sharing community model of the federation, in conjunction with a large role for the state, to have a substantially larger vertical fiscal gap than exists today. From a normative viewpoint, this would be a desirable outcome.

There are, of course, many arguments against such an increase in the vertical fiscal gap. Perhaps the easiest way to understand them is to consider the other end of the sharing-community spectrum, the *predominantly provincial sharing community* and its related arguments. To begin with, if provinces were the primary sharing community, the political goal of *assuring* reasonably comparable levels of services across the country would disappear. Thus, large conditional intergovernmental transfers for specific purposes, like health and social services, would be unnecessary. Moreover, it would be consistent with this view to focus less on the efficiencies and other benefits of centralized revenue collection and to concentrate more on the accountability and other benefits that flow from having the government that spends also be the government that taxes. Thus, the desired size of the vertical fiscal gap under this model would be considerably smaller than the current vertical fiscal gap and much smaller than that under a predominantly canada-wide sharing community model. The *dual sharing community* – the third model in the Banting-Boadway analysis – falls somewhere between these two.

The Séguin Commission's proposal to abolish the CHST and have the federal government reallocate tax room (for example, the GST) to the provinces is consistent with the predominantly provincial sharing community model of the federation. In effect, the size of the vertical fiscal gap would be limited to the size of the Equalization program, which we assume to be a given (in one form or another) in light of constitutional requirements.[21] This means that, under the predominantly provincial sharing model of the sharing community, the richest province or provinces would not receive any cash transfers from Ottawa. There would thus be no vertical fiscal gap between, say, the federal government and the provinces of Alberta and Ontario. In effect, all remaining federal transfers might then be thought of as reducing or eliminating differences in fiscal capacity among the provinces (reflecting Canada's equalization commitment). That is, their purpose would be to reduce or eliminate horizontal fiscal imbalances.[22]

From the preceding discussion, it should be clear that determining the desired size of the vertical fiscal gap is not a technical exercise but a normative one, which could lead to different results depending on how one views the nature of the Canadian sharing community, federalism, and the appropriate role for the state. To the extent that policy on intergovernmental transfers, at any point in time, somehow effectively reflects and fairly balances these competing views, then the idea of VFG as an accounting identity and VFG as a normative concept may coincide. When the provinces argue that the federal government is not contributing a sufficient share of health care funding and question the legitimacy of its role in setting the course of reforms, they are in fact claiming that there is an imbalance between the actual and desired level of VFG. But if provinces are able to deal practically with the problem, by raising more revenues on their own or by reducing low priority spending, then this difference between the actual and desired fiscal gap is not necessarily a case of vertical fiscal imbalance, notwithstanding provincial claims to the contrary. In that situation, if a revenue shortfall did occur, it would be due to the provinces' own budgetary decisions. However, if making budgetary adjustments is not an option that is practically available to provinces because the federal government is occupying an unduly large amount of tax room relative to its spending obligations (including transfers to provinces), and because citizens are demanding that provinces maintain or even enhance current expenditure programs, then the difference between the actual and desired VFG could indeed constitute evidence of VFI. This second interpretation reflects the provinces' position today. They view the current fiscal situation as a clear case of "vertical fiscal imbalance."

The concept of vertical fiscal imbalance, therefore, has to do with the idea that one order of government has less revenue (including the transfers it receives) than it needs and can readily raise to implement its expenditure responsibilities, while the other has more revenue than it needs (including what it may require for intergovernmental transfers). The problem with this definition is that it is very difficult to apply in a Canadian context. For instance, the first question that arises is whether VFI is even a meaningful concept in a federation such as Canada where both the federal and provincial governments have the constitutional right to levy taxes on all of the major tax bases – and in fact do so.[23] The response to this question is that, in practice, both orders of government – and governments of all political stripes – believe there are effective limits to taxation, and behave accordingly. Thus, if the overall tax burden (all levels of government combined) is equal to or exceeds the assumed limit, then having the constitutional power to tax is not of much value if, for practical economic or political reasons, it is not desirable to do so. In other words, despite the constitutional allocation of taxing powers, vertical fiscal imbalance can be a meaningful concept.

A second question has to do with how to delineate the expenditure responsibilities of each order of government. The spending obligations of Canadian governments today are more or less related to the responsibilities or jurisdictions laid out in the constitution, but the extent and the manner in which governments choose to fulfil these obligations are matters of public policy and democratic choice. They are also subject to change over time. Moreover, since the federal government can intervene in areas of provincial responsibility not only through intergovernmental transfers but also through its use of the direct spending power (for example, through transfers to individuals), it can be difficult to determine where its expenditure obligations end and where the fiscal imbalance begins at any point in time.

A related issue, given limited fiscal resources, is how one assigns priority among the various expenditure responsibilities of different orders of government. In times of war, this may be relatively easy to establish, but in peacetime there is no obvious way to do so other than through the political process. In effect, the order of government that believes it lacks the revenue required to meets its obligations will appeal to the public. If it can make a good enough case, then the public will somehow pressure the other order of government to transfer revenue to the government that is being shortchanged, or to vacate tax room. In the current context, the provinces claim that they lack the funds required to finance their large and growing expenditure responsibilities for health care and other social and educational services. The fact that the provinces have campaigned publicly for an adjustment to the allocation of revenues indicates that they believe they can win public support for their position. The fact that the federal government has increased its CHST transfer substantially over the last few years indicates that Ottawa has, up to a point, understood the power of their case.

Thus in spite of the complexities involved, the issue of vertical fiscal imbalance is a pertinent one. The question is how to identify VFI and measure it. Presumably, the imbalance would manifest itself in the relative fiscal outcomes of both orders of government over time. For instance, vertical fiscal imbalance could be an issue when one order of government is able to achieve structural fiscal balance or surpluses on a consistent basis while the other order of government is in a precarious fiscal position. We use the words "could be" because there is nothing automatic about these circumstances being symptoms of vertical fiscal imbalance. As already discussed, it is only when the order of government with the weaker fiscal structure is effectively precluded from correcting this weakness on its own (say because the fiscally stronger level of government has occupied too much tax room or has unilaterally reduced its share of joint-program funding) that a VFI can be said to exist. The next two sections of this chapter deal specifically with these issues.

Assuming a VFI does exist, it can be corrected in several ways. First, the order of government with the stronger structural fiscal balance can transfer cash to the other order of government. When this technique is used, the vertical fiscal imbalance shrinks but, of course, the vertical fiscal gap increases. Second, the government with the budgetary surplus can assume some of the expenditure responsibilities of the other order of government. Third, tax room can be transferred from the surplus order of government to the other. The second and third techniques have no effect on the vertical fiscal gap. Choosing among these methods, or combinations of them, is related to the normative issues discussed above concerning the desirability of a vertical fiscal gap. There is considerable historical precedent for all three methods in Canada.

There are other conceivable ways of dealing with a vertical fiscal imbalance. For example, the government in surplus position could commit to transferring a fixed percentage of revenues from a particular tax base to the other order of government. Assuming the federal government is the one with the surplus, a formal revenue-sharing scheme would preserve the administrative and economic advantages of centralized revenue collection and could also help to reduce the negative aspects of tax competition while ensuring that provinces have access to a certain share of aggregate revenues. These are significant advantages. A disadvantage with this approach, however, is that it would give provinces less fiscal autonomy than a transfer of tax room would. There is less precedence for this revenue-sharing method in Canadian experience, but it is used in a number of other federations.

To sum up, the size of the current vertical fiscal gap (that is, the level of intergovernmental transfers) does not tells us whether it is adequate or appropriate. And it tells us even less about whether there is a vertical fiscal imbalance above and beyond the observed or even the desired level of VFG. And this is what is at issue in the current debate. One's view of what constitutes an appropriate vertical fiscal gap for Canada will depend on what is perceived to be the appropriate role of the state in general, and that of the federal government in particular. Irrespective of these views, however, one would presumably also take into account the extent of VFI, if the latter could be ascertained.

VERTICAL FISCAL IMBALANCE: FROM CONCEPT TO APPLICATION

A number of Canadian studies produced since the early 1990s have attempted to quantify the extent of vertical fiscal imbalance between the federal and the provincial and territorial governments. These studies for the most part have taken a direct approach to the mismatch issue, based on a comparison of the structural fiscal balances of each level of government. In particular, Joe Ruggeri, Vaughan Chair in Regional Economics and Director of the Policy Studies Centre at the University of New Brunswick, has been publishing papers on this subject with his colleagues for a number of years.[24] More recently,

Ruggeri has updated some of this work at the request of provincial governments and produced new estimates. Many of the arguments put forward by the provinces on vertical fiscal imbalance are based on his reports.

The conceptual framework underlying Ruggeri's analysis was initially laid out in a paper by Ruggeri, Howard, and Van Wart in 1993. Their definition of structural fiscal balance focuses on the relationship between the built-in growth of existing expenditure programs and revenue sources for each order of government (1993a, 456). A structurally balanced fiscal system in this framework is one where the initial relationship between the built-in growth of spending and taxation is maintained through time. If it diverges, the fiscal system is deemed *structurally* unbalanced. Thus, in the absence of debt, structural balance can be defined simply as the maintenance of a balanced budget through time, which in turn requires that the growth rate of revenues and expenditures be equal (if they are not, the difference between the two is the measure of structural imbalance).

When deficit financing and debt are incorporated in the model, structural balance can be defined in one of two ways: (1) as a fiscal system that maintains constant deficit- and debt-to-GDP ratios; or (2) as one where the nominal value of the debt is kept constant, but its ratio relative to GDP falls over time toward zero. Assuming that the nominal interest rate is equal to the rate of growth of nominal GDP, maintaining structural balance under the first definition would require a balanced operating budget (i.e., revenues equal to program spending) and the same rate of growth in revenues and expenditures. Under the second definition, structural balance would require maintaining budgetary balance (i.e., revenues equal to program spending plus debt charges), that is, having an operating surplus which as a share of GDP is equal to the debt-to-GDP ratio times the nominal interest rate. If the nominal interest rate is greater than the growth rate of nominal GDP, the requirements for maintaining structural fiscal balance are more onerous, and *vice versa*. Under the first definition, an operating surplus equal to the level of debt times the difference between the interest rate and the growth rate of GDP would be required. Under the second definition, the surplus required is equal to the debt times the nominal interest rate plus the differential between the nominal interest rate and the growth rate of GDP. In a recent paper, Thomas Courchene (2002) describes the dramatic impact of the differential between the nominal interest rate and the GDP growth rate on the federal government fiscal position in the postwar period. For illustration, he notes that in 1994, when the interest rate was 3 to 4 percentage points above the GDP growth rate, an operating surplus of $20 billion was required just to keep the debt-to-GDP ratio constant.

For analytical purposes, Ruggeri, Howard, and Van Wart (1993a) prefer the first definition of structural imbalance (based on a constant debt-to-GDP ratio), because it allows one to distinguish between two sources of structural imbalance: that which is due to the initial mismatch between revenue and expenditure *levels* and that which results from the ongoing mismatch in revenue and expenditure *growth rates*. As the authors point out, each source of imbalance requires a different policy response. Whereas the first type of imbalance simply requires an adjustment in the level of revenue and/or expenditure, the second type could only be corrected by making structural changes on either the tax or expenditure side that would affect the built-in growth rates (for example, altering the tax mix or the rate structure, or changing program eligibility criteria). It is the second type of imbalance that is the focus of their analyses on vertical fiscal imbalance.

The basic methodology consists of projecting fiscal balances assuming steady economic growth and no change in government policy. The object is to examine separately the budgetary outcomes of the fiscal structures of the two orders of government in the absence of cyclical effects and discretionary government actions. In order to do so, the taxation and expenditure structures of each order of government in the base year are taken as given and their respective growth path projected based on the different built-in growth rates assigned to particular revenue sources and program expenditures. For each revenue and expenditure component the growth rate is assumed to be related in some particular fashion to growth in one or a combination of independent variables such as GDP, consumer price index (CPI), labour productivity, population growth, or aging.

The first column of Table 1 reports selected growth rates underlying Ruggeri's most recent estimates of vertical fiscal imbalance (Ruggeri 2001). These updated estimates incorporate significant policy changes implemented since the author's earlier report to provincial premiers in July 2000. The changes include income tax reductions by the federal and provincial governments and the CHST increases announced as part of the September 2000 Health Accord, as well as other spending initiatives and economic growth adjustments as of mid-2001. Based on Ruggeri's estimates, federal revenues are expected to grow an average of 4.1 percent per annum versus 3.6 percent for the provinces between 1999/2000 and 2019/20. Given that the federal government and the provinces share access to most of the main revenue sources, the discrepancy between the two in terms of overall growth in revenues stems primarily from two sources: 1) the federal government's greater reliance on the fastest-growing revenue source, the personal income tax (PIT) – 47 percent relative to 27 percent for the provinces; and 2) the significant share of provincial revenues (15 percent) that comes from slow-growing federal transfers. Ruggeri takes into account the effects of announced tax cuts and transfer increases in coming fiscal years, but after that assumes that PIT revenues will continue to grow at a rate of 1.25 times the growth in nominal GDP, and that CHST cash payments in real terms will only be kept constant at their 2005/06 level.

The opposite occurs on the expenditure side. Provinces have a relatively large share of their program spending in rapidly growing expenditure areas. Health and education, which combined make up for more than half of total provincial spending, are projected to grow at a faster rate than nominal GDP.[25] On the other hand, Old Age Security (OAS) is the only large federal expenditure program expected to grow rapidly, and it accounts for only 10 percent of total federal spending.[26] Transfers to provinces, which in aggregate account for 17 percent of total federal spending, are only projected to grow at a rate of 2.2 percent. Moreover, under the "no policy change" constraint, debt charges are assumed to remain constant. As a result, close to 25 percent of federal expenditures has a zero built-in growth rate (compared with less than 15 percent for the provinces).

Provincial spending is thus projected to grow at an average annual rate of 3.5 percent over the twenty-year period, whereas the corresponding rate for federal spending is 2.2 percent. Federal government revenues, on the other hand, are expected to grow almost twice as fast as its expenditures, while the provincial revenue growth rate is only marginally higher than that of expenditures. Ruggeri refers to these differential federal/provincial growth rates on the revenue and expenditure side as the *roots* of vertical fiscal imbalance. These growth rates are then applied to actual base-year fiscal parameters to project the budget position of the federal and provincial governments (Ruggeri 2001, 7). As Charts 1a and 1d show, relatively small growth rate differentials generate a substantial fiscal impact when projected forward ten and twenty years. According to Ruggeri's calculations, the federal surplus is expected to increase to $39 billion by 2009/10 and to triple to $126 billion ten years later, while the provinces will only manage to achieve budget balance in 2009/10 and a $5.5-billion surplus in 2019/20. The difference in the size of federal and provincial budget balances over

Table 1

SUMMARY OF ASSUMPTIONS IN RECENT STUDIES ON FISCAL IMBALANCE

	Ruggeri (2001)	Conference Board of Canada (July 2002)	Matier, Wu, and Jackson (2001)
Nominal GDP	4.7	4.2	4.3
Inflation	2.0	2.0	2.0
Interest rate on debt	7.0[1]	7.2	7.0
Federal revenues			
Total revenues	4.1	3.5	3.8
PIT	5.0	3.9	3.9
CIT	3.7	3.5	3.2
GST	4.7	4.0	4.7
Federal expenditures			
Total expenditures	2.2[2]	2.5	3.7
Program expenditures	2.9	3.9	4.7
OAS	4.6	4.2	6.2
CHST	1.9	4.5	4.1
Equalization	2.5	3.5	4.3
Provincial revenues			
Total revenues	3.6	3.4	4.1
PIT	5.1	3.8	3.9
CIT	3.7	3.3	3.4
RST	4.7	4.0	4.4
Provincial expenditures			
Total expenditures	3.5[2]	4.0	3.6
Program expenditures	4.0	4.1	4.4
Health care	5.3[3]	5.2	5.2
Education	4.5[3]	3.2	3.1

Note: The figures reported are the average annual percentage change over the period 2000/01 to 2019/20 in Matier, Wu, and Jackson and in the Conference Board of Canada, and average growth rates over the period 1999/2000 to 2019/20 in Ruggeri. The figures reported for Matier, Wu, and Jackson were calculated from data provided to us by the authors based on their alternative simulations incorporating announced revenue measures.

[1] In Ruggeri, the interest rate on the federal debt is assumed to fall slowly from 7.5 percent in 1999-2000 to 7.0 percent in 2005/2006 and remain at that level thereafter. For the provincial debt, it is assumed to decrease from about 8.9 percent in 1999-2000 to 8.25 percent in 2005/2006.

[2] Growth rates reported here for total expenditures and debt service at the federal and provincial levels correspond to the case in which surpluses are not used to reduce the public debt.

[3] The underlying growth rate, excluding announced changes, is 5.1 percent for health care and 4.2 percent for education.

Sources: G.C. Ruggeri. A federation out of balance: update. Department of Economics, University of New Brunswick, Fredericton. 2001; Conference Board of Canada. *Fiscal prospects for the Federal and Provincial/Territorial Governments.* July 2002; Chris Matier, Lisa Wu, and Harriet Jackson. Analysing VFI in a framework of fiscal sustainability. Working paper 2001-23, Department of Finance Canada.

Chart 1a

GOVERNMENT EXPENDITURES AND REVENUES—RUGGERI (2001)

(average annual growth rate)

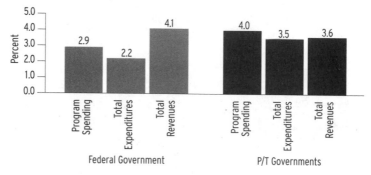

Chart 1b

GOVERNMENT EXPENDITURES AND REVENUES—CBoC (JULY 2002)

(average annual compound growth rates)

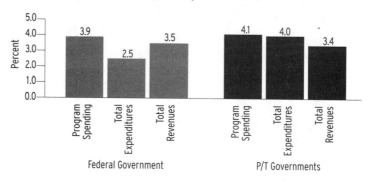

Chart 1c

GOVERNMENT EXPENDITURES AND REVENUES—MATIER, WU,

AND JACKSON (2001) (average annual growth rates)

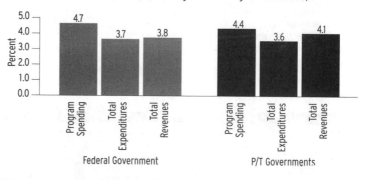

Chart 1d

PROJECTION OF FEDERAL AND P/T BUDGET BALANCES—RUGGERI (2001)

(billions of dollars)

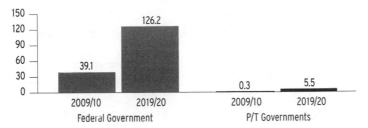

Chart 1e

PROJECTION OF FEDERAL AND P/T BUDGET BALANCES—CBoC (JULY 2002)

(billions of dollars)

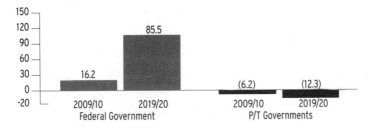

Chart 1f

PROJECTION OF FEDERAL AND P/T BUDGET BALANCES—MATIER, WU,

AND JACKSON (2001) (billions of dollars)

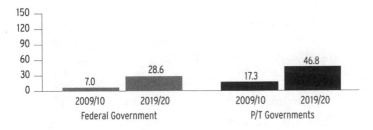

Sources: G.C. Ruggeri. A federation out of balance: update. Department of Economics, University of New Brunswick, Fredericton. 2001; Conference Board of Canada, *Fiscal prospects for the Federal and Provincial/Territorial Governments*, July 2002; Chris Matier, Lisa Wu, and Harriet Jackson. Analysing VFI in a framework of fiscal sustainability. Working paper 2001-23, Department of Finance Canada.

time is what Ruggeri describes as the *path* of vertical fiscal imbalance. According to his estimates, approximately 80 percent of the difference between the federal and provincial fiscal positions stems from the divergent growth paths on the spending side.

In his alternative scenarios, Ruggeri illustrates the precarious state of the provinces' fiscal position. For instance, he shows that adding half a percentage point to the annual growth rate of health care spending transforms small provincial surpluses into a string of growing deficits (up to $10 billion by the end of the twenty-year period). The size of federal surpluses provides a much greater cushion against unforeseen circumstances, a situation that, Ruggeri's estimates show, is further reinforced when allowing for a portion of these surpluses to go to debt repayment. An assumption that half of any surplus goes to debt repayment increases the federal surplus (relative to the base case reported in Chart 1) by $14.7 billion in 2014/15 and by $35.8 billion in 2019/20, at which point the federal debt would be eliminated. Since the option of paying down the debt is not widely available to the provinces (for lack of the necessary surpluses), this self-feeding mechanism leads to an even greater vertical fiscal imbalance.

The Conference Board of Canada (CBoC) (2002a), in a report prepared for the Commission on Fiscal Imbalance, uses a similar approach to project the public accounts of the federal and Quebec governments out twenty years to the year 2019/20. In July 2002 the Conference Board extended the study prepared for the Séguin Commission to cover all of the provinces and territories.[27] The Conference Board's results are based on its own long-term economic forecasts for basic macro-economic variables, as well as two separate forecasting models developed to estimate specific changes in per capita spending on health care and education. They also adopt a status quo benchmark with respect to fiscal and budgetary policy (except for measures announced in the 2000 and 2001 federal budgets and economic update). But in contrast to Ruggeri's work, their base case assumes that government surpluses in any given year are allocated entirely to debt repayment. As stated in the report, this assumption allows one "to evaluate the governments' room-to-manoeuvre and thus to indicate the degree of latitude available to them to implement new initiatives or, conversely, the budgetary actions needed to balance the books" (Conference Board of Canada 2002b, 28).

Table 1 (column 2) reports the Conference Board's estimates of average annual compound growth rates for selected variables. Estimates of budgetary revenues from direct taxes are calculated using the CBoC's personal income and

corporate profit forecasts, and revenues from indirect taxes are based on growth
in consumer spending or general economic activity. Other than recent budget
measures, federal program spending for the most part is assumed to grow in line
with two factors: growth in nominal GDP and the rate of growth of population
and inflation combined (the growth rate is the mean of these two rates). OAS
benefits are linked to projected demographic changes and indexed to inflation.
Growth in equalization payments is tied to growth in nominal GDP (in the same
way as observed in the past), and CHST payments increase as planned to
2005/06 and are then assumed to grow in line with population growth and inflation. While federal budgetary revenues are expected to increase by 3.5 percent
annually and program spending by 3.9 percent, the reduction in interest payments that follows from having budget surpluses used to pay down the debt has
a dramatic effect on the overall rate of growth of federal expenditures, which is
only 2.5 percent.

　　　Assumptions regarding growth in provincial and territorial revenues
and program spending are generally consistent with those for federal revenues
and spending. As mentioned earlier, health care and education spending are estimated separately. Health care spending is projected to increase at an average
annual growth rate of 5.2 percent over the twenty-year period (much faster than
the expected rate of growth of nominal GDP of 4.2 percent). Of the 5.2 percent,
2.1 percentage points per year is attributable to inflation, 1.7 to demographics
(population growth and aging) and 1.4 to real increases in the volume of services
provided due to technological change, broader access, and other factors.[28] As a
result, provincial health care spending is expected to increase from $63.5 billion
in 2001/02 to $166.5 billion in 2019/20, by which time it will represent close to
45 percent of budgetary revenues (compared to 32 percent currently). In the case
of education, spending is projected to increase by only 3.2 percent per year on
average, reflecting the decline in population in the relevant age groups. As Chart
1b shows, overall provincial and territorial program spending is expected to
increase at a slightly faster rate than federal spending (4.1 percent relative to 3.9
percent). However, since provincial and territorial governments collectively are
unable to reduce their interest charges due to ongoing deficits, their budgetary
expenditures increase by 4.0 percent per year over the twenty-year period, compared to 2.5 percent at the federal level.

　　　The main conclusion of the Conference Board report is that: "With current fiscal regimes in place, the vertical fiscal imbalance will widen in the future"

(2002b, 28). At the federal level, the results reveal a steady string of ever-growing budget surpluses reaching $16.2 billion in 2009/10 and $85.5 billion in 2019/20 (see Chart 1e). As a result, the federal government is able to pay down more than 90 percent of its interest-bearing debt by the end of the forecast period (from $589 billion to $53 billion) and see its annual interest charges reduced from $42 billion to $11 billion. The reduction in interest payments is largely responsible for the growing budgetary surplus and the fast decline in interest-bearing debt at the federal level.

Meanwhile, the combined budget balance of provincial and territorial governments is projected to remain negative throughout the forecast period, with the deficit peaking at $12.3 billion in 2019/20. By that time the aggregate provincial/territorial debt level will have increased by 54 percent from $251.5 billion to $386.9 billion[29] and the debt-servicing charges will be 3.5 times those borne by the federal government (Conference Board of Canada 2002b, 28). The CBoC report points to the expected rate of growth of health care expenses (5.2 percent) as particularly problematic given the expected average rate of growth (3.4 percent) in provincial and territorial budgetary revenues.

Researchers at the federal Department of Finance have also put forward their own analysis and estimates of vertical fiscal imbalance. The approach taken by Matier, Wu, and Jackson (2001) differs from the preceding two studies in three respects. First, they develop an indicator of vertical fiscal imbalance that incorporates explicitly the notion of fiscal sustainability; that is, the existing debt of each order of government is included directly in the measurement of structural fiscal balance. Second, they use a generational accounting framework that allows them to capture the impact of population growth and aging on all affected revenue sources and expenditure categories.[30] Third, based on their definition, a vertical fiscal imbalance is only deemed to exist if one order of government has fiscal room to reduce taxes or increase program spending and satisfy its intertemporal budget constraint, while the other order of government's fiscal structure is such that it would need to permanently increase taxes or reduce program spending to restore fiscal sustainability.[31]

A government's fiscal structure is considered to be sustainable if it satisfies its intertemporal budget constraint. This means that government debt must not grow faster than the rate of interest over time. In an intertemporal framework, this condition is satisfied if the present value of future operating budget balances (revenues minus program spending) equals the initial level of (net) debt. If a government's initial debt is larger than the present value of its project-ed primary balances, this constitutes a fiscal gap. If the initial debt is smaller than the present value of projected primary balances, the government has fiscal room at its disposal to implement new measures. Based on this model, a vertical fiscal imbalance exists only if one order of government is found to have fiscal room while the other suffers from a fiscal gap.

Matier and his colleagues estimate the extent of fiscal gap/room for each order of government based on long-term fiscal projections that take into account the effects of population growth and aging on government revenues and expen-ditures (using a generational accounting framework). The methodology used is the following: the first step consists of allocating GDP and each category of gov-ernment own-source revenues and program spending among 91 single-year age groups. Real average per capita levels for each age group are then assumed to grow at the same rate as productivity growth (the model assumes a constant annual rate of productivity growth of 1.5 percent and a constant rate of inflation of 2 percent). Using projections of population growth by age group, it is possi-ble to then project the growth of each fiscal variable. Thus, for the most part, the growth path for each revenue and expenditure category is determined by pro-ductivity growth, population growth, population composition, and inflation.[32] However, since productivity and inflation growth rates are constant, the key components determining different revenue and expenditure growth patterns are population aging and growth.

Table 1 (column 3) reports the underlying average annual growth rates for selected revenue sources and expenditure categories based on data provided by the authors. Although Matier et al. focus their analysis and conclusions on the results obtained in their benchmark case, the estimates reported here are those derived from one of their alternative simulations which takes into account feder-al and provincial tax measures announced in recent budgets and therefore pro-vides a better basis of comparison with the Ruggeri and the Conference Board studies. Total federal revenues are projected to grow at an average annual rate of 3.8 percent relative to 4.1 percent at the provincial level between 2000/01 and 2019/20. Their estimates suggest that overall, demographic change is of relative-ly little consequence for tax revenues.

Program expenditures are projected to grow at an average annual rate of 4.7 percent at the federal level and 4.4 percent at the provincial level. As expect-ed, the programs in which spending is skewed toward the elderly grow much faster relative to GDP than other less age-sensitive programs. For instance, in the benchmark case, the projected average annual growth rate of health expenditures from 2000/01 to 2019/20 is 5.1 percent. The authors observe that at this rate, provincial health spending as a share of GDP would rise from 6.1 percent in 2000/01 to 9.3 percent by 2040/41. Federal spending on Old Age Security is projected to rise even more rapidly at 6.2 percent per year over the next twenty years. In the case of education, an aging population has the opposite effect; spending is projected to grow at only 3.1 percent on average.

Based on these growth projections for revenues and spending, the authors calculate projected primary balances for both orders of government and estimate the size of the fiscal gap/room for each as an indicator of vertical fiscal imbalance. According to their estimates in the "announced revenue measures" case, the federal and provincial governments both have fiscal room equal to 0.33 percent and 0.30 percent (respectively) of GDP.[33] This suggests that both orders of government could permanently reduce taxes and/or increase spending by these amounts and still maintain fiscal sustainability. Consequently, they conclude that there is no indication of vertical fiscal imbalance. "Thus, the initial projected path of federal intergovernmental transfers is sufficient in this framework because it ensures that the provincial/territorial governments have the fiscal capacity to meet their projected spending in a fiscally sustainable manner" (Matier, Wu, and Jackson 2001, 24).

The results of the Matier et al. analysis produce opposite federal-provincial fiscal trends from those projected by Ruggeri and the Conference Board, with provincial revenues growing at a faster rate than federal revenues and federal program spending increasing more rapidly than provincial program spending (see Chart 1c). This somewhat counterintuitive outcome translates into projected budget surpluses that are expected to be higher at the provincial level ($17.3 billion by 2009/10 and $46.8 billion by 2019/20) than at the federal level ($7 billion by 2009/10 and $28.6 billion by 2019/20). However, this result is very much a function of the underlying assumptions and methodology used in their model. By having all real per capita/per age-group own-source revenues and spending grow at the same rate as productivity, the authors do not take into account the particular elasticities of different tax and expenditure categories (apart from those that result from population aging and growth). Their fiscal projections are entirely driven by changes in the age profile of the population. The advantage of such an approach is that it clearly highlights the relative effects of demographic change on particular revenue and spending categories for a given fiscal structure, all things being equal. But it also implies, for instance, that all social benefits (EI, OAS, social assistance, etc.) are not only indexed to inflation but are assumed to grow (in real terms and on a per capita basis) at a rate of 1.5 percent per year from their initial levels. Indeed, the same applies to all other spending categories and revenue sources. Thus, if we remove the age-profile effects, all categories of revenue (from income taxes to fuel and liquor taxes) and expenditure (from welfare benefits to defence spending) are projected to grow at the same rate. It can be argued that the same assumptions apply for both orders of government, thereby removing any potential arbitrariness in making selective assumptions about the relative growth paths of particular revenue sources and spending categories. However, it produces results that are somewhat removed from observed fiscal patterns in the past and from likely resource allocation in the future.

In the context of the vertical fiscal imbalance debate, the analysis produced by Matier and his colleagues is a useful contribution in the following sense. It broadens the debate by pointing out the need to take into account existing debt levels and the prudence factor required to ensure fiscal sustainability, when comparing the structural fiscal balances of both orders of government. It also advances the argument that vertical fiscal imbalance is only an issue if one order of government has excess fiscal room while the other suffers from a fiscal gap (as they define it). This reasoning is quite different from what is inferred in other studies, which is that there is VFI any time one order of government is in a more favourable structural fiscal position than the other. And finally the Matier et al. study produces estimates of the relative fiscal impact of population growth and aging on each order of government (all other things being equal). Other than these demographic effects, however, the study does not consider how, as a result of a different revenue mix and types of expenditures, the fiscal structure of each order of government is likely to evolve in the coming years. This is what is at the heart of the current intergovernmental debate, and it is the focus of both the Ruggeri and the Conference Board analyses.

These two studies also project fiscal balances based on the current fiscal structure of each order of government and assuming no policy change. Each attempts to model the particular growth path of each component of revenue and spending and its implications for future government budget balances. However, each draws quite a different portrait of the fiscal landscape. This is a classic example of "small differences that matter."

The Ruggeri results are driven by the following factors. On the revenue side, the relatively high projected growth rate for nominal GDP is a significant factor that affects the growth of certain tax revenues (in particular the PIT, which is assumed to grow 1.25 times GDP growth) and in turn favours the growth of federal revenues; at the same time the projected low rates of growth for federal transfers and other non-primary sources of revenue work in the opposite direction for provincial revenues. On the expenditure side, the Ruggeri model assumes relatively high rates of growth for health and education (representing half of provincial spending) and for OAS, but essentially assumes no real growth in the remaining categories.[34] This, combined with constant debt charges (which are larger at the federal level) and slow-growing federal transfers, results in a higher projected growth rate for provincial expenditures.

The Conference Board's estimates for revenue growth, which are based on their own macroeconomic forecast of projected growth in personal income, corporate profits, and consumption, among other factors, generate very different results than those reported in the Ruggeri study, with federal and provincial/territorial own-source revenues projected to grow at roughly the same rate (3.4 percent).[35] Overall federal program spending is expected to grow more rapidly than is assumed in the Ruggeri study, as it is partially linked to GDP growth in addition to inflation and population growth. Provincial/territorial program spending in aggregate is estimated to grow only at a slightly faster rate than federal program spending. The CBoC projected growth rate for education spending is considerably lower than the rate used by Ruggeri. The growth rates for total expenditures are not comparable since the Conference Board assumes all surpluses are allocated to debt repayment and debt charges are reduced accordingly, while the latter are held constant in Ruggeri's base case.

The results illustrate how important these small differences are when projected twenty years forward. Ruggeri's estimates of the difference between the built-in growth rates in federal revenues and expenditures generate a federal surplus of $39 billion by 2009/10 and $126 billion by 2019/20. When it is assumed that half of the federal surplus is allocated to debt, this surplus increases to $162 billion at the end of the twenty-year period. The Conference Board study, which assumes all surpluses go to debt reduction, also reports growing federal surpluses, but of a lesser magnitude at $16.2 billion in 2009/10 and $85.8 billion in 2019/20.

This overview of three studies on vertical fiscal imbalance in the Canadian context indicates that the results from such analyses need to be interpreted with caution. Since the fiscal projections are highly sensitive to the under-lying model specification and empirical assumptions, it is important to under-stand and take these into account. In each case the authors stress the fact that the results they present are *projections* of given fiscal variables in a given year based on assumptions about trends in economic and demographic variables and are not *forecasts*. This means that changes in the economic environment, which can and do have a determining and often long-term effect on revenue growth and partic-ular spending requirements, are not considered.

Moreover, these analyses are meant to examine and compare the *structur-al* rather than the *actual* balances inherent in the current tax and expenditure con-figuration. In order to do this, it is assumed that revenues and expenditures grow from their initial levels at a given built-in rate and that no policy change or adjust-ment takes place even if a pattern of cumulative surpluses or deficits emerges which creates its own set of fiscal dynamics. For instance, the Conference Board study indi-cates that in the absence of cyclical fluctuations and policy changes, the federal gov-ernment's current fiscal structure would likely produce a steady stream of budget surpluses even under fairly conservative assumptions about growth rates. But these surpluses can only materialize if economic growth is sustained, taxes are not further reduced, new spending measures are not implemented, and the entire surplus goes to debt payment, thus reducing debt charges as projected. However, as recent fed-eral budgets demonstrate, governments do adjust to both economic and fiscal cir-cumstances on an ongoing basis. It is therefore important to recognize that the fiscal position of both orders of government in any given year is inevitably the outcome of cumulative fiscal effects and adjustments to changing circumstances over a num-ber of years. For instance, any assessment of where we are now in terms of vertical fiscal imbalance has to take into account how federal-provincial fiscal relations have evolved over the years and how this history has affected the relative fiscal positions of each order of government.

FEDERAL AND PROVINCIAL PUBLIC FINANCES: RETROSPECTIVE AND PROSPECTIVE

The current fiscal position of both orders of government has been greatly influenced by the evolution of federal-provincial fiscal relations over the past several decades. This influence stems from the manner in which major national social programs were first established in the postwar years, the changes in the respective role and relative importance of each order of government that have taken place over time, and the various channels through which the fiscal status of one order of government affects that of the other.

Looking back on this history one observes that intergovernmental fiscal relations in Canada have essentially been in a continuous state of flux and adjustment. It is not clear that a state of vertical fiscal balance was ever achieved which could in turn be seen as a benchmark from which we have somehow derogated. Also, while there is clear evidence of structural fiscal imbalance over significant periods of time for both orders of government, the situation may or may not have been related to vertical fiscal imbalance issues. Indeed, notwithstanding the effects of cyclical fluctuations, the recurrence of substantial budget deficits or surpluses over a considerable length of time would indicate either: (a) a failure on the part of the government involved to make the necessary revenue or expenditure adjustments to achieve sustainable budget balances; or (b) an inability to do so because of a structural imbalance between revenue-raising capacity and expenditure responsibilities. The issue of vertical fiscal imbalance only comes into play in the second instance and only to the extent that the budgetary stance or actions of one order of government affect the other or in some way limit its capacity to adjust to its own circumstances.

An overview of the evolution of Canadian public finances and federal-provincial fiscal relations over the last four decades provides a useful historical perspective on the current vertical fiscal imbalance debate.

The Growth of the Welfare State and the Rise of Provincial Governments

One of the main characteristics of the Canadian federation is the degree to which it is decentralized. As in many other industrialized countries, there was a dramatic increase in the size of the public sector in Canada in the decades following the Second World War as governments laid the foundations of the welfare state and took on a more active role in the economy. What was particular in the Canadian case was that most of that increase occurred at the provincial level where constitutional responsibility for health, post-secondary education, and social assistance has been assigned. Thus the establishment of major social programs not only resulted in a rapid expansion of the role of provincial governments but also led to a significant increase in their importance relative to the federal government. In little more than a decade, the provinces became the dominant player in terms of public expenditures.

Charts 2 and 3 illustrate the trends in the relative size of the two orders of government over time and the repercussions on both expenditures and revenues. It is important to note that the data consist of current revenues and expenditures on a National Accounts basis (that is, they do not include investments in fixed capital, inventories, and net capital transfers). The reader should also note that the data for the provincial and local levels of governments have been consolidated in order to focus exclusively on the fiscal relationship between the federal government and the provinces. Since the division of responsibilities between provincial and local governments varies significantly from province to province, provincial grants to local governments are difficult to treat in a consistent fashion.[36] Moreover, the local government data include not only municipalities, but also universities, schools, and hospitals, which are relevant to this discussion.

As Chart 2a shows, the size of the public sector as a share of GDP essentially doubled from 22 to 44 percent between 1957 and 1982.[37] The provincial/local government sector, which grew from 9 to 26 percent of GDP during that period, accounted for about 80 percent of that increase. As for the federal government, the figure shows the rapid and substantial decline from wartime expenditures.[38] By 1957 the federal government's own expenditures had settled at about 14 percent of GDP and they remained in that range until the recession of the early 1980s when spending reached 18 percent of GDP. However, federal own-expenditures do not include transfer payments to the provinces, which were an important catalyst for the development of provincial social programs. Indeed, much of the growth in provincial expenditures coincides with the implementation of major cost-sharing transfer programs. These include the *Hospital Insurance and Diagnostic Services Act* in 1957; the various federal grants implemented in the 1950s to share the cost of provincial programs of social assistance to the blind, the aged, the disabled, and the unemployed, which were eventually combined and extended as part of the Canada Assistance Plan in 1966; the *Medical Care Act* in 1966; and various funding provisions for post-secondary education beginning in the early 1960s. The Equalization program, introduced in 1957, also increased the ability of recipient provinces to establish social programs.

Chart 2a also shows a levelling-off of public sector spending and even a slight decline throughout most of the 1980s, followed by a significant upswing that coincides with the recession of the early 1990s when government expendi-

Chart 2a

**FEDERAL AND PROVINCIAL/LOCAL GOVERNMENTS' EXPENDITURES
FOR OWN-PURPOSES, 1945-2000 (as % of GDP, National Accounts)**

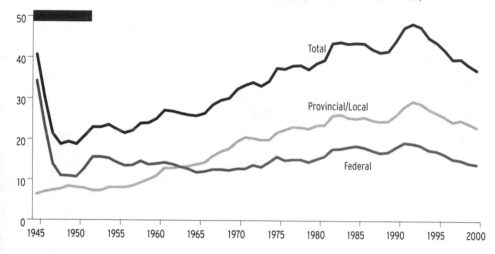

Chart 2b

**FEDERAL AND PROVINCIAL/LOCAL GOVERNMENTS' OWN-SOURCE REVENUES,
1945-2000 (as % of GDP, National Accounts)**

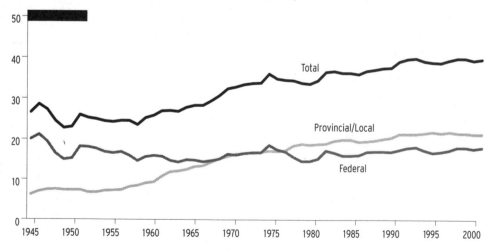

Source: Statistics Canada, Cansim matrices 6581, 6582, 6585, 8629, and *National Income and Expenditure Accounts*, STC 13-531.

tures peaked at 48 percent of GDP, again with most of the increase taking place at the provincial/local level. The extent of the spending restraint efforts that followed in the 1990s is also evident. Aggregate public spending dropped from 48 percent of GDP in 1992 to 37 percent in 2000 (back to 1980 levels), a reduction of 11 percentage points overall (6 percentage points of GDP at the provincial/local level and 5 percentage points at the federal level).

Chart 2b shows the trends on the revenue side. The pattern in the first decade or so after the war reflects the Wartime Tax Agreements whereby provinces had agreed to have the federal government collect personal and corporate income taxes and succession duties in return for tax rental payments. These payments continued (with some modifications) for most provinces until 1957, at which time the federal government gradually began shifting income tax room back to the provinces leading up to the federal-provincial tax collection agreements in 1962. As part of this process, Ottawa purposively reduced its income tax rates to enable provinces to raise theirs without imposing an overall increase on taxpayers. The small decline in federal revenues (relative to expenditures) in the immediate postwar years reflects the fact that the federal government accumulated large operating surpluses in order to pay down a substantial amount of war-related debt. As was the case with expenditures, we see the effects of the rapid growth of the public sector, and here again most of the increase is at the provincial/local level. Notwithstanding a marked decline between 1974 and 1979 (a drop of 2.4 percentage points), the federal government's own-source revenues have remained more or less in the range of 15-19 percent of GDP since the early 1950s. Provincial/local revenues (excluding federal transfers), on the other hand, doubled from 8.5 percent to 17 percent of GDP between 1957 and 1972, and continued to increase over the next two decades, levelling off at 22 percent of GDP in 1992.

Overall, revenue growth more or less kept pace with expenditures until the mid-1970s and then rapidly lost ground and failed to recover in spite of significant increases during the economic recovery in the 1980s. Between 1981 and 1992, expenditures rose from 40 to 48 percent of GDP, while revenues only increased from 37 to 40 percent, resulting in a significant shortfall that had detrimental long-term effects on public finances. Although Chart 2 suggests that this revenue shortfall occurred only at the provincial/local level, this does not reflect the actual impact on the respective governments' budget balances. As will be shown further on, the fact that expenditures at the provincial/local level are partially funded through revenues raised by the federal government and transferred to the provinces under various fiscal arrangements produced a very different outcome than is apparent here. Finally, while expenditures declined sharply after 1992, revenues as a share of GDP remained relatively constant, having apparently reached a plateau at that level.

Chart 3 reports the changes in the shares of current public expenditures and revenues by level of government over the past several decades.[39] Chart 3a shows the dramatic reversal in the relative importance of each order of government which took place between 1953 and 1971. The federal government, which accounted for 68 percent of public expenditures at the beginning of the period, saw its share reduced to 39 percent by 1971, while provincial/local governments' own expenditures had grown to 61 percent. These federal/provincial ratios have remained remarkably stable ever since (38/62 percent in 2001). The pattern is similar on the revenue side. The federal/provincial-local shares of own-source revenues went from 72/28 percent in 1952 to 44/56 percent in 1978 and have also remained in that range ever since (46/54 percent in 2001).

The Role of Federal Transfers

As already mentioned, federal transfers played an important role in the initial establishment and development of major social programs at the provincial level. Given that, with the exception of the Equalization program put in place in 1957, most of these were initially cost-sharing grants, their relative size and growth rate was very much related to the magnitude and expansion of the social programs in question. Between 1950 and 1962, specific-purpose transfers and equalization payments quickly supplanted federal tax rental payments to the provinces under existing tax arrangements as these were being phased out.[40] By 1959 federal transfers represented 23 percent of provincial/local government current expenditures, and they remained in the general range of 21 percent until 1975 (see Chart 3a). The marked increase in 1958/59 reflects the implementation of hospital insurance and Equalization, which were introduced in 1957. As for the increase in 1969-71, it follows the introduction of the Canada Assistance Plan (CAP), medicare, and fiscal arrangements for post-secondary education in 1966/67. In 1970 these five transfer programs accounted for 87 percent of federal transfers to the provinces.

As Chart 3a shows, the relative importance of federal transfers to the provinces has been in steady decline from the mid-1970s onward, dropping from

Chart 3a

FEDERAL AND PROVINCIAL/LOCAL GOVERNMENTS' SHARE OF GOVERNMENT SECTOR
EXPENDITURES (National Accounts), 1945-2000

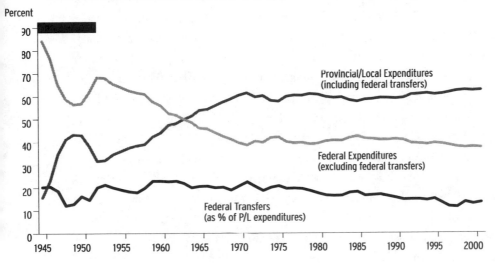

Chart 3b

FEDERAL AND PROVINCIAL/LOCAL GOVERNMENTS' SHARE OF GOVERNMENT SECTOR
REVENUES (National Accounts), 1945-2000

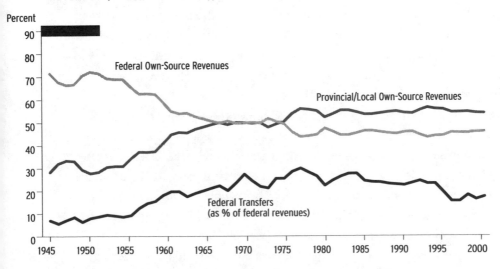

Source: Statistics Canada, CANSIM matrices 6581, 6582, 6585, and *National Income and Expenditure Accounts,* STC 13-351.

21 to 15 percent of provincial/local government expenditures by 1995 to a low of 11.4 percent in 1998. The 1977-82 drop in cash transfers coincides with the conversion from cost-sharing grants for health and post-secondary education to block funding in 1977. Under Established Programs Financing (EPF), approximately half of the value of the previous transfers for health and education was shifted permanently to the provinces as tax room. The other half was converted to a block fund transfer, which was initially set to grow in line with GNP rather than according to provincial spending in these areas. The latter had been growing at a faster pace than the economy and in the case of health care has continued to do so at an average rate of 0.8 percent higher than the rate of growth of GNP since 1977. (More details on EPF are provided in the following chapter.) The further decline from the mid-1980s to the mid-1990s came as a result of a series of measures imposed by the federal government to curb the growth of transfer payments in a context of rapid deterioration of its own finances. This process began in 1982. Equalization underwent important changes with new ceiling and floor provisions and the replacement of the ten-province standard with a five-province standard as the benchmark for entitlement. The EPF growth formula was also amended such that the escalator would no longer apply only to the cash transfer but to the combined value of the tax and cash transfer. Since the value of income tax points grows at a faster rate than the economy, this significantly reduced the rate of growth of the cash transfer, which from then on was calculated as a residual. This was followed in subsequent years by a number of reductions in the EPF escalator, culminating in a freeze from 1990 to 1994. The 1990 federal spending restraint measures also included a 5-percent annual growth limit on CAP payments to Ontario, Alberta, and British Columbia (the cap on CAP). However, the drop in the relative size of federal transfers from 1995 to 1998 was even more dramatic. This reflects the impact of the ten-province freeze on CAP payments in 1995/96 and the cuts (in excess of 30 percent over two years) associated with the introduction in 1996 of new block-funding arrangements under the CHST to replace CAP and EPF. Moreover, it is important to note that these cutbacks in federal transfers took place in a context of significant reductions in provincial spending, which fell from 29 to 24 percent of GDP between 1992 and 1997. As we can see, the impact of the cuts had been partially reversed by 1999.

Chart 3b traces the evolution of federal transfers from the federal goverment's perspective. Transfers as a share of current federal revenues rose sharply from 10 percent in 1957 to 27 percent in 1971, with a marked upswing between

1969 and 1971. After 1971 transfers as a share of federal expenditures (not shown) experienced a steady decline, similar to that shown as a share of provincial/local budgets in Chart 3a. Between 1971 and 1998, transfers to provinces as a share of federal expenditures dropped by approximately 11 percentage points to 15.6 percent. The somewhat different trend reported in Chart 3b for transfers as a share of revenues is a function of the significant revenue shortfall at the federal level that persisted from the mid-1970s to the mid-1990s.

Structural Fiscal Imbalance

A number of factors and issues need to be considered in order to assess whether or not vertical fiscal imbalance is a problem in Canada. First, it is important to have a sense of the relationship between each order of government's own-source revenues and expenditures. Significant discrepancy between the two over time could be an indication of structural fiscal imbalance. Second, a comparison of the relative fiscal position of each order of government might also indicate whether a situation of vertical fiscal imbalance exists, for instance, if the difference between revenue-raising ability and expenditures at one level is related to an opposite set of circumstances at the other level. But structural fiscal imbalance can also be due to other factors unrelated to VFI. The imbalance may be the result of policy (i.e., the budgetary impact of policy decisions on either the revenue or expenditure side of the ledger) or it may be structural in nature (e.g., the budgetary impact of a recession or a rise in interest rates). If there is evidence of a vertical fiscal imbalance, then one needs to look at the role of intergovernmental transfers and other policy factors in reducing or increasing that imbalance.

Charts 4a and 4b compare the relative fiscal balances of the federal and provincial/local governments in terms of their own revenues and expenditures (FFBEX and PFBEX) and including net federal transfers (FFBIN and PFBIN) over the last five decades. Again it is important to note that the data only include current transactions.[41] From the federal government's perspective, FFBEX indicates the difference between current own-revenues and expenditures (excluding transfers to the provinces) as a percentage of expenditures (also excluding transfers). For most of the period under consideration, the data indicate the extent to which the federal government raised revenues in excess of its own spending needs. The large federal revenue balances in the early postwar years (ranging from 40 to 52 percent of own-expenditures between 1946 and 1951) were used to reduce the federal debt from levels in excess of 100 percent of GDP to less than 40 percent

by the mid-1950s. In the period that followed, the federal government gradually began shifting tax room back to provinces and established major cost-sharing
transfer programs. By the early 1970s, federal revenue balances were still in the
30 percent range. This could be viewed as reflecting the extent of the vertical fiscal gap at that time, a gap that was essentially eliminated as all excess revenues
were transferred to the provinces (see FFBIN). However, as Chart 4a shows, 1974
marked a definite turning point, with a significant five-year drop in federal revenue levels followed by a substantial and prolonged deterioration of the state of
federal finances. In most years from 1982 to 1995, revenues were not even sufficient to cover the federal government's own spending and debt charges. The
strength of the post-1995 turnaround is equally noteworthy, with current revenue balances once again in the 30-percent range.

Chart 4b tracks the fiscal position of the provincial/local governments
with and without federal transfers. PFBEX represents the percentage of provin-
cial/local current expenditures not covered by own-source revenues. While in
most years during the 1950s and 1960s the provinces are within a range of 5 percent of fiscal balance, the revenue shortfall increases steadily beginning in 1969,
reaching a high of 26 percent in 1992 before returning to a 5-percent level in
1999.

A very different picture emerges when one looks at the relative fiscal balances of both orders of government in the presence of federal transfers. FFBIN and
PFBIN represent federal and provincial/local budget balances (based on current
transactions) as a percentage of expenditures, with net federal transfers included
as part of federal expenditures and provincial revenues, respectively. With federal
transfers to supplement their own-source revenues, provincial/local governments
consistently recorded current budget surpluses in the range of 5 to 18 percent of
expenditures until the mid-1970s, when their fiscal position also suffered a
marked deterioration (see PFBIN, Chart 4b). Over the following twenty years they
struggled to maintain budget balance and ended up posting a deficit on their current transactions almost every year (except for two) from 1980 to 1995.
Compared with the 1980s recession when the federal government bore the brunt
of the economic downturn, the impact of the 1991/92 recession was mostly felt at
the provincial level as deficit levels reached almost 12 percent of expenditures.

The federal government has fared much worse by comparison (see
FFBIN, Chart 4a). From a surplus position in the 1940s and 1950s, federal current budget balances dropped markedly in 1957/58, although deficits remained

Chart 4a

FEDERAL GOVERNMENT'S FISCAL BALANCE, EXCLUDING AND INCLUDING FEDERAL CASH TRANSFERS, 1945-2000

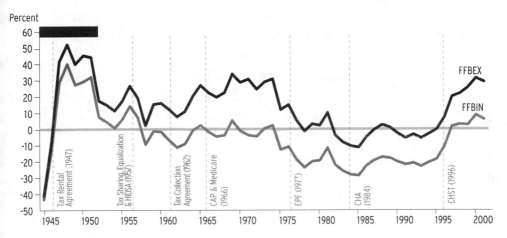

FFBEX = [REV - (EXP - TR)] / (EXP - TR) x 100
FFBIN = (REV - EXP) / EXP x 100

Chart 4b

PROVINCIAL/LOCAL GOVERNMENTS' FISCAL BALANCE, INCLUDING AND EXCLUDING FEDERAL CASH TRANSFERS, 1945-2000

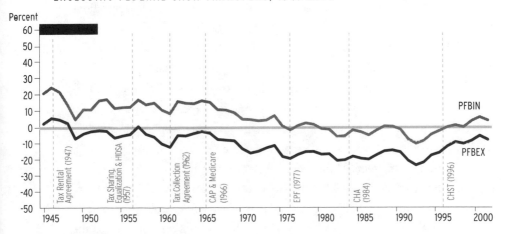

PFBEX = [(REV - TR) - EXP] / EXP x 100
PFBIN = (REV - EXP) / EXP x 100

Source: Statistics Canada, CANSIM matrices 6581, 6582, 6585, and *National Income and Expenditure Accounts*, STC 13-531.

within a range of 5 percent of expenditures for most of the next 15 years. The federal government's fiscal position took a definite turn for the worse in the mid-1970s. By 1978 the revenue shortfall had reached 24 percent of current expenditures. The situation improved considerably over the next three years as current deficit levels dropped by half to less than 12 percent in 1981, but the subsequent recession had a dramatic impact on federal finances. By 1985 federal current deficit levels had reached the highest level yet since the end of the war, with current expenditures exceeding revenues by close to 29 percent. Moreover, by that time the federal government had been running substantial deficits on its operating budget (in the order of 1 to 4 percent of GDP for the better part of a decade), which meant that revenues were insufficient to cover program spending let alone the debt charges, which were also increasing rapidly. Spending reductions and tax increases implemented over a number of years beginning in 1982 only succeeded in bringing the level of the deficit down to 17 percent of expenditures by 1988. In the following years the situation at the federal level would once again regress as the economy went through another recession, although this time the relative fiscal impact was more pronounced at the provincial/local level. The data also show that, even with relative deficit levels almost double those found at the provincial/local level, the federal government finally managed to restore budget balance in as little as four years.

Chart 5a shows how this actually played out in terms of overall budgetary balances (including capital transactions) for both orders of government. Except for a few years in the 1950s, when the federal government was still in the process of shifting tax room back to the provinces, provincial/local governments combined had better fiscal outcomes throughout most of this period. For the federal government, this translated into modest budget deficits in most years up until 1974. However, given that it maintained an operating surplus almost every year in a context where the rate of growth of the economy was consistently in excess of the rate of interest, this was not a problem. Indeed, the difference between the rate of growth of GDP and the rate of interest during this period of time was increasing steadily from approximately 4 percentage points in the early 1960s to a peak of close to 7 percentage points in 1974. As a result, even if the federal operating budget balance had been zero, the federal government's debt-to-GDP ratio would have still continued to fall rapidly (Courchene 2002). In fact, the debt-to-GDP ratio dropped 17 percentage points between 1960 and 1974 – from 31 percent to a postwar record low of 14 percent (see Chart 5b).

Chart 5a
FEDERAL AND PROVINCIAL/LOCAL GOVERNMENTS' BUDGET BALANCE, 1946-2001
(as a % of GDP, National Accounts)

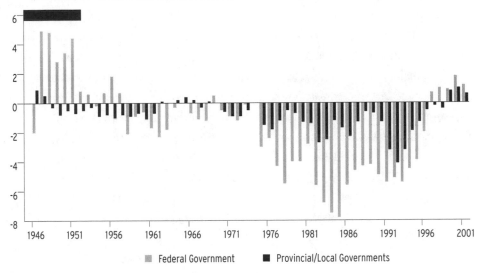

Federal Government   Provincial/Local Governments

Chart 5b
FEDERAL AND PROVINCIAL/LOCAL GOVERNMENTS' NET DEBT, 1946-2001
(as a % of GDP, National Accounts)

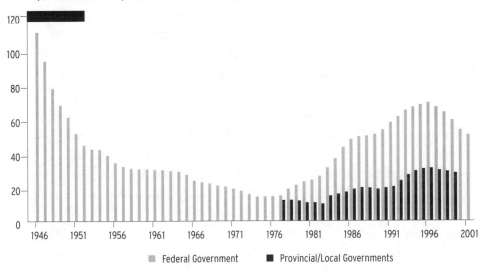

Federal Government   Provincial/Local Governments

Source: Statistics Canada, CANSIM matrices 3198, 3199, 6581, 6582, 6585, 8629, and *National Income and Expenditure Accounts*, STC 15-531.

However, as Courchene points out in his analysis of Canada's fiscal turn-around in the 1990s (2002), a combination of policy and structural factors in and around 1974 dramatically altered the fiscal dynamics that had prevailed in 1950s and 1960s. Courchene refers in particular to the federal government's decision in 1972 to index the personal income tax against inflation[42] while at the same time indexing many transfer programs for inflation, a measure which caused a simultaneous drop in revenues and upward shift in expenditures. But macroeconomic factors and a failure to adjust to a new fiscal environment are singled out as the main culprits. The change in fiscal dynamics began with the first oil shock in 1973/74, which provoked slower economic growth and higher interest rates and reversed the favourable pattern described in the preceding paragraph. The GDP growth-interest rate differential thus began to decline, and it continued to do so at an even faster rate as a result of the second oil shock in 1979 and the 1981/82 recession. By 1984 the rate of interest exceeded the rate of economic growth, and five years later the difference was over 4 percentage points.[43] This in turn meant that running small operating deficits was no longer consistent with a falling debt-to-GDP ratio. Indeed, progressively higher operating surpluses would be required to achieve budget balance. Not only did the federal government fail to make this adjustment, it also ran substantial deficits on its operating budget from 1975 to 1986 (see Chart 6).

The combined effects of higher interest rates, slower growth, and ongoing operating deficits had devastating consequences on federal budget balances and debt-to-GDP ratio (see Chart 5). These results can be seen as evidence of deep structural fiscal imbalance under any definition. By 1985 the federal deficit had reached its highest level since the war at 7.8 percent of GDP (up from 2.4 percent in 1976), and the level of debt had more than tripled from its 1975 level to 43 percent of GDP. Moreover, the debt-to-GDP ratio continued to climb over the next decade up to 69 percent of GDP in 1996, this in spite of significant operating surpluses in most years, beginning in 1987. As Chart 6 illustrates, operating surpluses of close to 2 percent of GDP prior to the 1990s recession were more than offset by the debt-servicing charges, which at that point were in the order of 5 to 6 percent of GDP.

The provinces fared relatively better than the federal government throughout the 1980s. For instance, while their deficits doubled through the 1980s recession, they tripled at the federal level. Ongoing budget deficits never-theless caused their debt-to-GDP ratio to double over the decade (see chart 5).

Chart 6

FEDERAL GOVERNMENT OPERATING AND BUDGETARY BALANCE, 1945-2000
(as a % of GDP)

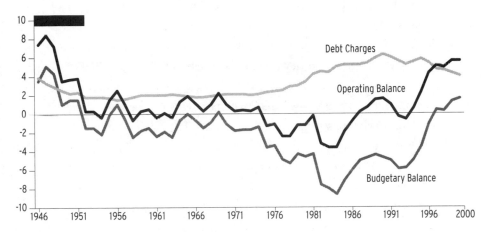

Source: Department of Finance Canada. Fiscal Reference Tables, various years.

The real setback, however, came in the 1990s. With the combined impact of the 1990s recession and the freeze in federal transfers, provincial/local deficits climbed from $4.8 billion in 1989 to over $28 billion (4.1 percent of GDP) in 1992. This time it was the provinces that bore the brunt of the recession. More than 70 percent of the fiscal impact took place at the provincial level (Courchene 2002). The 1990 federal measures to scale down the revenue stabilization program and the capping of CAP payments (social assistance) to the three richer provinces were major factors in explaining the larger impact on the provinces compared to the previous recession. This was particularly the case in Ontario where the effects of the economic downturn were most strongly felt. As a result the provinces saw their combined debt-to-GDP ratio increase from 20 to 30 percent in five years.

The fiscal turnaround for Canadian governments took place in two stages. The first stage was marked by the dramatic drop in budget deficits, beginning in 1994. The federal government managed to eliminate a deficit of close to $40 billion (5.4 percent of GDP) in four years, while the provinces went from a deficit of $23 billion (3.2 percent of GDP) to a surplus of more than $7 billion in 1999. The second stage occurred in 1997, which marked the end of two decades of continuous increases in the level of federal debt as a share of GDP, following a four-year run-up in the operating surplus to 5 percent of GDP (Chart 6). This was also a turning point, although much more modest, for the provinces. The pace and extent of the fiscal recovery were due not only to the significant restraint measures undertaken by both orders of government but also to a return to a more favourable macroeconomic environment. By 1997 the negative difference between the rate of economic growth and the rate of interest, which had slowly begun to decline in the first half of the 1990s, was falling rapidly. And by 1999/2000, the rate of growth finally exceeded the rate of interest for the first time since 1984, with positive consequences in terms of the requisites of structural fiscal balance. This return to favourable fiscal dynamics, combined with the fact that the federal government has continued to run large operating surpluses ($59 billion or 5.6 percent of GDP in 2000/01) and managed to make payments on the debt, has had a significant impact on the debt-to-GDP ratio, which dropped from 69 percent in 1996 to 50 percent in 2001.

Vertical Fiscal Imbalance in Retrospect

In the preceding overview, we have described the rapid and constant evolution of fiscal relations between the two orders of government since the Second World War. While intergovernmental fiscal relations have played an important role, it is also clear that structural factors have been the dominant factor affecting public sector fiscal balances for the past twenty-five years. Both orders of government faced the same dramatic change in fiscal dynamics post-1974, but the federal government's fiscal structure was evidently more vulnerable to a changed fiscal environment. Its failure to adjust was a reflection of both weakness on the revenue side and inherent rigidities on the expenditure side, including a lack of control on the growth of large budget items such as social programs based on universality and cost-sharing transfers. The substantial vertical fiscal imbalance, which had enabled the federal government to foster the establishment and development of major provincial social programs in the areas of health, welfare, and post-secondary education in the previous two decades, quickly vanished and gave way to a situation of deep structural fiscal imbalance at the federal level. Large operating budget deficits and rising debt levels became chronic. By the early 1980s, it was the federal government that was complaining of a vertical fiscal imbalance in favour of the provinces as it began to implement increasingly effective measures to control the growth of intergovernmental transfers.

The provinces' fiscal position also deteriorated during this period but remained more or less under control until the recession in the early 1990s. It was at that time that the impact on the provinces of federal spending restraint measures became most apparent. The combined effects of the ongoing freeze on EPF transfers, the 5-percent annual limit on growth of CAP payments for social assistance to Ontario, Alberta, and British Columbia, the scaled-down federal revenue stabilization program, and Unemployment Insurance (UI) reforms translated into a much larger fiscal impact on the provinces as they faced the second recession in little over a decade. The effect of these changes was structural – they affected the provinces' fiscal balances both on the revenue and on the expenditure side and made them more vulnerable than in the past to unfavourable economic circumstances.

Both orders of government came out of the recession with unprecedented and unsustainable levels of debt and deficits and took drastic action. The provinces, one after another, had already begun to cut back spending, focusing for the most part on public sector wage freezes, cutting welfare benefits and/or eligibility, closing hospital beds, and shifting costs and responsibilities to the municipalities. The federal government also followed suit with cuts to the federal civil service, a program review process to reduce operating costs, and some transfer of responsibilities to the provinces. However, its most significant deficit-cutting measures came after 1995 with the introduction of the CHST and the associated $6-billion cut in cash transfers to the provinces, and the 1996 reform in UI (renamed Employment Insurance). The budgetary impact of the EI reforms resulted both from new measures to further reduce benefits and limit eligibility and from the decision to withhold corresponding adjustments to contribution rates. This has allowed the federal government to collect contributions of between $5 and $7 billion in excess of benefits paid each year since 1995.

According to the 2001 federal budget, federal program spending as a share of GDP fell from 17.5 percent in 1992/93 to 11.3 percent in 2000/01, while for the same period combined provincial-territorial spending fell from 20 percent to 15.1 percent of GDP (Department of Finance 2001, 191). Presumably the provinces would have been able to balance their budget a few years earlier had it not been for the transfer cuts. As it turned out, they only managed to achieve an overall surplus in 1999. The situation differs quite considerably across provinces, however. For instance, provincial governments posted a combined budgetary surplus of $11.5 billion in 2000/01. But as Table 2 indicates, Alberta ($6.4 billion) and Ontario ($3.2 billion) accounted for the bulk of that. For fiscal year 2001/02, the ten provinces combined reported a budgetary deficit of

Table 2

PROVINCIAL GOVERNMENTS' CURRENT FISCAL STATUS

	Deficit (-) or Surplus (million $) 2000/01	Deficit (-) or Surplus (million $) 2001/02	Debt Charges As a % of Total Revenues 2001/02	Net Debt (million $) 2001/02	Net Debt As a % of GDP 2001/02	Forecasted Deficit (-) or Surplus (million $) 2002/03
Nfld	-33	-64	15.5	5,674	40.8	-93
PEI	-7	-15	10.9	1,050	30.7	29
NS	-199	-106	18.5	11,538	46.3	1
NB	33	37	12.7	6,519	32.3	21
Que	500	22	14.4	81,970	35.9	0
Ont	3,192	58	14.3	110,507	25.1	0
Man	26	54	6.1	7,041	20.1	13
Sask	58	1	10.2	7,010	21.2	45
Alta	6,388	772	3.5	-5,043	-3.4	724
BC	1,498	-1,233	3.3	13,376	10.3	-4,400
10 Provinces	11,456	-474	11.4	239,642	22.2	-3,005

Source: The first three columns are public accounts data from Department of Finance Canada, Fiscal Reference Tables, 2002. The fifth column is calculated using provincial GDP at market price from Statistics Canada, CANSIM matrices 9001 to 9010. Forecast deficits or surpluses for 2002/03 are from the 2002 provincial budgets.

$474 million overall. Four provinces were still in deficit, while the remaining provinces were only in surplus by a very slim margin and the outlook for 2002/03 is not encouraging.

THE FISCAL CONTEXT AND THE FISCAL IMBALANCE DEBATE IN 2002/03

Even though the provinces have more or less succeeded in balancing their budgets in recent years, the fiscal position of the federal government appears significantly stronger at the present time than that of the provinces. It has managed to run operating surpluses in excess of 4 percent of GDP since 1996 and even made substantial payments on the debt ($46.7 billion). The *2002 Economic and Fiscal Update* indicates that the government expects operating surpluses to remain well above $40 billion in coming years (Department of Finance 2002). More importantly, these projections take into account federal commitments in 2000 to increase transfer payments to the provinces by $23.4 billion and cut taxes by $100 billion over five years, as well as other spending measures announced since. Moreover as a result of declining debt levels and lower interest rates, the share of revenues allocated to debt-servicing charges, while still considerably higher than that of the provinces, has been reduced to less than 22 percent from 36 percent in 1993/94. Finally, given the much better than anticipated performance of the economy, the federal government's 2001 fiscal outlook calling for balanced budgets and no surplus over the next three fiscal years turned out to be overly pessimistic. For instance, the surplus recorded for 2001/02 was $8.9 billion and was also expected to be in that range for 2002/03.[44]

In many ways the current fiscal environment resembles that which prevailed prior to 1974 in terms of the requirements of structural fiscal balance, although there is still some uncertainty as to how the relationship between the rate of economic growth and the rate of interest is likely to evolve in coming years. The main difference of course is the current level of federal debt, which is still substantial and will require a greater degree of fiscal prudence. However, as events in recent years demonstrate, any continuing progress on that front will quickly translate into a sizable fiscal dividend. Also, many of the measures undertaken by the federal government over the past two decades to achieve the levels of operating surplus required to restore fiscal balance have been structural in nature. For instance, there is no doubt that the federal government is now much better positioned than it was in the mid-1970s in terms of controlling the rate of growth of its expenditures. It is no longer tied to cost-sharing transfer arrangements with the provinces, most transfer programs to individuals are now needs-tested or have clawback provisions, and the coverage of employment insurance has been substantially reduced. On the revenue side, the surtaxes and de-indexing provisions of personal income tax have been removed, but Ottawa still benefits the most from this source of revenue, which continues to grow at a faster pace than the economy.

The provinces' fiscal position, on the other hand, is more precarious. They only recently restored budget balance (all provinces combined) in 1999 and were back in deficit in 2001/02. For provinces with balanced budgets, surplus levels are best described as modest. Even a relatively mild economic slowdown could mean a return to deficits for many of them as the budget balance forecasts reported in Table 2 suggest. Indeed, both Alberta and British Columbia show a marked deterioration in their fiscal outlook. And although the provinces have a lesser debt burden, they have not made nearly as much progress as the federal government in reducing their combined debt-to-GDP ratio, which has only declined by 5.5 percentage points since 1997 compared to 19 percentage points for the federal government. More importantly, the same structural changes that have made the federal government less vulnerable on the expenditure side have had the opposite effect on the provinces. As the last recession showed, they have become much more vulnerable to an economic downturn. Finally, there is also evidence that provincial cuts to health care imposed in the early and mid-1990s did not fundamentally alter the cost-drivers in the system. In the last few years, health care costs have once again started to grow at a faster rate than the economy and are expected to continue to do so, given the high cost of many technological and medical improvements, rising public expectations, and an aging population. It is in this context that the issue of vertical fiscal imbalance arises.

Summary

The structure of federal public finances is at present stronger than that of most provinces. This appears to have been the case since the mid-1990s. For most of the preceding twenty years the opposite was true. These shifts are integral to the history of Canadian federalism. They occur with changing economic circumstances and changing revenue and expenditure policies of both orders of government.

While the stronger state of federal finances can be viewed as an indication of vertical fiscal imbalance, as we have seen in this chapter, assessing the extent of the imbalance is another matter. The relative fiscal strength of the federal government arises from a dramatic turnaround in fiscal dynamics over the past decade. Recent budgets have succeeded in reversing an entrenched pattern of growing operating deficits and rising debt levels and interest charges, making way for substantial budget surpluses, reduced debt levels, and declining debt charges. With the provinces in a more precarious fiscal position, the prospect of ongoing fiscal dividends at the federal level and ever-rising health care costs at the provincial level inevitably raises issues of resource allocation. This in turn, however, opens up a much larger debate regarding appropriate levels of public debt, tax burden, and other competing claims on the public purse. It is in this context that VFI issues must be considered and resolved as matters of political assessment and policy choice. Such a deliberation must consider the public sector as a whole and how to best capture the advantages of a federal system. Inevitably this also implies a re-examination of the federal role in funding health care, a task we undertake in the following chapter.

NOTES

1 See Department of Finance Canada (1995b). Numbers are derived by subtracting Equalization line from the cash transfers line in the table on page 13. Note that the anticipated effects of the CHST on the cash transfers to the provinces changed over time because of changes in the estimated value of the tax point component of the transfer.

2 The spending cuts had a direct effect and may have also contributed to reduced borrowing costs as debt instruments were rolled over. The strength of the United States economy, and the related growth of Canadian exports to that market, was probably an even larger factor.

3 See Department of Finance Canada (1995b), "The Canada Social Transfer."

4 Provincial and Territorial Premiers (1995, 2).

5 Ibid.

6 See Provincial and Territorial Finance Ministers (1997, 6).

7 Ibid., 8.

8 Ibid., Executive Summary, i.

9 Provincial and Territorial Finance Ministers (1998).

10 First Ministers (1997).

11 Provincial and Territorial Premiers (1998).

12 Provincial and Territorial Premiers (2000).

13 First Ministers (2000b).

14 See Provincial and Territorial Finance Ministers (2002).

15 These excerpts are from Provincial and Territorial Finance Ministers (2001, 4-6).

16 These paragraphs are drawn from the summary of the report. See Commission on Fiscal Imbalance (2002, viii-ix).

17 The Department of Finance first released a paper entitled *The Fiscal Balance in Canada* in August 1999, presenting initial counter-arguments to the provinces' claim of a VFI. This document was subsequently expanded and updated in April 2002 (see *The Fiscal Balance in Canada: The Facts*). The federal government's perhaps more formal response to the ongoing VFI controversy can be found in a document produced by the Privy Council entitled *Fiscal Balance and Fiscal Relations between Governments in Canada* (May 2002).

18 Department of Finance Canada (April 2002), *The Fiscal Balance in Canada: The Facts*.

19 See Government of Canada (2002), *Fiscal Balance and Fiscal Relations between Governments in Canada*.

20 The concept of horizontal fiscal imbalance relates most directly to these differences in revenue-generating capacity resulting from significant disparities in regional economic circumstances. But inevitably in the Canadian context, the objective of providing "comparable levels of services" also brings into consideration differences among provinces related to need and costs of delivery.

21 Note that the Séguin Commission calls for a strengthened Equalization system. That would have the effect of increasing the vertical fiscal gap if its proposals were implemented on this point. Of course, if all of its recommendations were implemented, the net effect would be a significant reduction in VFG.

22 While Equalization is specifically designed to reduce horizontal fiscal imbalances, the CHST is another matter. Although it is designed primarily as a VFG-related transfer, it has a significant redistribution effect. This is due to both its design as an equal per capita transfer financed out of general federal revenues and the method used to calculate the cash transfer (i.e., as a residual after subtracting the value of the EPF tax points from the total entitlement). Eliminating the CHST would therefore exacerbate horizontal fiscal imbalances.

23 The personal and corporate income taxes and the GST/retail sales taxes now account for 80 percent of federal tax revenues and 64 percent of provincial/territorial tax revenues. In addition both levels

of government also collect payroll taxes, fuel taxes, and tobacco and liquor taxes.

24 See Ruggeri (1998, 2001); Ruggeri and Howard (2000); Ruggeri, Howard, and Van Wart (1993a); Ruggeri, Van Wart, Robertson, and Howard (1993b); and Ruggeri, Van Wart, and Howard (1995).

25 The estimated built-in growth rate of health spending is based on CPI growth plus the rate of growth of population plus an aging factor and an additional cost pressure factor of 1.2 percent per year. Education spending is assumed to grow at a rate .9 times nominal GDP growth.

26 Most of the remaining federal and provincial spending categories are assumed to remain constant in real terms or, in the case of the wage component, linked to a combination of the rate of growth of inflation and labour productivity.

27 See Conference Board of Canada (2002b). This report was released following the submission of our work to the Romanow Commission. We have since then updated this section of our report using the latest Conference Board estimates for the provinces and territories as these provide a better basis of comparison with the other two sets of estimates analysed. This update does not change in any way our conclusions from this exercise.

28 As measured by a trend variable in the forecast model.

29 Although as a percentage of GDP it will have decreased from 23.3 to 16.4 percent.

30 The authors point out that "the 'growth ratio' approach [as used by Ruggeri] to projecting government revenue and spending – only indirectly and somewhat partially – incorporates the structural demographic determinants of revenue and spending. The projected rate of GDP growth incorporates assumptions about population and employment growth and these components enter into most of the revenue and spending categories. In some cases, such a federal OAS payments and provincial health spending, there is an attempt to incorporate, more explicitly, the impact of demographics. However, the remaining spending categories and all revenue categories capture only the impact of population growth and do not account for the changes in the age structure of the population on spending and revenue" (Matier, Wu, and Jackson 2001, 12).

31 The authors also point out that a VFI indicator based on the differential between the fiscal balances across levels of government implies that a vertical fiscal balance can only exist in a situation where those fiscal balances are equal (See Matier, Wu, and Jackson 2001, 8-9).

32 The main exceptions relate to intergovernmental fiscal arrangements. Equalization payments are projected to grow in line with nominal GDP. CHST payments are set to increase as announced in recent budgets to $21 billion in 2005/06, and then are projected to grow at an annual rate of 3.5 percent based on the average annual rate of increase in CHST cash over the period 2001/01 to 2005/06.

33 The results in the benchmark case (i.e., prior to incorporating recently announced tax reductions) are much larger, with fiscal room estimated at 2.11 percent of GDP at the federal level and 1.21 percent at the provincial. According to the authors' estimates, announced reductions in the personal and corporate income tax along with other recent tax measures (e.g., cuts in EI contribution rates at the federal level) reduce the overall average revenue growth rate over the first twenty years from 4.4 to 3.8 percent for federal revenues and from 4.3 to 4.1 percent for the provinces.

34 Except for the wage component, which is partially adjusted for increases in labour productivity.

35 Revenues are also lower than Ruggeri's estimates, reflecting the lower projected average growth rate for nominal GDP.

36 It can also be argued that the local government sector can essentially be viewed as an administrative arm of provincial

governments (they have no constitutional status and their policy directives and mandate come from the province in many instances).

37   We used GDP at market price (income-based).

38   The defence expenditures of the federal government went down from $2891 million (67.5 percent of total expenditures) in 1945 to $847 million (28.4 percent of total expenditures) in 1946 and $227 million (10.7 percent of total expenditures) in 1947. They went back up to $1157 million (37.3 percent of total expenditures) in 1951 and $1800 million (41.9 percent of total expenditures) in 1952 (Source: STC 13-531 *National Income and Expenditure Accounts*).

39   Data for 2001 in Charts 2 to 4 are preliminary estimates.

40   Under the 1947 Tax Rental Agreement and the 1957 Tax Sharing Agreement, the National Accounts include personal income taxes as federal revenues and show the payments to provincial governments as intergovernmental transfers. However, for the corporate income tax, the provincial share is presented as provincial revenue. Starting with the 1962 Tax Collection Agreement, personal and corporate income taxes collected by the federal government on behalf of provincial governments are presented as provincial revenues. As for the Quebec abatement, the National Accounts do not include it as federal revenues.

41   Cansim data do not provide sufficient detail on capital transactions, which are reported on a net basis and therefore cannot be properly allocated between revenue and expenditures.

42   This was introduced as part of a tax reform package that also included substantial new tax expenditures.

43   As Courchene points out, monetary policy and the exchange rate appreciation also exacerbated the situation (2002).

44   In January 2003, the Conference Board of Canada announced that it expected the federal government to post a surplus of $8.7 billion for 2002-03 and $11.2 billion for 2003-04 in the absence of new spending measures.

CHAPTER 4

FEDERAL HEALTH CARE FUNDING:
TOWARD A NEW FISCAL PACT

HARVEY LAZAR, FRANCE ST-HILAIRE,
AND JEAN-FRANÇOIS TREMBLAY

CONTEXT AND ISSUES

The long-standing dispute between Ottawa and the provinces regarding the role of the federal government in funding health care has been greatly exacerbated by rapidly rising health care costs since the mid-1990s. For many years following the enactment of the federal *Hospital Insurance and Diagnostic Services Act*, 1957 (HIDSA), the federal *Medical Care Act*, 1966, and related provincial legislation, expenditures on provincial health care services grew more rapidly than the rate of economic growth and the rate of increase in spending in other provincial programs. While provinces were able to exercise considerable restraint on their health expenditures during the first half of the 1990s, the rate of growth of health care spending has since then spiked again.

This recent increase in provincial health care costs has re-ignited political debate about the financial sustainability of Canada's universal, publicly insured health care system. As discussed in chapter 3, it has also given rise to a broader debate on the issue of fiscal imbalance between the two orders of government. In the case of health care, provinces have been demanding that the federal government cover a larger share of their costs.[1] Through the *Canada Health Act* (CHA), the federal government effectively requires provinces to operate a universal, accessible, portable, and publicly administered system of medical and hospital insurance.[2] Regulations under the Act also allow Ottawa to financially penalize provinces if they introduce or allow user charges or facility fees as a way of raising revenues or controlling use. From the provinces' viewpoint, the federal government exercises far too much influence over provincial policy choices,

given the relatively small amount of funding it provides. In their view, if Ottawa
wants to remain a player at the health policy table, it will have to ante up considerably more money.

In this chapter we examine the debate over the federal role in financing
health care for Canadians by assessing the current federal contribution to health
care relative to current provincial health care costs and to the federal contribution in the past. We also propose alternative federal funding options for the
Canadian health care system. In so doing, we acknowledge that there is no consensus within Canada about the appropriate federal role in health care. Rather, as
Keith Banting and Robin Boadway have described in chapter 1, there are a number of competing views based on different definitions of the sharing community
within the federation.[3] We delve further into their alternative conceptions of the
federal role and propose funding options that might be appropriate under each
of the three models they discuss.

Provincial Health Care Costs

Provincial spending on health as a share of total provincial program
spending varies widely across the country, ranging from 32 percent in Alberta to
43.5 percent in Ontario (see Table 1). For all provinces, however, health care is
the largest item in their operating budget. Moreover, the pressure to spend more
is very strong and growing across the country.

One should be cautious, however, when comparing data on health
spending across provinces. For instance, the province that devotes the largest share
of its budget to health care does not necessarily spend more on a per capita basis
than the other provinces. To illustrate, Table 1 shows that even though Ontario
devotes a larger share of its program spending to health care than all other
provinces, it spends less than most in per capita terms. Nor does the growth of
health spending as a share of provincial expenditures mean that provinces are allocating too much money to their health ministries. For one thing, the growing share
of health spending in some provinces has as much to do with cutbacks in other
programs as with increased outlays for health. It may also be the case that the need
for additional public spending in health care is greater than in other parts of the
provincial public sector. What is not in dispute, however, is that provincial health
spending has in fact risen sharply since 1997 after flattening in the first half of the
1990s (Figure 1). Clearly, the financial pressures from health ministries are making it more difficult for finance ministers to meet the needs in other policy areas.[4]

Table 1

PROVINCIAL GOVERNMENTS' HEALTH SPENDING
AS A PERCENTAGE OF PROGRAM SPENDING, 1975-2001

	Nfld	PEI	NS	NB	Que	Ont	Man	Sask	Alta	BC	Can
1975	23.4	22.6	27.3	22.4	29.6	30.8	30.2	25.3	25.1	26.6	28.4
1980	25.1	24.0	26.6	26.7	27.5	32.7	31.9	26.5	23.2	30.8	28.7
1985	28.2	27.7	31.2	28.7	29.4	34.4	31.2	27.7	23.8	31.1	30.2
1990	29.8	26.3	33.2	29.9	29.7	36.2	35.2	34.1	30.1	34.6	32.8
1995	30.0	28.8	31.3	31.5	29.4	35.0	35.8	33.9	30.0	33.4	32.3
2000	37.1	29.9	38.2	32.4	32.1	42.8	40.4	36.4	31.3	38.6	36.9
2001	38.6	32.4	38.6	35.1	32.2	43.5	41.2	39.0	32.0	41.3	37.8
$ per capita	2,551	2,066	1,967	2,125	2,077	2,146	2,436	2,210	2,331	2,479	2,212

Note: Program spending refers to total provincial government expenditures less debt charges, calculated in current dollars.
Percentages for 2001 are only forecast. The numbers for Canada include territorial governments.
Source: Canadian Institute for Health Information (CIHI), Preliminary Provincial and Territorial Government Health Expenditure
Estimates, Table A.4.

Figure 1

PER CAPITA HEALTH EXPENDITURES, CANADA, 1975-2001 (Current $)

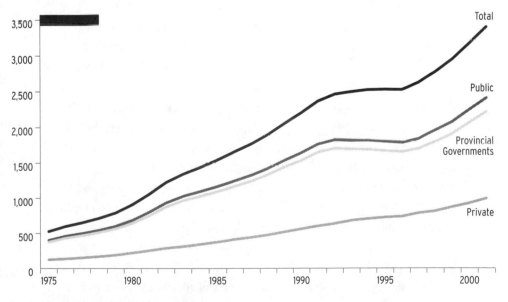

Source: Canadian Institute for Health Information

Thus, even if the level and growth of expenditures on provincial health services were satisfying the public that their health care needs would be adequately met in the future, the sheer magnitude of this spending would still pose serious challenges for provinces in their budget-making process. But much of the Canadian public appears to lack confidence that the current system of public health insurance is affordable in the medium term and hence is politically sustainable. There is also a perception among many Canadians that the quality and availability of health services have been deteriorating in recent years.[5]

All of these concerns have led provincial governments to undertake extensive analyses of the underlying factors driving health care costs and ways of getting them under better control. These were discussed in other reports for the Romanow Commission.[6] Suffice it here to observe two points. The first is that provincial governments are in receipt of many recommendations about how to better control costs, be it through primary care reform, more cost-efficient purchase of pharmaceuticals, or techniques for managing demand and encouraging more patient treatment on an outpatient or home-care basis. The second is that provinces are looking for additional sources of revenue to meet their needs. It is the revenue side of the equation that is the focus of this chapter.

The Federal Contribution to Health Care Funding

The history of federal financial contributions to provincial governments to maintain a universal publicly insured system is discussed in considerable detail below. It is important to recall it was the federal government that, to varying degrees, helped persuade provincial governments to introduce hospital and medical insurance between 1958 and 1970 through cost-sharing incentives.[7] For every dollar a province spent on insurable hospital and medical services, the federal government paid around 50 cents.[8] If a province chose not to join in these arrangements, its residents would effectively be subsidizing, through the federal taxes they paid, the residents of the provinces that did participate. Therefore, for practical reasons, provinces could not afford to remain outside such arrangements. A block transfer replaced the federal cost-sharing formula in 1977 through the *Federal-Provincial Fiscal Arrangements and Established Programs Financing* (EPF) *Act.*[9] The Canada Health and Social Transfer (CHST) in turn replaced that financing instrument in 1996. At the time of EPF, Ottawa decided to "pay for" some of its fiscal contribution through the transfer of equalized tax points to the provinces in combination with a cash component.

During the first year of EPF, the total federal transfer for health (cash plus tax points) is estimated to have represented 41 percent of total provincial health expenditures with the cash component at 25 percent.[10] Although current estimates of the cash component vary widely, the federal share of provincial health care spending for 2001/02 was, according to some reports, only 12 percent. This represents a slight increase from the 11 percent estimate for 1999, but it is still significantly lower than the provincial estimate of 16.5 percent for 1994/95, the year before the CHST was implemented. While it is not always clear what level of federal health funding would be considered fair by the provinces, their position has in general tended to be that Ottawa should restore its cash funding to the pre-CHST share of provincial spending by 2004/05. The federal contribution would then be expected to grow annually on the basis of an agreed formula. This increase in funding for health care, of course, should not come at the expense of that portion of the CHST notionally allocated for social assistance and services and for post-secondary education. In this wider context, the overall federal CHST cash contribution would thus have to rise to 18 percent of provincial costs for all the services that CHST is intended to cover, namely, health care, social assistance and services, and post-secondary education.

Following the very large cuts in cash transfers to the provinces implemented in 1996 with the introduction of the CHST ($6 billion over the next two years), the federal government slowly began to reverse the course set more than twenty-five years before when it initiated a series of progressively effective measures to reduce the burden of transfer payments. The first decision Ottawa took in this regard was to reduce the potential impact of measures announced in its 1995 budget plan on the provinces by setting an $11-billion CHST cash floor guarantee in the 1996 budget and raising it to $12.5 billion in the 1998 budget. Then, in its 1999 and 2000 budgets and again in September 2000, the federal government announced significant increases in CHST transfers to provincial governments. (The September 2000 announcement of additional increases in transfers for health was interpreted by many as a way for the federal government to reduce the profile of health care financing as a sensitive issue in the general election campaign that followed.) Some of these increases were presented as one-time injections of funds, while others were built into the CHST base. Under current federal law, CHST cash transfers are scheduled to increase annually until 2005/06, when they will reach $21 billion. While there is disagreement between

Ottawa and the provinces as to whether these increases have restored cash transfers to their pre-CHST levels, there is no doubt that the cumulative impact of these increases has been substantial.

From September 2000 until the release of the report of the Commission on the Future of Health Care in Canada in late 2002, the federal government balked at further increases, at least in part because it appeared unconvinced that more federal money would improve the financial sustainability of provincial health care systems. The concern was that additional federal funding would take the pressure off the provinces to implement the reforms that were nesessary but politically difficult to achieve. Ottawa worried that additional cash transfers would be largely passed on to existing health care providers (physicians and nurses, in the main) and in no significant way lead to reforms that were desirable from the perspective of fiscal sustainability or quality of care.

The current situation is thus one in which the federal government is contributing about $5 billion less annually under CHST than provinces believe to be fair and reasonable (not all of which is dedicated to health care). Provinces are also critical of the fact that the 1999 and 2000 transfer increases provide no guarantees for the long run, since there is no explicit escalator provision beyond 2006.

This intergovernmental dispute about the size of the federal cash transfer to the provinces for health care has become linked in recent years to a broader dispute about whether there is a "vertical fiscal imbalance" in Canada between federal and provincial governments. What is meant by vertical fiscal imbalance (VFI) has been discussed and analysed in some detail in the previous chapter. Essentially, the provinces argue that the amount of revenue they are collecting is insufficient relative to their expenditure responsibilities, whereas the federal government is collecting more revenue than is necessary relative to its spending responsibilities. This "imbalance," they claim, should be corrected through the transfer of additional tax room or cash to the provinces. When provinces make this argument, they point to their increasing health care costs as one of the main factors leading to this imbalance. The federal government, for its part, dismisses the provinces' argument, suggesting instead that the finances of both orders of government are in reasonable shape and that if the provinces indeed require additional revenues, they should increase their own taxes. Provincial governments have the constitutional right and political freedom to do so. Instead, Ottawa points out, some provinces have been lowering their tax rates and then calling on the federal government to make up for their revenue shortfalls.[11] The origins of this dispute, however, are also very much related to the role that the federal government has played historically in financing health and health care programs in Canada.

A HISTORICAL PERSPECTIVE ON THE HEALTH CARE FINANCING IMPASSE

The Expansionary Period

J ust as it is important to examine the evolution of intergovernmental fiscal relations as a backdrop to the recent fiscal imbalance debate (see chapter 3), it is also useful to provide some historical perspective on the role of the federal government in financing health care in Canada. Indeed the current controversy regarding the appropriate federal role in shaping the future of health care in Canada – and the related financing dispute – can only be understood by examining how Canadian governments reached the current impasse.

The federal government's interest in promoting public health insurance dates back to a pledge of the federal Liberal Party in 1919.[12] This commitment remained on the back-burner in the interwar years but was revived in the context of Ottawa's wartime planning for the postwar peace. Thus, in 1942 the federal government appointed an Advisory Committee on Health Insurance. Its ideas were carried forward in the subsequent Marsh Report on "the principal matters involved in the consideration of comprehensive social security legislation for Canada."[13] The Marsh Report examined the link among the various elements of social insurance, constitutional and administrative issues, and questions related to financing.[14]

Nation building was also an important objective of the government in Ottawa at that time. When it introduced its social security proposals in its Green Paper, the dominion government stated three purposes. The first two were to provide a network of protection for the Canadian people that "justif[ied] itself on social and humanitarian grounds" and would "buttress the economy as a whole in times of stress and strain." The document then declared: "Less tangible perhaps, but in some ways most important of all, they [the social security proposals] would make a vital contribution to the development of our concept of Canadian citizenship and to the forging of lasting bonds of Canadian unity."[15]

In other words, elements of the Canada-wide sharing community described in chapter 1 were already embedded in the policy orientation of that era. The words "social union" were not part of the lexicon then, but the dominion government saw the idea of the country as a sharing community as a concept upon which to build. This document helped define Ottawa's approach to social security and to federal-provincial fiscal relations in the postwar period.

The federal government included proposals for public health insurance on the agenda of the Dominion-Provincial Conferences on Reconstruction in 1945 and 1946. Specifically, the federal government undertook to assist the provinces in setting up an approved health insurance scheme and to pay for 60 percent of its operating costs. Since, under this proposal, Ottawa was to remain the only government to tax personal and corporate income and inheritances, it suggested that provinces pay for their share of operating costs (40 percent) through a poll tax on all residents. Ottawa's sweeping Green Paper proposals for social security and related tax-sharing arrangements encountered stiff resistance, however, from the governments of Ontario and Quebec in particular.

As for its specific proposals on public health care insurance, the resistance of the largest provinces meant that the federal government once again had to wait to implement its agenda. In the meantime, however, Ottawa judged that it would be easier to eventually secure provincial support for such a major health initiative if provinces had the necessary physical and service infrastructure to provide health care programs.[16] To this end, it began in 1948 to issue National Health Grants to the provinces for hospital construction, general public health, tuberculosis control, mental health, professional training, cancer control, and public health research. The transfers for hospital construction and cancer control required matching provincial dollars, while the others were non-matching. All had some form of cap. The National Health Grants marked a significant step in the evolution of a comprehensive health system, even though this initiative was initially introduced on a piecemeal basis (Smiley 1963, 8-10).

While the federal government was encouraging provincial investment in health, some provinces began to move forward with their own hospital insurance plans. The Government of Saskatchewan instituted a premium-financed plan in 1947. When Newfoundland entered Confederation in 1949, it already had a government-financed health plan. At that time, Alberta provided hospital coverage for polio and maternity cases and, beginning in 1950, the province assisted municipalities that wished to establish their own prepaid hospital plans. In 1954

British Columbia replaced its premium-based health plan with a plan that was financed through a sales tax and general revenues.

While the provinces initially rejected the federal government's Green Book proposals, intergovernmental dialogue continued with respect to the underlying objectives. In 1955 a standing committee of federal and provincial ministers of finance and health was set up to study a national health insurance scheme. Finally, after much deliberation, "general agreement between the federal and provincial governments was reached" (Smiley 1963, 32). In April 1957 Parliament passed the *Hospital Insurance and Diagnostic Services Act*. Under its provisions, federal grants-in-aid or transfers were to be paid to provinces with universal, publicly administered insurance plans for acute hospital care, including in-patient and outpatient services. The plan, which was to come into effect when six provinces with a majority of the Canadian population were willing to participate, was not yet in place when the Liberal government of Louis St. Laurent was defeated in the 1957 general election. There was wide support for HIDSA among federal MPs at that time, however, and, at the urging of the provinces that had already implemented hospital insurance schemes, the legislation was amended by the Progressive Conservative government led by John Diefenbaker in 1958 to allow for the entry of the five provinces that were ready – Saskatchewan, Newfoundland, Alberta, British Columbia and Manitoba. By 1961 all provinces had joined.

The federal financial contribution to the provinces under HIDSA was set at 25 percent of the national average per capita cost plus 25 percent of the individual province's per capita costs, less any direct charges to patients for services, multiplied by the province's population. As a result of this formula Ottawa covered a little over 50 percent of costs in provinces with below-average per capita costs, and it paid for a little less than 50 percent in provinces with costs above the national average. Thus, the financing scheme featured some implicit equalization.

As for the provinces, they chose to pay for their share of the costs in a number of different ways, including earmarked sales, income and property taxes, premiums, and general revenues.[17] Alberta and British Columbia also imposed co-insurance or deterrent charges on patients at a rate of $1-2 per day.

Not all hospital services were covered by HIDSA. In particular, treatment for mentally ill and tubercular patients was excluded, as were long-term convalescent services, unless they were provided in facilities that were licensed as hospitals by a province – in which case their costs were deemed sharable (Canada 1956-57, 3123). Capital depreciation and interest on capital debt were also excluded from federal cost sharing. To qualify for cost sharing, HIDSA required that insured services be made available to all provincial residents under uniform terms and conditions. Provinces also agreed to maintain adequate financial records in accordance with federal regulations.

Although the Government of Quebec was a signatory to HIDSA, during the years in question it was engaged in an ongoing dispute with the federal government regarding the overall tax-sharing arrangements in the federation and the legitimacy of the federal spending power. This dispute ultimately led to the *Established Programs (Interim Arrangements) Act*, which was passed in 1965. Under the provisions of this law, provinces could opt out of two categories of federal programs. For the first category, which included HIDSA and health grants, tax point abatements were available. In the case of provinces that chose to opt out of these programs, the federal government abated fourteen equalized personal income tax points to the province for HIDSA and one equalized tax point for health grants. For the second category, cash compensation was available for provinces that offered programs similar to those supported by the federal government. The hospital construction program was in this grouping. Only Quebec availed itself of these opting-out arrangements.

While these legislative provisions altered the form of the federal-Quebec financial arrangements, they did not change the policy content. Thus, for any program from which Quebec had opted out, it had "to undertake to continue the program along the same lines as the joint program for a specified interim period ranging from two to five years and to submit 'information and accounts in the form and manner prescribed in the authorizing instrument' as well as 'permit such federal inspection and audits as are necessary for the purposes of the opting-out agreement.'"[18] In effect, Quebec had to account for insurable hospital expenses, since the federal legislation stipulated that if the equalized abatement provided more than the federal contribution would have been had the province not opted out, a cash recovery would be made. Conversely, if the equalized abatement fell short, Ottawa would make an additional payment to the province. The federal government and the provinces subsequently renewed this opting-out arrangement for the 1967-72 period and beyond.[19] It should also be noted that these abatement arrangements marked the beginning of the confusion regarding the value of the federal contribution to the provinces for health care.

As HIDSA was being enacted, some provinces were calling for a more comprehensive hospital cost-sharing scheme, one that would cover most of the excluded services referred to above. Given the dominant federal role in taxation at that time, provinces were also asking Ottawa to pay for more than half of insurable expenses.[20]

In 1962 the Government of Saskatchewan introduced a publicly insured medical care plan for residents of that province. Then, in December 1966, Parliament passed a bill to authorize the federal government to contribute funds for medical services provided under provincial medical care insurance schemes that met certain conditions. To qualify for federal cost-sharing for medical care as of 1967, provincial plans had to be comprehensive (cover costs for both general practitioners and specialists), universal (cover at least 95 percent of residents within two years, and not impose more than a three-month waiting period on new residents), accessible (provide reasonable access to insured services), publicly administered (be administered and operated on a non-profit basis by a public authority), and portable (make benefits available to insured persons temporarily absent from the province and to individuals who move to another province until such time as the second province would provide coverage).

Under the *Medical Care Act*, the federal government committed to pay each province half the national per capita costs of providing insured services multiplied by the average number of insured persons in that province in the year in question. By calculating the payment only on the basis of national per capita costs rather than on the basis of combined national and provincial per capita costs as with HIDSA, an even larger element of implicit equalization was included in the federal funding arrangements for medicare. Newfoundland and Nova Scotia, the first provinces to join the plan, entered in April 1969. By November 1970 all the remaining provinces had joined, including Quebec, which was the last to come on board.

As with HIDSA, provinces were free to raise their share of the funding as they saw fit. Some provinces relied exclusively on general revenues. Others imposed premiums (with relief for low-income families) or earmarked taxes, usually combining the premium or tax for medical care and hospital insurance.

The Era of Fiscal Restraint and the Decline of the Federal Contribution to Health Care Funding

Publicly insured hospital and medical services were introduced to improve the economic and social security of Canadians as part of the revolution in thinking in the aftermath of the Great Depression and the Second World War that gave rise to the welfare state. The overarching goal was to provide Canadians a better future.

The inauguration of these services also fundamentally changed the role of the public sector in Canada. It put government at the centre of a web of relationships involving individuals, families, churches, charities, and the private sector. It also created a new relationship between government and health providers. And it made government much larger in financial terms.

For the federal government, the last result was the most significant; Ottawa's expenditures rose dramatically. Thus, within a few years of implementation of the *Medical Care Act*, Ottawa began to express concerns about the high cost of its share of health care services. A large proportion of federal program spending was being determined by the provincial expenditure budgets for hospital and medical services and other cost-shared programs for welfare and post-secondary education. Transfers to the provinces as a percentage of federal expenditures were increasing dramatically, having risen from 9.5 percent of federal spending in 1955 to over 24 percent of federal expenditures in 1973.[21] To curb this trend, the federal finance minister announced in the June 1975 budget speech that the growth of federal transfer payments for medicare would be limited to 14.5 percent, 12 percent, and 10 percent for 1976/77, 1977/78, and 1978/79, respectively. The relevant legislation was subsequently amended to apply only to the first two years.[22]

The cost-sharing arrangements also raised difficulties for provinces. Donald Smiley traced provincial concerns back to the federal-provincial conference of July 1960 (1963, 12-14). By the early 1970s, provincial governments were generally worried about the effects that cost sharing might have on their own priorities. Programs that were half-funded by federal transfers were more likely to be allocated incremental funds than programs that were fully funded by provincial treasuries.[23]

Federal worries about uncontrollable federal expenses and provincial concerns about the distortion of their resource allocation process generated intense federal-provincial dialogue in the 1970s, leading ultimately to a new set of financing arrangements for joint programs. As already noted, the 1977 *Federal-Provincial Fiscal Arrangements and Established Programs Financing Act* rolled the two health and post-secondary education cost-sharing programs into a single block transfer. The base year for determining the amount of the new federal transfer was 1975/76.

The EPF transfer consisted of a combination of tax and cash contributions. The transfer of tax room was set at 13.5 personal income tax points and one corporate income tax point.[24] The provincial receipts from the tax points were equalized to the national average so that they had close to the same value for all provinces, including those with less than average fiscal capacity. The size of the cash transfer was initially set equal to 50 percent of the national average per capita federal contribution for the three programs in the base year (1975/76), plus a small dollar amount, multiplied by provincial population and adjusted by an escalator linked to the rate of growth in per capita Gross National Product (GNP).[25]

The *Established Programs Financing Act* marked a fundamental change in Canadian fiscal federalism in respect of health care and post-secondary education. It ended cost sharing, thus giving the provinces more incentive to manage health and education costs efficiently and leaving them with much more flexibility to determine their own priorities. No longer would the provinces have to maintain books that the federal government could audit. At the same time, EPF also removed the federal government from its direct involvement in provincial hospital and medical services. This reduced Ottawa's ability to ensure that the principles that had underpinned public hospital and medical insurance would be maintained. For those who believe that a strong federal role is essential in maintaining Canada-wide social programs, it was a setback. For those whose conception of the federation gives more weight to provincial autonomy, it was a large step toward the classical federalism that they preferred. (The implications of these differing views have been discussed in more detail in chapter 1.) In terms of the present discussion, however, the main point is that EPF represented a milestone in the history of public health insurance in Canada. And while the EPF arrangement was federal legislation and not a formal contract among governments, it was nevertheless the product of prolonged and intensive federal-provincial negotiations in which Ottawa worked hard to achieve agreement with the provinces. The result, unlike the CHST, was not presented as a *fait accompli* sprung on unprepared provinces in the context of a federal budget.

The changes in funding arrangements for health care and post-secondary education under EPF were also a major factor adding to the *fiscal confusion* that persists to this day regarding the size of the federal contribution to provincial health care programs that had begun with the Quebec abatement. Thus, it is necessary to pause at this point and clarify what the federal financial role was immediately before the end of cost sharing.

At the time, the federal share of *insurable* hospital and medical costs was roughly 50 percent, if the tax points abated to Quebec in 1965 are included. As mentioned earlier, the federal share was somewhat higher in low-cost provinces and vice versa. The share of *total* (not just insurable) hospital and medical costs was somewhat lower, however, given that several categories of hospital and medical services were not eligible for cost sharing. Moreover, provinces were incurring health costs outside of the hospital and medical care areas, notably for public health and other services. Based on available data, it is estimated that the federal share of provincial health spending *prior* to EPF was in the 41 percent range.[26] In the first year of EPF, the notional value of the federal *cash* transfer for health as a share of provincial health spending was 25 percent according to one estimate[27] and just under 27 percent according to another.[28] For purposes of this discussion, we settle on 26 percent. Again the reader should bear in mind that this percentage relates to total provincial health expenses, not just health expenses that had been cost-shared prior to EPF. If the federal cash contribution in the first year of EPF is compared to what had previously been sharable costs, then the federal share in that year is equal to well over 26 percent.

Our objective here is to shed some light on the share of provincial health care expenses that was covered by the federal government when cost sharing was ended. The federal share, at that time, was not necessarily a "fair" share. But it was a proportion that reflected 30 years of federal-provincial bargaining that had begun with the federal government Green Paper proposals in 1945 and the provinces' initial rejection of them. In recent debates on health care financing there are occasional references to the fact that Ottawa used to pay 50 percent of provincial costs, but that is not a valid benchmark – for two reasons. First, the 50 percent federal share pertains only to what were sharable costs at the time. Second, under EPF the provinces were given additional tax room that converted approximately half of the value of pre-EPF transfers into own-source revenues for the provinces. Therefore, from that point on, the only relevant benchmark is the cash portion of the transfer. Thus, for those who believe that Ottawa should return to its traditional share of total provincial health spending, the appropriate benchmark is around 26 percent.

Both the federal and provincial governments expected that the value of the 1977 EPF tax transfer to the provinces would grow faster than GNP, whereas the federal cash contribution was legislated to grow in line with the rate of increase in GNP. It was also expected that provincial health care costs would grow faster than GNP, which was part of the reason for transferring fast-growing tax points to the provinces. For both reasons, it appears that federal and provincial governments recognized that the federal cash contribution would likely shrink both as a share of provincial health spending and as a share of the total EPF compensation. Therefore, while we by no means exclude 26 percent as an appropriate benchmark for the federal cash contribution, for today's circumstances, we would suggest that this number is best considered as the upper end of a range of possible options.[29]

With the severe recession of the early 1980s and the continuing deterioration of federal finances as context, the federal government amended the EPF legislation in the early 1980s, even though provinces had expressed general satisfaction with the 1977 arrangements (Perry 1997, 260). From the provinces' perspective, a major advantage of the 1977 funding provisions was that they provided long-term stability, which enabled them to make their own long-range plans. At the same time, as noted in the preceding chapter, by the early 1980s the federal fiscal position had worsened much more than that of the provinces, and there was great pressure on Ottawa to take fiscal action. But despite expressed federal concerns, provincial governments were reluctant to voluntarily give up their privileged fiscal position. In the event, for 1982/83 and subsequent years, federal legislation reset the value of the EPF per capita entitlement (cash plus tax transfer) based on the national average per capita federal contribution in 1975/76 with the growth escalator (a three-year compound moving average of GNP growth per capita) applying to that amount rather than the cash portion only, as had been the case since 1977. Under the new formula, the total EPF compensation was to be the same in per capita terms for all provinces (whereas under the initial formula, the cash and tax components grew separately, which meant that total per capita compensation varied among provinces). The per capita cash contribution was to be calculated by subtracting the per capita value of the equalized tax points for each province from the established per capita entitlement. An important consequence of applying the growth escalator to the total entitlement rather than to the cash component was that the federal cash payment was significantly reduced in comparison to what it otherwise might have been.

These new transfer arrangements were then subjected to Ottawa's anti-inflationary "6 and 5" program in 1983/84 and 1984/85, but this only applied to the notional post-secondary education component, not health care. While the federal action may well have been justified by the worsening fiscal situation, it is important to point out that, unlike the 1977 arrangements, the new EPF provisions that took effect in 1983 did not have provincial concurrence. Ottawa imposed them unilaterally and, in this sense, the early 1980s also marked a turning point in federal-provincial fiscal relations. As will be seen below, a case can be made that a return to the more collaborative approach to federal-provincial/territorial fiscal relations that prevailed up to that point would be helpful in improving the outlook for public health insurance in Canada.

At the same time as the federal government was reducing the rate of increase in EPF transfers for fiscal reasons, it was also increasingly concerned about the erosion of the principles stipulated in the *Hospital Insurance and Diagnostic Services Act* and the *Medical Care Act*. These principles remained in force when EPF was enacted in 1977, and Ottawa expected provinces to preserve the key Canada-wide elements of the two programs. But, there were no enforcement measures or penalty provisions available to the federal government in the event that provinces breached them. By the early 1980s, faced with ongoing cost pressures and often-difficult negotiations with provincial medical associations, some provinces began to allow physicians to employ extra-billing and hospitals to impose user fees. In the 1981 federal budget the federal finance minister expressed his concern about these trends. He also restated several federal goals in relation to health care, including: greater visibility for the federal financial contribution, increased accountability to Parliament, greater emphasis on minimum levels of performance, a greater federal voice in provincial administration, and assurances of adequate provincial funding (Perry 1997, 260). This statement is of interest here because it clearly indicates the federal government's intention to sustain its influence in public health insurance at the outset of a long period of fiscal restraint. Provinces resisted the federal initiative, and this difference of opinion, which was not resolved through negotiation, ultimately led to the passage of the *Canada Health Act* (CHA) in 1984 (again without provincial concurrence). The CHA enacted the broad principles for the provision of public health care in Canada that still apply today, and it also authorized the federal government to withhold EPF payments in the event of extra-billing or user charges. In terms of the financing needs and options discussed in this paper, the latter provision is very significant because it makes it impractical (or has to date) for provinces and territories to use fees of this kind to manage demand or to increase revenues.[30]

From the early 1980s until the introduction of the Canada Health and Social Transfer in 1996, the federal government tightened its transfers to the provinces on several other occasions, as its own fiscal position worsened. The EPF growth escalator was set at 2 percentage points less than the rate of growth of per capita GNP from 1986/87 to 1989/90 and was expected to be scaled down yet another percentage point for 1990/91, although this reduction was pre-empted by the 1990 federal budget announcement that per capita entitlements were to be frozen at the 1989/90 level. This freeze was subsequently extended into the mid-1990s.

In 1994/95, the year before CHST came into effect, cash payments to provinces in respect of insured health services under EPF (as notionally calculated at that time) were $8.1 billion, or just over 16 percent of total provincial health care outlays.[31] Thus, as a result of both the high rate of growth in health spending in the years prior to CHST (notwithstanding the fiscal restraint provinces exercised in the early 1990s) and the EPF tightening by Ottawa, the cash share of federal contributions had fallen from 26 percent of provincial health expenses just before EPF was introduced to around 16 percent just before CHST came into effect. For those who consider that the appropriate benchmark for a "fair" federal cash contribution today is an amount equal to its pre-CHST share, the 16 percent figure might be the one to use. Just as we suggested above that 26 percent represents the high end of a conceivable range, however, we think that 16 percent is at the low end if Ottawa is to sustain its political position as a major player at the national health policy table. As the events we have just described indicate, federal and provincial governments were unable to agree on the federal policy role in health care in the early 1980s, at a time when Ottawa's cash contribution for health care was much larger and the fiscal benefits from the tax transfer were still fresh in the minds of the provinces. It seems unrealistic to expect, therefore, that a 16 percent funding share would provide the federal government with the political legitimacy it needs to sustain its policy role in 2003 and beyond. (As noted above, provinces have argued that a figure of 18 percent is the pre-CHST benchmark but this estimate is linked to the combined amount of EPF and Canada Assistance Plan (CAP) cash transfers as a share of a wider basket of provincial expenditures.)

In the run-up to the 1994 federal budget, the federal finance minister cautioned his provincial counterparts that federal cash transfers to the provinces would have to be further reduced. He effectively gave them one year's notice that some fiscal action would take place. The 1995 budget announced that new fiscal arrangements were to be introduced the following year along with additional cuts in transfer payments.

The Current Controversy over the
Federal Financial Contribution for
Health Care

In the context of the present chapter, the main implications of the changes in transfer arrangements under the CHST are twofold. First, by folding CAP, the only remaining cost-sharing program, with EPF into a single block-funding instrument, the federal government gained full control of the rate of growth of its contributions to provincial social programs and a greater capacity to effect reductions. Second, the fact that federal transfer payments for health, post-secondary education, social assistance, and social services are now combined under a single block grant (which still carries the tax-point and entitlements features of EPF) has made it even more difficult to decipher what Ottawa effectively contributes to each of these programs. In recent years, there has been a change in direction, with the federal government once again committing to transfer increases over five-year horizons and making explicit attempts to earmark new funding mostly for health care. Table 2 summarizes the history of the CHST to date.

What is relevant for our purposes here, however, is the impact of the CHST on Ottawa's *cash* contribution to the provinces for health care. As is well known, the federal government continues to calculate its share of provincial health care, post-secondary education, and social programs on the basis of the value of the 1977 tax transfer, associated Equalization, and cash. Provinces have long challenged the federal position on this point. One of the more persuasive provincial analyses of this issue was set out in the 2000 report of the provincial and territorial ministers of health.[32] We won't restate their case in detail here. In summary, the position of the provinces and territories is that the tax points that were transferred twenty-five years ago cannot reasonably be held to be a federal contribution today. After all, for the last quarter-century, it has been the provinces that have levied the relevant taxes, not Ottawa. When Ottawa asserts that these provincial tax revenues are a federal contribution, it simply confuses the facts and hampers public deliberation on the future funding of these crucial public services. We find these arguments convincing.

There is, however, a major qualification to our support for the provincial position. It is that the current share of federal cash transfers for provincial and territorial programs for health care alone – or for health care, post-secondary education, and social assistance and services programs combined – cannot fairly or reasonably be compared to the pre-EPF 50 percent federal cash share. This is,

Table 2

THE HISTORY OF THE CHST, 1995-2000

1995	Budget announced that EPF and CAP transfers would be replaced by the CHST, with entitlements allocated among provinces in the same proportion as combined EPF and CAP transfers in 1995/96. Total entitlements (cash and tax transfers) were set at $26.9 billion for 1996/97 and $25.1 billion for 1997/98. Cash transfers were to be calculated as the difference between the total entitlement and the value of the tax transfer for each province.
1996	Budget announced a cash floor of $11 billion per year. Total entitlements were fixed at $25.1 billion for 1998/99 and 1999/2000 and then set to grow at GDP less 2 percent, GDP less 1.5 percent and GDP less 1 percent for the next three years. New allocation formula was moving halfway to equal per capita entitlements by 2002/03.
1998	Cash floor was increased to $12.5 billion for years 1997/98 to 2002/03.
1999	Budget announced additional CHST funding of $11.5 billion over five years, earmarked for health care and allocated on an equal per capita basis among provinces. Allocation formula to move to equal per capita transfers by 2001/02.
2000	February budget announced the creation of the CHST Supplement Fund of $2.5 billion, allocated on an equal per capita basis among provinces. Provinces to draw their share any time between 2000/01 and 2003/04. Additional funding, announced in September, of $21.1 billion over five years, including $2.2 billion for early childhood development, resulting in cash transfers equal to $15.5 billion for 2000/01; $18.3 billion for 2001/02; $19.1 billion for 2002/03; $19.8 billion for 2003/04; $20.4 billion for 2004/05; and $21.0 billion for 2005/06.

Source: Adapted from Department of Finance Canada, budget documents; and Standing Senate Committee on Social Affairs, Science and Technology, *The Story So Far.* Vol. 2 of *The Health of Canadians – The Federal Role. Interim Report* (Ottawa: Queen's Printer for Canada, March 2001).

of course, because Ottawa transferred tax room to the provinces in 1977 to replace a large part of its cash contribution. This bears repeating because when provincial spokespersons occasionally use the 50 percent figure as a benchmark for an appropriate federal contribution today, they are being as misleading as the federal government is when it continues to claim the 1977 tax transfer as an ongoing federal transfer.[33] The provinces' argument that the federal government has re-occupied tax room it vacated in 1977 is also irrelevant, because the federal government had the constitutional and political right to do so and it presumably assumed the political price for imposing these tax increases.

What this ongoing intergovernmental dispute demonstrates, more importantly, is that there is a need to re-establish an appropriate benchmark for the federal CHST cash contribution for provincial health care programs at a level that informed Canadians would consider "fair." While there may be no objective basis that would point toward a particular number, there is at least some rationale to the 16-26 percent range we have identified, even though, for reasons already stated, the 16 percent figure seems much too low to be sustained politically for any length of time.

Before giving our view as to what might be considered a fair federal government contribution to provincial health care, however, we try to clarify how much Ottawa is now paying. What share of provincial health care costs is Ottawa currently bearing with its CHST cash contribution? Unfortunately, there is no single correct answer to this question. Or, stated differently, there is a range of possible answers to this question.

To provide these answers, we proceed as follows. First, we estimate the percentages of CHST cash that can be attributed to health care based on different rationales. Second, we apply these percentages to the $18.3 billion in CHST cash for 2001/02 in order to determine the amount of CHST cash contribution to provincial health care expenditures in that year. Third, we compare these CHST cash amounts for health care to total provincial health care spending in 2001/02.

The first step is to establish the percentage of CHST cash that can be seen as representing federal health care funding. There are at least five ways of dealing with that issue. From a first perspective, the CHST can be seen as a block transfer that can be used by the provinces however they see fit. The transfer goes into each province's general revenue fund and there is no effective way of tracing the federal dollars to any particular provincial program. In provincial hands, the money is fungible. When the federal government declares the funds to be for health, post-secondary education, and social assistance and services, it is really only perpetuating a myth. No fixed share of the CHST base transfer is assigned to health care – or indeed to any other provincial program – and there is therefore no way of determining what percentage of provincial health care spending Ottawa covers. From a second and somewhat different perspective, the CHST may be thought of as being used by the provinces for its stated purposes only, which include health, post-secondary education, and social assistance and services. But even with this different starting point, there is still no effective way of determining which shares are allocated for each of the stated purposes. The money remains fungible across this basket of services. From a third perspective, one can notionally divide the CHST among its various purposes using the allocations from the cost-sharing era and carrying them forward (which is the approach Ottawa has used for many years). From yet a fourth perspective, the method of notional allocation can be modified to take account of the fact that increases in the CHST since 1999 have been intended mainly to supplement provincial health care budgets. Thus, according to this fourth perspective, the current share of CHST cash that is notionally allocated to health care is greater than the share for health care based on the third perspective. Examining the current allocation to provincial expenditures among the relevant program categories introduces a fifth way of dealing with this question. Under this perspective, we calculate the share of provincial spending for health care as a percentage of provincial spending for health care, post-secondary education, and social assistance and services and infer that the resulting percentage is the federal CHST cash share for health care. These perspectives are summarized in Table 3.

In our view, there is no clear-cut or objective basis for arguing that any one of these methods is evidently superior to the others. Each has its merits and weaknesses. The third, fourth, and fifth perspectives result in estimates of the health component of CHST of 43 percent, 50 percent, and 68 percent, respectively.[34]

The second step in estimating Ottawa's current contribution consists of applying these three percentage shares to the $18.3 billion allocated to CHST for 2001. This generates federal CHST cash contributions for health care in the order of $7.9 billion, $9.1 billion, and $12.4 billion, respectively. As this analysis of different (and each partially valid) perspectives – and the fairly wide range of estimates it produces – should make clear, *there is no single number and no right number that objectively represents the federal CHST cash contribution for provincial health services.*

The final step entails comparing the amounts in the last column of Table 3 to the estimated $68 billion in total provincial health care spending in 2001. Based on these calculations, it can be argued that CHST cash notionally covered between 12 and 18 percent of total provincial health care spending in that year, depending on which of the allocation perspectives one prefers.

It is interesting to compare our estimates of the federal cash share to recent estimates put forward by the provincial and territorial governments and by Ottawa. According to the report of the provincial and territorial ministers of health released in August 2000, federal cash transfers had dropped to a level of just over 10 percent of provincial health care costs in 1998/99 following the introduction of the CHST. However, as a result of the 1999 and 2000 budget increases, they were projected to rise to almost 14 percent in 2000/01 (Provincial and Territorial Ministers of Health 2000, 19). In a more recent document released on 25 April 2002, the provincial and territorial finance ministers stated that the cash component of CHST was equal to 14 percent of provincial-territorial health care and social costs in 2001/02 (Provincial and Territorial Finance Ministers 2002). (The 14 percent number appears to include provincial costs for primary and secondary education that were never eligible for cost-sharing. If the provinces had excluded expenditures on primary and secondary education, the number might have been closer to 17 percent.) In any case, the provincial and territorial finance ministers claim that in 1994/95 (pre-CHST), federal cash transfers under EPF and CAP represented 18 percent of this same basket of provincial social expenditures. If the 18 percent share had been preserved, this would have entailed a CHST cash contribution in the order of $23.5 billion for 2001/02, or $5.2 billion more than the actual federal cash outlay that year. Of this $5.2 billion, around $2.2 billion would be attributable to health care, if one assumes that 43 percent of the federal transfer is for health, or $3.5 billion if the 68 percent allocation estimate is used.

Not surprisingly, the federal view is different. In a document dated 29 April 2002 (Department of Finance Canada 2002b), Ottawa argued that calculations of the federal share of provincial health care spending should take account of the 1977 tax transfer and the flexibility inherent in a block fund. It also made the argument that a share of Equalization payments can be allocated to health care, and it drew attention as well to federal direct spending on health. In a subsequent document a few weeks later, the federal government produced a pie chart showing the federal share of provincial health spending at 40 percent (with 15 percentage points from CHST tax points, 14 percentage points from CHST cash, and 11 percentage points from Equalization).[35] For the most part, however, Ottawa focuses on the absolute increase in the size of its cash transfer in recent years, not on the share of provincial costs that it covers. This approach is understandable, given that CHST is purposively not a cost-sharing instrument.

To recap, our estimates indicate that CHST cash notionally covered between 12 and 18 percent of provincial health care spending in 2001/02. These percentages are not far from the provincial estimates, although they are much different than the federal calculations. This is not surprising, given that Ottawa usually chooses to include the value of the tax transfer in its estimates and has even begun to include a portion of Equalization payments. It is also worth noting that

Table 3

FIVE PERSPECTIVES ON FEDERAL CHST CASH TRANSFERS
TO PROVINCES FOR HEALTH CARE

Perspective	Implicit Share of Federal CHST Cash Transfer Targeted for Health Care	Estimated Share of $18.3 Billion in CHST Cash for Provincial Health Care in 2001/02
(1) Block funding: general revenues	Can't be determined	Not applicable
(2) Block funding: social programs	Can't be determined	Not applicable
(3) Notional shares: cost-sharing era	43 percent	$7.9 billion
(4) Notional shares plus earmarked health transfers	50 percent	$9.1 billion
(5) Provincial program allocation	68 percent	$12.4 billion

Source: Authors' calculations.

adding an amount of $2.2-3.5 billion to satisfy provincial claims in respect of health care would have raised Ottawa's share of funding to between 15 and 23 percent. These estimates can also be examined in relation to the 16-26 percent benchmark range proposed earlier as the basis for determining a "fair" federal cash contribution, a subject we return to later in this chapter.

By this time, the reader may be understandably frustrated by the ambiguity and complexity involved in answering what at first glance is a simple question: How much is the federal government contributing to provincial health care programs? And both orders of government have been making the issue even more obtuse by recent initiatives in their quarrel of numbers. As already noted, provinces, for example, have begun to include their spending on primary and secondary education as part of social program expenditures when calculating the share of provincial costs covered by the federal CHST cash contribution. Primary and secondary education were never cost-shared by Ottawa and it is hard to see how their inclusion helps to clarify what is already a very complex issue. Moreover, provinces have been implying recently that a fair federal contribution would be equal to half of their costs. The federal government, on the other hand, is now including a portion of its Equalization payments as part of its overall contribution to provincial health care funding, although this argument had not been part of the federal position in the past. This new perspective is unlikely to help clarify matters. While it can be argued that the unconditional Equalization payments must be paying for some share of provincial health programs among recipient provinces, their explicit purpose is to fulfil the federal government's constitutional obligation to enable provinces with lower fiscal capacity to provide comparable services (overall) at comparable levels of taxation. Clearly, the dispute about numbers has escalated to a point where it has become difficult even for the most careful analyst to follow. And it most assuredly makes the arcane world of fiscal federalism even less transparent than it was just a few short years ago.

Concluding Observations

There are number of key observations that follow from this tortuous tale of events and developments in federal-provincial fiscal relations pertaining to health care. The first is that there is, and has been for some time, an imbalance between the federal government's cash contribution to provincial health care and the amount of policy influence it seeks to exert. Since 1999 the federal government has redressed the imbalance somewhat through improvements in the CHST. At the same time, however, it has also been attempting to discredit the idea that any imbalance remains, by claiming that its contribution to the provinces is larger than what strikes us or the provinces as reasonable. As for the provinces, they occasionally seek to overstate the imbalance by ignoring entirely the significance of the 1977 tax transfer under EPF. Having worked through the rhetoric on both sides, however, the impression of a policy/funding disconnect remains.

Second, and related to this first point, there is evidently an urgent need to secure intergovernmental agreement (we stress the word agreement, about which more below) on what would constitute a "fair" federal cash contribution to provincial health care. As we have demonstrated, there is simply no objective basis for determining what share of provincial health care costs CHST cash covers or should cover. Meanwhile, the federal-provincial conflict on what Ottawa's cash contribution is and should be is highly damaging to the cause of health care reform in Canada. This counterproductive dispute is both hindering and detracting from the provincial planning process at a time when important reforms are required. It is unhelpful as well to the functioning of the federation and therefore does not in any way serve the public interest.

Ambiguity is often a useful device for securing agreement on a contentious issue. It enables both parties to an agreement to put their own spin on it and somehow claim victory. In this case, however, ambiguity is harmful. Both parties must come to *agree* not only on what Ottawa's share of funding of provincial health care costs is, and should be, but also exactly how it is to be measured. Otherwise, within months of a new fiscal arrangement, provinces will claim that the new transfer amount is too small and the federal government will argue the opposite. In other words, unless the two orders of government can *agree* explicitly on what goes into the numerator and denominator when calculating the percentage of provincial health care costs covered by the federal government's transfer, the best that can be hoped for is a series of brief ceasefires in an ongoing federal-provincial dispute. And that dispute will continue to hamper both health care reform and intergovernmental relations. What is required, therefore, is essentially the equivalent of a peace treaty.

The third observation is that there is a disconnect between the expressed public desire for federal-provincial cooperation on public health insurance, on the one hand, and the way in which the federal government has made decisions regarding its financial contribution, on the other. Without being naïve regarding the cost-sharing agreements of the 1950s and 1960s, and the 1977 EPF arrangements (hard negotiations were involved), it is fair to say that they were the product of a prolonged and genuine intergovernmental dialogue. In contrast, the experience since then has been one of Ottawa acting largely unilaterally. At the same time, the federal government may not be entirely responsible for the current unilateral process. During the years of escalating federal budgetary deficits (from the very late 1970s to the mid-1990s), provinces may have viewed federal proposals for reductions in planned rates of increase in transfers as efforts to co-opt them into sharing the political blame for unpopular federal decisions. They may have thus preferred to be seen as the victims of federal budgetary measures, despite knowing that federal fiscal restraint was necessary. However the blame is allocated, the current dynamics of intergovernmental fiscal relations are not conducive to effective intergovernmental relations on health care issues. A return to more collaborative federal-provincial relations will be in order if Ottawa wishes to use fiscal arrangements to encourage a Canada-wide approach to health care reform.

This last point on Ottawa's unilateral approach is also linked to the issue of predictability raised earlier, and brings us to our fourth observation: a formal growth escalator for the federal health care cash contribution is needed. Under current arrangements, the law sets annual CHST payments until 2006. But there is no explicit provision as to what is to come after 2006. Nor is there a set of principles that would provide general guidance to the provinces as to what they might expect. This lack of explicit arrangements regarding the longer-term federal cash contribution unduly and unnecessarily complicates the task of long-range planning for the provinces at the very time when predictability is most essential, namely, when provinces are attempting major reforms. The requirement for a built-in growth escalator will need to be addressed in the context of any new fiscal arrangements pertaining to health care.

A fifth and final observation is that the current impasse around health care financing and how to calculate the federal contribution erodes the quality of Canadian governance. The public has no idea how much Ottawa contributes to provincial health care because contribution levels can be (and are) calculated in many different ways. Transparency is absent. Accountability is confused. Thus, regardless of which direction the two orders of government eventually take with respect to the future of health care in Canada, it is essential that they find a way to extract themselves from this unproductive and ultimately futile battle.

DETERMINING A "FAIR SHARE" BENCHMARK FOR FEDERAL HEALTH FUNDING

In this section we make some suggestions for determining what might be considered a fair federal cash contribution for health care. For a number of years, the federal government used the notional allocation of 43 percent to identify the health component of CHST. Although provinces were not required to approve this number, they appeared to have tolerated it. But when provinces began to base their political claim for more CHST dollars heavily on their escalating health care budgets, and Ottawa agreed to CHST increases mainly or exclusively for health care purposes, the 43 percent allocation began to lose its saliency.

As already observed, there is no objective basis for preferring the 43 percent, 50 percent, or 68 percent allocation as the health component of the CHST, although the 43 percent number now seems to be the one that is least grounded in reality. A number close to the middle of the range (i.e., 55 percent) is arbitrarily adopted here as a base for other calculations and to illustrate new financing options in the remainder of this chapter. Based on this assumption, the federal cash contribution for health care in 2001/02 amounted to just over $10 billion of the $18.3 billion in CHST cash payments that year. This is equal to a little under 15 percent of provincial health care costs, which is less than the 16-26 percent minimum-maximum range proposed earlier.

We have already suggested that 16 percent is too small a share to be politically sustainable. As for the upper end of the range, on the other hand, it could be argued that a federal cash share in excess of 25 percent of provincial health care costs would in some sense result in the federal government contributing twice for the same provincial expenses. Ottawa was paying for one-half of insurable hospital and medical costs before EPF. When Parliament enacted EPF, the federal government converted about half of its share of funding of insurable provincial health costs into a transfer of tax points. In our view, it is neither fair nor reasonable for the provinces to negotiate with the federal government to transfer tax points to them so that they can cover more of their own health costs, as they did in the 1970s, and then imply that the federal government should pay the same share in cash as it did before the tax room was transferred, as occasionally happens today.

In discussing possible fair-share benchmarks, we make a distinction between what might be a fair federal cash contribution under current *Canada Health Act* conditions and what might be fair in the event of more substantial conditions that limit provincial flexibility and imply further costs. Under current conditions, a figure of 20 percent strikes us as a reasonable and politically sustainable compromise.

We also proceed on the assumption that an appropriate federal share should be linked to total provincial health care costs, not just to costs that were eligible under the pre-1977 cost-sharing regime. Two reasons have led us to this position, although we acknowledge that a case can be made for the opposite point of view. The first and main reason is that provincial hospital and medical costs would be much higher today than they are now if provinces had not invested as much as they have in home care and pharmaceutical programs (programs that were not cost-shared). It seems inappropriate to ignore this fact in determining a fair federal share. Second, the early federal proposals to the provinces on health care went well beyond medical and hospital costs, and it was always implied that full health care coverage was the long-term federal plan. As a point of reference, the reader will recall that the federal cash contribution in the immediate aftermath of EPF was equal to 26 percent of total provincial health care spending.

In the event that a new funding agreement on health care is reached between the federal and provincial governments, there might be a case for increasing the federal contribution beyond the 20 percent benchmark. In particular, if the conditionality of the federal transfers were to become more restrictive or demanding from the provinces' perspective (even assuming that these new conditions were the outcome of an intergovernmental agreement), then the case for moving toward, or even to, a 25 percent share would be much stronger. At the same time, other factors might also influence the choice of a "right" number. For example, direct federal spending on health research and information, public health, and Aboriginal health are likely to provide payoffs in terms of improved quality and efficiency in Canada's health care system. It could be argued that these kinds of federal spending should be taken into account in any negotiation of the benchmark for the federal funding contribution to provincial health care.

If the 20 percent benchmark had been in force in 2001/02, it would have added $3.5 billion to the federal CHST cash contribution. An amount in this order of magnitude is not inconsistent with the historical federal role, and we speculate that it is large enough to secure the federal government a seat at the table, should that be Ottawa's wish. For our purposes in the remainder of this chapter, this amount is arbitrarily rounded up to $4 billion. This is our *base case,* the minimum we suggest is required to sustain any significant role for the federal government in the health care area. And we use it as a starting point to help illustrate some further options. Under more demanding or enhanced CHA conditions, the $4 billion would probably have to increase, but determining a precise amount is difficult, given the range of possible changes to the CHA. The larger federal contribution might be necessary for two reasons. First, the enhanced conditions might impose added costs on provincial delivery systems. Second, if the federal government was strongly determined to obtain new conditions, provinces would sense a bargaining opportunity. At the upper end of the proposed range, the federal cash contribution for 2001/02 would have been $17 billion (25 percent of $68 billion), adjusted downward perhaps to reflect some direct federal spending. In short, under alternative scenarios in which CHA conditions are strengthened, the increase might be in the range of $4.5 (half a billion above the $4 billion base) to $7 billion. These scenarios are summarized in Table 4.

Again, we do not argue that these are the "right" numbers for an enhanced federal cash contribution but rather that they do reflect a reasoning

Table 4

SCENARIOS FOR THE FEDERAL CONTRIBUTION
TO PROVINCIAL HEALTH CARE SPENDING, 2001/02

	20 percent	25 percent
Federal share of provincial health care costs		
Required federal contribution	$14 billion	$14.5-$17 billion
Additional federal contribution in 2001/02 above notional $10 billion	$4 billion	$4.5-$7 billion

process that takes into account some of the considerations that strike us as relevant. Of course there are other factors to consider that have more to do with the "how to" rather than the "how much" side of things. For instance, it seems clear that the federal government worries that additional federal transfers may do too little to improve either the quality of care or the fiscal sustainability of provincial health care systems. The concern is that additional funds will flow in large measure into the compensation package of current health care providers without contributing to the health care reforms that provinces are trying to achieve but that are politically difficult for them to secure. To reduce this risk, increased federal funding should be accompanied by other actions that enhance the probability that provinces will be successful in their reform efforts. We cannot design the elements of such a risk-reduction strategy but will state its purpose, which is for Ottawa to become a more genuine partner of the provinces by helping them to overcome the difficult political obstacles to the health care reforms they are seeking to implement.

The idea of Ottawa as "a more genuine partner" of the provinces is admittedly vague. The tangible ways of breathing life into such a partnership would have to be worked out among the affected governments. However, it would probably require that Ottawa be willing to absorb some of the political heat that would otherwise be directed exclusively at provincial governments. If provinces could count on federal political support when they embark on politically difficult reforms (for example, primary care reform), this support would at least assure them that they have a powerful ally. Provinces might then be able to say to local interests that are resisting proposed reforms: "We have no choice.

National policy requires us to do it." or, "We are sorry but federal funds are not available for that purpose." This strategy fits well with opinion polls that indicate that the Canadian public wishes both orders of government to work together to help make public health insurance viable.

At the same time, this idea of partnership is not intended to imply that all provinces need to make the same reforms in the same way. Individual provinces have much more direct knowledge of their health care system than does Ottawa. They also have the constitutional and operational responsibility for delivering health care (with some exceptions). Our idea is therefore not for the federal government to dictate provincial reform initiatives or become involved in the way delivery systems work but that it be available as an ally in helping to make provincial reform objectives a reality.

Several of the considerations we have highlighted can be summarized neatly using an analogy suggested by Claude Forget. At the moment the federal government is contributing financially to provincial health care programs like a bondholder. Like a bondholder, it is in the health care business with a fixed financial commitment only, sharing neither the fiscal risks of uncertain future costs nor the political risks of alienating powerful interests. Nonetheless, Ottawa wishes to retain its place at the policy table as if it were an equity shareholder, casting votes on crucial issues. By re-basing its financial contribution, and working politically in partnership with the provinces to make it easier for them to achieve their reform goals, the federal government would be better able to justify its continued status at the policy table. Recent federal investments in health research and information can be seen, in this regard, as important down-payments on this partnership role.

FEDERAL FINANCING OPTIONS

We have taken two different scenarios into account in considering the future of the Canadian public health care system. The first scenario assumes that there will not be an expansion of the current system and that efforts will be focused instead on consolidating core services and programs and on improving the financing and the quality of the care provided by Canada's hospital and medical insurance programs. We call this the improved status quo or *maintenance* scenario.

The second scenario assumes that the main emphasis of future reforms will be to broaden the publicly insured system to cover a wider range of services, including possibly pharmacare or home care, or both. This we refer to as the *transformation* scenario. Of course, the financing objectives and the best use of fiscal instruments would differ considerably in each scenario. We present these considerations and the resulting federal financing options in the next two sections.

In discussing the role of the federal government in health care in chapter 1 of this volume, Banting and Boadway argue that the extent of this role would differ significantly depending on the view of the federation and the definition of the sharing community that was espoused. Thus in the discussion that follows, we outline an appropriate federal role in financing health care for each of the three models of the sharing community identified in their analysis: (1) the *predominantly Canada-wide sharing* model, (2) the *predominantly provincial sharing* model, and (3) the *dual sharing* model that lies between. There is substantial support within the country for all three conceptions of the federation. But each has different implications for the federal role in financing the health care system and the degree of policy flexibility available to the provinces, and so we treat each separately.

Before turning to financing options under each of these models, in both the maintenance and transformation mode, we lay out a number of principles or points of departure that guided us in all of the considerations set out below. For the most part, these principles are based on the preceding analysis, and they are repeated here mainly to reinforce the weight that we attach to them.

First, the options presented are not premised on the existence of a vertical fiscal imbalance, but reflect the view that there is a need to overcome the discrepancy between the federal government's desired policy role in health care and the extent of its financial contribution.

As indicated in the preceding chapter, the structure of federal public finances is currently stronger than that of the provinces. While the difference in fiscal prospects between the two orders of government can be interpreted as evidence of a vertical fiscal imbalance, assessing the extent of the imbalance is another matter. In chapter 3, we describe the limitations and conceptual difficulties involved in producing such estimates. We conclude that while ongoing federal surpluses are indeed a likely scenario in coming years, the fact is that decisions regarding the use of these surpluses will have to take into account numerous and legitimate competing claims on these resources – be they debt or tax reduction or new spending needs, including increasing transfers to the provinces and in particular the level of federal contribution to health care. Ultimately, we do not need to define the magnitude of any fiscal imbalance mainly because we believe that the discussion about federal health financing should focus on another type of imbalance, that between the federal government's desire to have a substantial role in health care policy and its unduly modest financial contribution.

Second, as already noted, we suggest that the size of the increase in the federal cash transfer should be linked to the nature of the federal conditions associated with the transfer. The more the conditions restrict the scope for provincial flexibility and control, the larger the transfer should be.

Third, the process of reaching a new fiscal agreement between Ottawa and the provinces should be based on the pre-1980s model of intergovernmental negotiation, not on the unilateral approach of recent years. While this will require changed behaviour on the part of the federal government, it will also require that provinces bargain in good faith. It is simply unrealistic to expect that the federal government can sustain its policy role over time unless its fiscal relationship with the provinces becomes more collaborative.

Fourth, a substantial improvement in federal funding should be associated with new coordinated provincial-federal strategies that will make it easier for provincial governments to successfully implement the health care reforms they want. To this end, a new political partnership among the provinces and with Ottawa may be essential.

Fifth, a new fiscal pact between federal and provincial governments must enhance the transparency of the federal contribution to health care, if the federal government is to continue to make transfer payments to the provinces. To this end, we support a separate block transfer for health and a precise agreement between governments as to how each order of government is to interpret the federal transfer. Any effort toward greater transparency would also require that the issue of the 1977 EPF tax transfer be set aside once and for all.

The case in favour of a separate health transfer is not one-sided. By splitting the CHST into two or three block funds, there would be less money in each of them than there is in a combined transfer. Consequently, from a federal perspective, there would be less leverage to enforce the conditions of the transfer. Perhaps more important, in a context in which health care has high priority, the end result could be a much enhanced federal contribution for health care and much less generous federal payments to provinces for social assistance or post-secondary education. At the same time, a separate health transfer improves the visibility of the federal contribution and may result in greater accountability. If the federal government is inclined to reduce or be restrictive in respect of cash transfers for social assistance and post-secondary education, separating the transfers at least allows everyone to be aware of this and to hold the federal government accountable for its decision. On balance, the case for a separate Canada Health Transfer (CHT) seems strong.

We also hold to the view that the health block fund should have a built-in growth escalator that is predictable and that corresponds to a certain degree to the growth in provincial health care costs. The escalator should have the following characteristics. First, the overriding goal of an escalator should be to provide provinces with a reasonable measure of predictability regarding the growth in transfers. Second, the escalator should be set out in law and be based on an indicator that is expected to grow at a rate that is similar to the anticipated growth rate in national health care costs. The escalator might be linked to changes in GDP or to growth in income tax revenues. Implicit in this last point is a judgment that a return to an explicit cost-sharing agreement does not offer enough benefits to be worth the disadvantages it entails (for instance, the administrative costs of determining which provincial expenses are eligible for sharing, the administrative costs of audit, the political downside of such federal intrusion, and the potential distortion of the provincial resource allocation process). Third, with appropriate notice (say, two or three years), it should be possible to adjust the escalator if the trend in the rate of growth in provincial health care costs changes. Fourth, the legislation should allow Ottawa a necessary degree of flexibility in the face of an unexpected financial crisis.

The federal government will understandably be concerned that an escalator with the above characteristics would weaken its control of its expenditures. At the same time, if Ottawa wishes to continue to play a major role in national health care policy, it seems only reasonable that it assume some of the related risks. And provinces would still have a significant interest in managing health costs efficiently given that, under all conceivable fiscal arrangements, they would pay the lion's share of costs. We deal with this issue of risk more fully below.

Sixth, the requirements for asymmetrical arrangements between the provinces and the federal government depend on the vision of the sharing community that is embraced. The scope for opting out of federal conditions is greatest in the *predominantly provincial sharing* model. In the *dual sharing* model, the federal government might be somewhat more flexible with respect to non-participating provinces than it would be under the *predominantly Canada-wide sharing* model. For example, for a province that does not opt in, the federal government could still make transfer payments as long as the money was used for provincial health programs and met the conditions that apply to the hospital and medical services. The emphasis on uniformity or harmonizing of services is strongest under the *predominantly Canada-wide sharing* model of the federation. For provinces that participate in the national community, the asymmetries that now exist in relation to hospital and medical services would shrink in a maintenance scenario. Under a transformation strategy, the federal government could play "hard ball" with non-participating provinces and decline to transfer funds until a reluctant province decides it can no longer afford to stay out, as was the case in the early days of hospital insurance and medicare.

In the options that follow, we focus mainly on the parameters identified below, although we occasionally address additional factors and considerations as they arise:

> The form of the transfer (cash *versus* tax *versus* other options)
> The nature of the transfer (whether conditional or not, whether cost sharing or block funding)
> The size of any increase
> The escalator provisions
> Considerations related to equalization

Maintenance Context

The options presented in this section apply in the maintenance context where the principal objective of health care reforms is to improve the financing and quality of currently insured services (for CHA purposes). The different types of fiscal federalism arrangements that might fit best under the three models of the sharing community in this scenario are examined in turn. In each case our objective is to present options that improve the fairness of the federal contribution while facilitating provincial reform objectives. The result is three distinct sets of policy options, but they are perhaps best viewed as points on a continuum and as illustrations of the range of possible policy choices.

Predominantly Provincial Sharing

Under this particular conception of the federation the province is the principal community for sharing and redistribution. This model nevertheless rests within the framework of the constitutional provisions for equalization. As Banting and Boadway note in their chapter, section 36(2) of the *Constitution Act* states that provinces should all be able to provide reasonably comparable levels of public services at reasonably comparable levels of taxation. Thus, even in the predominantly provincial sharing model, some national redistribution is required. However, it is not the job of the federal government to ensure inter-personal equity among all Canadians in respect of health care. It satisfies its constitutional obligations in relation to health care mainly, if not exclusively, through Equalization. As we will describe below, the main implication of this model for the future funding of health care is a realignment of revenues between federal and provincial governments.

A) *Form, nature, and size of transfer* The federal financial contribution for health care under this model could be in the form of cash, tax room, or a share of a particular federal revenue base. While all three are conceivable, the cash transfer option is the one that is the least suited to this vision of the sharing community. In what follows, therefore, we focus only on the other two options.

The first option entails a transfer of tax room from the federal government to all provinces as a replacement for the health component of the CHST, or the entire CHST, perhaps along the lines proposed by the Quebec Commission on Fiscal Imbalance. The size of the transfer would be negotiated between federal and provincial governments. Based on our earlier analysis, the tax transfer could be equal in value to the current federal cash transfer for provincial health care (around $10 billion) plus up to another $4 billion annually. We say "up to" $4 billion because it would make little sense to maintain the *Canada Health Act* and all of its conditions under this model. Without the conditionality of the CHA, provincial autonomy and flexibility would be increased and thus the case for a smaller transfer of tax room rather than the full $14 billion might reasonably be part of the negotiations. (The focus here is on the health component of CHST but if the entire CHST were to be eliminated, the size of the tax room transfer would be correspondingly larger.)

An important question, under the predominantly provincial version of the sharing community, is what would happen to the Canada-wide system of publicly insured hospital and medical services if this vision prevailed. The answer is that it would depend mainly on the political will of provincial governments. All provinces have repeatedly declared their support for the five principles of the *Canada Health Act*. This option would put that support to the test since Ottawa would lack the teeth to enforce its provisions, suggesting that the CHA should in fact be removed from the federal statute books. Tom Courchene, a few years ago, wrote about a Canadian social union whose principal partners would be the provincial governments (Courchene 1996, 3-26). This option would also test the Courchene scenario.

To the extent that the transfer of tax room entailed income tax points, one unfortunate possible side effect would be the erosion of the federal-provincial income tax collection agreements and the tax harmonization associated with those agreements. This is a risk because the capacity of the federal government to effect this harmonization is linked to a continuing federal occupancy of a substantial share of total income tax room and this share would be reduced under this option. Another downside of this approach is that it would put additional strain on the federal Equalization program (about which more below). These particular drawbacks could be avoided, or at least mitigated, by transferring to the provinces a tax base other than the income tax (such as GST).

A second (and preferred) option would be a federal-provincial/territorial revenue-sharing arrangement. Under this approach, the federal government would pay a pre-determined share of a specified federal revenue base to the provinces as its fair-share contribution for health care. In collecting the revenues, the federal government would have the option of labelling the share to be transferred to the provinces as revenues collected on behalf of the provinces for health care. An advantage of this option is that it would maintain the size of the federal tax take and the importance of the federal role as a tax collection agency. Thus, it does not entail the risks to tax harmonization referred to above. From the viewpoint of equalization, this approach also has advantages, as will be discussed below. The disadvantage of revenue sharing, as compared to a transfer of tax room, is that it is vulnerable to changes in federal tax policy. Thus the revenue base under this option is somewhat less secure for the provinces.

Even under the predominantly provincial sharing model of the federation, a revenue-sharing arrangement could provide efficiency (in addition to sharing) advantages, since it could be made conditional on portability and mobility provisions being respected. With a tax transfer, this would be difficult to enforce.

The federal government would have to put in place an alternative mechanism that would enable it to maintain this aspect of the internal economic union. That mechanism could be a relatively small cash transfer (for example, a transfer equal to a quarter or a third of the value of the tax transfer considered under this option). In that eventuality, the $14 billion tax transfer envisaged above might have to be reduced to, say, $10 billion, with the rest provided as a cash transfer.

B) Escalator considerations This issue does not arise under the tax room and revenue-sharing options in the predominantly provincial sharing model. In each case it is up to the federal government to choose a tax base (whether to be transferred or shared) that will grow at a rate that resembles the growth in provincial health care costs, at least to some significant degree.

C) Equalization considerations Implementing a tax room transfer could have some adverse effects from the viewpoint of almost all provinces, including those that receive Equalization. One reason is that current CHST payments are based on an equal per capita entitlement, with the cash transfer calculated as a residual. This means that transfers to provinces are fully equalized to the level of the highest province. Under the tax transfer option, the equalization associated with the tax point transfer would almost certainly be limited to the current five-province standard. Thus, the allocation of revenues among provinces would be much less equal than it was under the CHST.

A second consideration is that with the end of CHST, the only remaining major federal transfer program would be Equalization and, if additional tax points were equalized, that program would grow. The consequence is that the wealthiest provinces would no longer receive large federal transfers, while the other provinces would receive even larger payments under Equalization than they now do. This change may leave the Equalization program more vulnerable to political attack from those who view such inter-provincial redistribution as undesirable. (With the CHST, the federal government can defend Equalization by discussing the two major transfer programs as a package and pointing out the benefits they bring to all provinces.)

Under the tax transfer option, it would be possible for the federal government to adjust the equalization associated with the tax room transfer to take into consideration differences in need among provinces that result from demographic and geographic differences. The case for doing so is weaker here than under the other two models of the sharing community. Even under this model, however, such a needs-based adjustment would help to ensure that the allocation of federal funds took account of the fact that demographic and geographic factors may impose higher costs on some provinces than others.

A needs-based adjustment could also be implemented under the revenue-sharing option. Alternatively, the allocation of shared revenues could be designed to replicate the current equal per capita allocation under CHST. In any event, the formal Equalization program would not grow. Revenue sharing is thus a more attractive option from an equalization perspective.

D) *Other considerations* While the predominantly provincial model of the sharing community does not require any changes in the direct federal role in health and health care, it would be entirely consistent with this vision for the federal government to carve out for itself a much enhanced role in health areas that leaves provincial health care services untouched. The Senate Committee categorizes the federal roles in health and health care, excluding transfers to provinces, as follows: research and evaluation (funding for innovative health research and evaluation of innovative pilot projects); infrastructure role (support for the health care infrastructure and the health infostructure, including human resources); population health role (health protection, health and wellness promotion, illness prevention, and population health); and service delivery role (the direct provision of health services to specific population groups, including Aboriginal peoples) (Standing Senate Committee on Social Affairs, Science and Technology 2001b, X). The federal government could assume a much larger role in these broad areas, as a way of assuring Canadians that the decision to end the CHST (should this be the option that is pursued) and to leave decisions about Canada-wide standards to the provinces was made in pursuit of a different vision of the federation, and was not an abdication of interest in the health or health care of Canadians. Indeed, given the evidence that health protection and wellness promotion are instrumental to long and healthy lives for Canadians, these would be logical areas in which Ottawa might choose to play an enhanced role both because of the potential economies and spillovers. Similarly, given that improvements in evidence-based health care require better information systems than are in place today, it makes sense that these costly systems not be duplicated across the country. Once again, there is a strong rationale for greater federal leadership in this area.

Dual Sharing

This model of the sharing community is perhaps closest to the current situation in the country. It features a countrywide framework that defines some basic parameters of major social programs but leaves room for provincial variation in program design and delivery. It acknowledges the coexistence of both complementary and competing visions of the federation.

A) Form, nature, and size of transfer Perhaps the main difference between this model and the predominantly provincial sharing model is that the federal government retains an important role, in cooperation with the provinces and territories, in preserving and improving the Canada-wide publicly insured health care system. For this reason, it is important that the federal government continue to transfer a considerable amount of money to the provinces to help them meet the costs of delivering health care. The transfer payments would remain conditional on the principles and other rules of the *Canada Health Act* being respected, with appropriate sanctions for non-compliance.

While federal CHST dollars flow into provincial governments' general revenues and can be allocated by provinces as they see fit, when Ottawa transfers this money its purpose is to support provincial efforts for health, social assistance and services, and post-secondary education. What is confusing when the federal government talks about this transfer, however, is that it cannot be precise about the share of the transfer that is for health care and the share that is for other purposes. This is not by accident: CHST as a block fund is in fact intended to leave provinces with the flexibility to allocate the transferred funds as they see fit.

In the context of a continued substantial role for the federal government in health care, this ongoing ambiguity is not helpful. Our key argument here is that the federal transfer should be redesigned to clarify what is the federal government's contribution for health care without reducing provincial flexibility. As long as the federal transfer is not based explicitly on cost sharing, that is, as long as it is a block fund, whether it be a single block or not, provinces have this flexibility. They can use a block fund transfer for its stated federal purpose, say, health care, but they can also use it for any other purpose. Even with funds being fungible in this fashion, as discussed earlier, there would be advantages to having the CHST split into two or three block transfers. It would then become clear, to citizens and others, how much Ottawa is transferring to the provinces specifically for health (and for other purposes), and, even though provinces would be effectively free to use the money as their own priorities required, greater public accountability might ensue. Also, from a federal government viewpoint, visibility would be somewhat improved. In short, for the dual sharing community, we suggest a separate Canada Health Transfer (CHT).

As for the size of a new CHT, the notional $10 billion base (the estimated health component of CHST in 2001/02) together with an adjustment of $4 billion as suggested earlier, is an appropriate starting point under existing CHA conditions.

It is also possible, under this model, that CHA conditions would be modernized to include considerations like quality, timeliness, affordability, and accountability. To the extent that this occurred, it might be necessary to go beyond the $14 billion. However, we envisage any additional conditions as emerging from a federal-provincial negotiation that is based on mutual respect of constitutional competencies, not unilateral federal imposition. Thus, moving the base amount beyond $14 billion would not be a *quid pro quo* for Ottawa's imposition of extra conditions but rather, to the extent that it were true, because the added conditions imposed further costs on the provinces. Since we have no way of knowing the actual costs of these hypothetical additional conditions, we arbitrarily assume that the upper end of such a cost increase would be $2 billion. The total CHT transfer in this context would be in the range of $14-16 billion.

The simplest way of allocating such a transfer is on an equal per capita basis, but this would reduce the share being transferred to the poorer provinces relative to the current CHST arrangements. As noted in our discussion on the predominantly provincial sharing model, all provinces except the wealthiest one currently receive more cash per capita now than the latter. This issue is discussed below under Equalization considerations.

B) Escalator considerations We propose a built-in escalator for the CHT that would be carefully designed to reflect the growth in national per capita health care costs. This might entail a formula based on GDP or tied to personal income tax revenue increases.

It is unrealistic to expect that the federal finance ministry would commit to an enhanced health transfer with a built-in escalator unless it had some freedom to alter the terms of the arrangement in the face of a financial emergency. The relevant legislation might therefore provide for some form of federal flexibility. At the same time, it is also unrealistic to expect that provincial governments would support such a provision unless the conditions under which it could be exercised assured them of fairness in the way that the federal government allocated expenditure reductions between federal programs and provincial transfers. Thus, the legislation might prescribe that the percentage reduction in federal transfers to the provinces should be no greater than the percentage reduction in other federal program spending.[36]

C) *Equalization considerations* The CHST equalizes in two distinct ways. First, since the total CHST per capita entitlement (tax and cash) is equal across the country, nine provinces receive more cash per capita than the province with the highest fiscal capacity. This is an important form of equalization. Second, the cash transfer is paid out of general federal revenues, and wealthier provinces contribute more to federal coffers on a per capita basis than do the less wealthy provinces.

In the context of a dual sharing model, in principle we can think of no reason to weaken the equalizing properties embedded in the CHST. Yet as a result of a shift to an equal per capita cash transfer, most provinces would see their *share* of the total transfer decline relative to the current allocation of transfer payments under the CHST. (In effect, they would lose the benefit of having their transfer revenues equalized to the level of the richest province because the value of EPF tax points would no longer be relevant in calculating transfer payments to provinces.) Therefore, the case for adjusting the federal cash contribution to reflect demographic and geographic differences is even stronger for the dual sharing model than it is for the predominantly provincial sharing model. In the predominantly provincial sharing case, we argued that such a needs-related component could be associated with the transfer of tax room or the revenue-sharing arrangement to make it easier for provinces with greater than average needs to meet their obligation to provide a reasonably comparable level of services at reasonably comparable levels of taxation. The case for adjustment is stronger under the dual sharing model because provinces are also subject to certain national conditions that might make it even more difficult for them to meet this challenge. To take an extreme hypothetical example: if all provinces were required to provide comprehensive hospital services, and one province had a very old population and another a very young population, an equal per capita transfer would make it relatively harder for the province with the old population to meet its obligation, and vice versa.

This option does not mean that poorer provinces would lose all of the benefit associated with the equal per capita entitlement (and unequal per capita cash) under the CHST. They would not, however, directly obtain these particular equalization advantages through the CHT (except to the extent that the inclusion of a needs-based component happened to benefit the provinces that have less fiscal capacity). Nonetheless, they might be able to recoup these benefits through the allocation formula devised for the non-health component of the CHST. This could be a separate Canada Social Transfer (CST). If this transfer were allocated wholly or in part on a basis that reflected real differences in welfare incidence across the country, the provinces with higher welfare rolls would receive relatively more cash per capita than the provinces with lower rates of social assistance. Indeed, having the separate CST dedicated solely to social assistance and services might make sense, especially as the federal government has been spending on post-secondary education in recent years through alternative instruments (Canada Research Chairs, new funding for research granting councils, and Millennium Scholarships, for example) (see Hobson and St-Hilaire 2000). It is unclear whether an equal per capita transfer that was adjusted for differences in need among provinces would achieve a greater or lesser degree of equalization than is now implicit in the CHST. This would depend on the outcome of the needs-based adjustment.

D) *Other considerations*   Under the dual sharing model, we argue that at least $4 billion (and conceivably as much as $6 billion) annually should be added to the federal contribution to provincial health care programs under a new CHT in the maintenance scenario. It is unlikely, however, that the federal government would accept a reform of this magnitude, regardless of what we consider to be its inherent fairness, without some *quid pro quo*. There are two conditions that Ottawa might want. The first is some assurance that the re-basing of the federal financial contribution is the new "permanent" deal and that it will *not* be seen as just another improvement in transfers heading inexorably, even if in the very long-term, toward a 50 percent federal CHT cash contribution. As noted previously, a 50 percent federal cash contribution is not a relevant benchmark given the 1977 tax transfer under EPF, whereas a cash contribution in the order of 20-25 percent of provincial expenditures would be consistent with the federal government's historical role in funding health care. Using the language suggested above, the federal government might justifiably insist on a peace treaty, not just a ceasefire. The second is an assurance of visible improvements in the kind of "quality of service" items referred to in the communiqué on health emanating from the 11 September 2000 First Ministers' Meeting (for example, "access to 24/7 first contact health services" and reduced "waiting times for key diagnostic and treatment services"), or at least tangible initiatives that ensure such improvements. This might entail having some of the increases in funding initially tied to specific provincial initiatives, say for five years, with the funds subsequently being rolled over into the CHT base.

With regard to the direct federal role, the same considerations that were raised under the predominantly provincial sharing model apply here.

Predominantly Canada-Wide Sharing

This concept of the sharing community is at the opposite end of the continuum relative to the predominantly provincial sharing perspective. It sees Canada as a whole as the primary sharing community for Canadians in matters related to health care and requires strong countrywide standards with respect to the kinds of services and redistribution policies that should be available across the country.

In this model, a relatively precise package of health care services would be provided by provincial governments all across the country, and these services would be more or less equally accessible and of similar quality. While it may be impractical to think that a person living in northern Quebec or northern Ontario can have as easy access to certain specialized services as someone living in the Montreal or Toronto areas – and this is equally true for northerners and southerners in other provinces as between provinces – the same minimum package of services with the same standards is provided for under this model.

A) Form, nature, and size of transfer Implementing this vision of the sharing community would require a substantial increase in the conditions associated with the federal health transfer to the provinces – the new Canada Health Transfer – since there would be a much greater commitment to uniform health care services across the federation. Questions thus arise as to how governments would determine what would be contained in the Canada-wide package of services, the ease of accessibility rules and any other conditions that may be required, and how to enforce whatever is decided. Fortunately, the Social Union Framework Agreement (SUFA) provides some guidance. The introduction of substantive new health care conditions attached to a CHT is analogous to introducing a new Canada-wide program, and Ottawa would need to satisfy the SUFA rules to that effect. In turn, this would provide provinces with considerable bargaining power that they might be expected to use to ensure that the new conditions met their needs as well as Ottawa's. For example, they might wish to negotiate some clear understanding of how the federal government would interpret key terms like "covered services" or "accessibility." We also believe that the full 25 percent federal CHT cash contribution would be essential in this case. Under this benchmark, for instance, the federal cash contribution for health care in 2001/02 would have been $17 billion (and possibly even more given that additional provincial costs likely would have been incurred under increased standards).

One place where we consider the SUFA rules too weak is in relation to the minimum level of provincial support required for such an initiative to proceed. In this scenario, we suggest a 7/50 rule (at least two-thirds of the provinces representing at least one-half the population) is the minimum threshold needed. In some sense, if that measure of provincial support is not available, then the support for this vision of the sharing community may also be lacking.

B) *Escalator considerations* The same considerations apply here as in the dual sharing model.

C) *Equalization considerations* Given the sharing principles involved, we believe the case for a needs-based adjustment to the per capita contribution is strongest under this model of the federation. In other respects, the considerations are similar to those in the dual sharing model.

D) *Other considerations* It would be consistent with this view of the sharing community to convert CHT from a block fund to a cost-sharing transfer. Cost sharing would certainly give the federal government more leverage to achieve its goals. However, we think that this would be a retrograde step in intergovernmental relations, not to mention the possibility that all the difficulties that led to EPF in 1977 (problems for Ottawa in controlling its costs, potential distortion of provincial resource allocation, and administrative headaches regarding what is eligible for cost sharing) would reoccur. We do not recommend it. In other respects, the points made in the dual sharing case also apply here.

Transformation Context

This section presents the federal financing options that would be appropriate in a context where a broadening of the Canadian health system was judged to be a priority and it was decided to extend the range of services covered. From a legal point of view, this decision could entail amendments to the CHA or entirely new legislation that would supplement the CHA and deal only with the newly covered services. There are a variety of political considerations that would influence the choice of legislative strategy. This chapter does not attempt to analyse them. Rather, we arbitrarily assume, for analytical purposes only, that the newly covered services would be included in the CHA. But if an alternative legislative strategy were preferred, this would make little difference in terms of the financing options discussed below.

As a starting point it is assumed under this scenario that a decision would be made in implementing the recommendations of the Romanow Commission's final report to include pharmaceuticals, home care, or both, wholly or in part as newly covered Canada-wide services. The main concern in setting out potential options under this scenario is what the federal government can or should do financially to make this happen. From the perspective of fiscal federalism, how does Ottawa ensure that these new services are provided? And how can it do so in a way that is fair to provinces and fiscally sustainable?

We consider these questions only with respect to two of the three sharing community models. (We doubt that the transformation scenario is consistent with the predominantly provincial sharing model and therefore exclude it from our analysis.)[37] But before we do so, an important proviso is in order. It must be recognized that the potential demand for insured health care services is almost limitless. Thus in the context of a broadened CHA, in one fashion or other, a fiscal cap or constraint will have to be enforced by governments, either directly or indirectly. Determining what this constraint should be is beyond our mandate. In the real world, the political process will determine the outcome, and one would expect the claims of the health care system on the public purse to be in competition with demands for tax reductions, a strengthened military, farm relief, and various other pressures with respect to social services and education. Our analysis is based on a hypothetical example of extended insured health services and therefore can only provide a general indication of the magnitude of the costs involved. The more important aspect of this analysis is to indicate the ways in which the tools of fiscal federalism can be used to facilitate the introduction of the expanded health insurance provisions envisioned in the hypothetical example.

Thus, for illustrative purposes, we include both home care and pharmacare under a broadened CHA. We do not know with certainty what these would cost (the definition of insured services is crucial) but, based on a quick examination of available data and choosing a figure for purposes of discussion, we assume here that together they would amount to $16 billion annually (three-quarters for prescription drugs and one-quarter for home care). We further assume that, while physician and hospital services would still be completely covered, the newly insured services under the CHA would only be partially (perhaps half) covered. Note that provinces are already covering, to varying degrees, some prescription drug and home care costs.[38] Thus, the new insurance requirement (i.e., 50 percent coverage) would not imply an additional $8 billion in provincial costs. (In fact, if each province were already covering exactly one-half of prescription drugs and home care, the incremental cost to them would hypothetically be zero.) We arbitrarily assume that, in total, the incremental costs to the provinces to secure partial (50 percent) coverage of the extended benefits would be half of that amount, that is $4 billion. Among the reasons why provinces would incur added costs, we note three. First, there is unevenness in current provincial coverage of drugs and home care, with some provinces offering relatively little coverage. For those provinces, there would be substantial incremental costs. Second, part of the costs that provinces currently incur is for coverage that, in respect of certain client groups, exceeds the 50 percent coverage that the new CHA would require. But for other client groups there may be no existing coverage, and thus providing the latter with 50 percent coverage would add to provincial costs. Third, the new CHA public insurance coverage might trigger additional demand. In other words, in addition to what provinces and individuals or families are now paying for insured home care and pharmaceuticals, $4 billion might be required to ensure that all provinces cover half of the costs. We repeat that these hypothetical numbers are for illustrative purposes only, and additional research and analysis on a province-by-province basis would be required to provide accurate estimates.

Of course, our purpose here is not to provide the detailed design of newly extended health programs. Rather, we are laying out some principles for consideration should such a scenario become a possibility. Based on our earlier analysis, we believe the following fiscal federalism principles should guide the implementation of extended CHA insurance coverage:

> Initially, the extended coverage should be financed through a separate block fund (or funds). But this separate funding should be maintained only until provinces have some experience with the new programs and they are deemed established. Once experience/maturity is achieved, the separate block fund (or funds) should be folded into the main CHT suggested above.
> During the initial phase, the separate block fund (or funds) should increase annually based on a growth formula that reflects the rate of growth in provincial expenditures for these new programs. However, there should be no explicit cost sharing.
> In general, the conditions associated with the extended insured services should be similar to those that apply to hospital and medical insurance.

Predominantly Canada-wide Sharing

We begin by discussing the predominantly Canada-wide sharing model. In the tranformation scenario, the federal government would extend the current health insurance arrangements to include some or all of uninsured services. Following our hypothetical case, the extended coverage includes 50 percent of the costs of the $16 billion in prescription medications and home care services. It is assumed that the actual incremental costs to provinces would have been $4 billion in 2001/02.

Given the provincial governments' current concerns over escalating health costs and their position that there is a vertical fiscal imbalance in Canada that favours the federal government, it seems highly improbable that provinces, as a group, would be willing to sign on to such new expenditure obligations. How, then, might Ottawa encourage provinces to agree to cover such costs as part of their publicly insured health care programs? The answer is that it might be able to do so if there was no net cost to the provinces. Put differently, if this were a high priority for the federal government, it might have to pay disproportionately to secure provincial compliance.

A) Form, nature, and size of transfer This scenario entails both extended health insurance (additional covered services) and a much greater degree of similarity of coverage across provinces (associated with the predominantly Canada-wide sharing model). Thus, insured services and conditionality are both increased relative to the current context. This requires a federal cash transfer, not a tax transfer.

While the case for cost sharing is strongest under this model of sharing, we maintain that the benefits of block funding outweigh the benefits of cost sharing. (The reasons for this were noted earlier and are not repeated here.) We also suggest that there should be separate block funds, as noted above, for the extended services (pharmacare and home care) until these programs are well established and governments have a reasonable sense of the costs involved and their rate of growth. Finally, we propose an equal per capita grant as the appropriate instrument, subject to some equalization considerations that will be discussed below.

One way to secure provincial agreement for such extended services would be for the federal government to pay for 100 percent of the assumed incremental costs to the provinces, that is, the $4 billion referred to above. While we lack the data to be precise, it is likely that this would create windfalls for some provinces, whereas others would more or less break even. More to the point, detailed knowledge of all aspects of provincial programs for home care and pharmaceuticals would be required in order to determine the minimum amount of the federal transfer needed to make this proposal fiscally attractive to the provinces. In practice, this would entail extensive information exchange among governments and prolonged negotiation. In any case, given that the $4 billion is a hypothetical number, it is possible that figure might have to be increased to ensure that no province is at a fiscal disadvantage as a result of the extension, although it is also possible that it could be reduced. We understand, of course, that the federal government might be very reluctant to pay all of the costs of new programs. Short of doing so, however, it may be very difficult to persuade provinces in the present context.

Thus under this scenario and this model of the sharing community, the combined cost of the CHT and the transfers for newly covered services could be as high as $21 billion (including the current $10 billion federal contribution, up to $7 billion associated with the predominantly Canada-wide sharing model for maintenance, and around $4 billion for the newly covered services). Note that in these circumstances, the share of provincial health care costs financed by the federal government would likely exceed 25 percent.

B) Related strategic considerations By now it will be clear that this scenario implies very large expenditures on the part of the federal government and that it would also impose substantial new obligations on the provinces. For this type of scenario to become reality, it could require widespread public support. But even with this level of support, it could not happen without the federal government deciding that such an initiative was really its highest fiscal priority and without the provinces feeling assured that it would not make them more vulnerable fiscally. This would no doubt entail a difficult and lengthy negotiation, in which both orders of government would attempt to maximize their goals at minimum cost.

Again in this case we would argue that SUFA-type rules regarding joint planning between federal and provincial governments are appropriate, given the magnitude of such an extension, but with the higher 7/50 threshold for provincial support. Without this level of concurrence, adequate national support for such an initiative might be lacking.

In the context of this transformation scenario – which would include both more stringent Canada-wide standards and broader insurance coverage – the question arises as to whether the enhanced federal financial contribution proposed in the maintenance scenario should be combined with the increased funding envisaged for new services to improve federal leverage in achieving broadened health coverage. Indeed, it might make sense for Ottawa to try to leverage all the additional funds ($11 billion) to convince provinces to accept the broadened scope of the CHA. In other words, while we have developed separate financing rationales for the enriched maintenance context ($7 billion) and the transformation context ($4 billion), the federal government, were it in the transformation mode, might well view the amount as a single envelope to be used to win provincial support.

Conversely, provinces would likely seek the opposite. They could well demand more federal funding for services covered under the current CHA before considering any broadening of insurable services. However, at this point, one can only speculate on these dynamics and the likely outcome of the negotiation process that would unfold.

What is certain, on the other hand, is that the provinces will want to minimize the risk that on some future occasion the federal government will act as arbitrarily as it did in respect of both the cap on CAP and the CHST. Provinces will want assurances that Ottawa will continue to pay its fair share as the future unfolds and will not unilaterally change the funding deal five or ten years down the road. On this point, a proposal from Richard Zuker merits attention. Zuker proposes an approach that borrows from the federal-provincial decision rule for amending the Canada Pension Plan legislation.[39] Based on this idea, whatever the new federal-provincial fiscal agreement for extended health insurance coverage,

Ottawa would legislate that it would not amend its financial commitment without the consent of seven provinces representing 50 percent of the population. While one Parliament cannot legally bind another, it would be politically very difficult for a new Parliament to unilaterally breach this kind of commitment.

What might Ottawa get in return? It might convince the provinces to legislate provincial health care acts based on an agreed model bill. The model would enshrine the scope and principles of the new CHA. The provinces would commit not to amend their legislation without the agreement of the federal government and at least six other provinces (comprising half the Canadian population). All provinces claim to support the principles of the current CHA; provinces that agreed to a broadened CHA might find it attractive politically to be seen to be implementing and enforcing their own legislation. Of course, in this case too, a future legislature could amend such legislation.

C) Escalator considerations It is suggested that a separate growth formula be used for the transfers associated with newly insured services until such time as the pattern of growth in these services becomes relatively predictable. This escalator should reflect growth rates in Canada-wide (all-province) costs for the new programs. For the first few years, until the pattern of growth in provincial costs became clear, the escalator might require several adjustments; thus it would effectively behave as a cost-sharing instrument. Eventually the CHT escalator would apply, as the separate block fund (or funds) is integrated into it.

D) Equalization considerations An equal per capita grant, as already seen, redistributes revenues from provinces in which taxpayers pay more federal taxes than the national average to those whose taxpayers pay less. This redistribution effect helps to equalize fiscal capacity. But, of course, this approach focuses on assuring equal levels of service across provinces. An equal per capita grant would not address the fact that some provinces have costlier health care needs, due to the presence of older and perhaps more rural populations. As we indicated under the maintenance scenario, the predominantly Canada-wide sharing vision is the one in which the case is strongest for adjusting the equal per capita grant to take account of differences in need.

E) Other considerations Even if the federal government were to assume most of the costs of an extension of universal publicly insured health care services, it should not be the delivery agent. In addition to the obvious constitutional objections, there are also more pragmatic considerations that motivate this judgment. The main one is that the health care system should be seamless. The various forms of intervention (medical, pharmaceutical, and surgical, for example) and modes of delivery (hospital, long-term care, and home care) should be managed as part of a coherent whole. The provinces should therefore remain the jurisdiction with broad management responsibility.

Finally, depending on the fiscal situation of the federal government, Ottawa would have the option in this scenario of offsetting its large costs by levying an added tax – call it a health premium. For individuals who would be paying lower premiums to private insurers for drug and home-care coverage, the result would be smaller private and larger public insurance payments. For some without existing private coverage, taxes would be higher and coverage enhanced. The tax policy implications of such a move are well beyond the scope of this chapter. The point we are making is that to the extent that Canadians continue to find a public health insurance system attractive and are willing to pay more taxes to ensure its viability, this option may be worth considering. It is thus not inconceivable that a part of the incremental cost of the predominantly Canada-wide sharing model in a transformation context would be covered through additional tax levies.

Dual Sharing

The dual sharing model resembles most the current balance that exists in the social policy roles of both orders of government and the extent of countrywide sharing that prevails. Under this model in a context of transformation, we start from the same principles and hypothetical scenario as described above. The main difference is that there is not as stringent a requirement that Ottawa "enforce" countrywide norms and standards for the enhanced services as there is in the predominantly Canada-wide sharing model.

A) Form, nature, and size of transfer   Under this model, a federal cash transfer would remain the appropriate instrument for promoting the extension of insured services. It is much harder, if not impossible, to enforce conditions with a transfer of tax room. For reasons discussed above, a separate block transfer (or transfers) in respect of the newly insured services seems appropriate to us, at least initially.

As for conditionality, the scenario is consistent with a modernization – and perhaps expansion – of CHA conditions, but is expressed in broad and general terms, since there is a weaker commitment to uniformity of health care services from province to province than there is in the predominantly Canada-wide sharing model. There is considerably more room for individual provinces, working from certain basic principles that are applied Canada-wide, to interpret or adapt those principles to correspond to local conditions and preferences.

The size of the transfer would be consistent with the amount set out in the case of the predominantly Canada-wide sharing model. Thus, for 2001/02, it would add a hypothetical $4 billion onto the $14-16 billion associated with dual sharing under the maintenance scenario.

B) Related strategic considerations   Many of the considerations raised under the predominantly Canada-wide sharing model also apply here. The main difference is that the provinces have much more scope to determine how to implement their obligations under the CHA, perhaps as much as they have today. Given the lesser constraint on provincial operational discretion, the 7/50 standard might be unduly onerous for federal action. The SUFA requirement for majority provincial support, meaning at least six provinces, might suffice for some, but our view is that there should be compliance with the 50 percent of the population requirement.

C) Escalator considerations   Our comments regarding the predominantly Canada-wide sharing model also apply here.

D) Equalization considerations   The existence of an equal per capita mechanism would mean that the CHT would help equalize fiscal capacity across provinces. The same would apply to the equal per capita contribution for the newly insured services. The case for adjusting the equal per capita grant to reflect needs is similar to that under dual-sharing in the maintenance scenario.

E) Other considerations   Our comments regarding the predominantly Canada-wide sharing model also apply here.

Table 5 below summarizes the financing options under the three models of the sharing community, in both a maintenance and transformation context, that were presented in this part of the chapter.

A FRAMEWORK FOR RENEWAL

W hile the federal-provincial dispute over the federal role in funding health care in recent years has focused almost exclusively on the issue of fiscal imbalance between the two orders of government, our main conclusion is that what is really at issue is the imbalance between the role the federal government appears to want to play with respect to the countrywide dimensions of health care policy and its financial contribution to the Canadian health care system. In our view, Ottawa's current level of funding is insufficient, particularly if it wishes to continue to exercise its influence on the future direction of the system. As things stand now, a disproportionate share of the financial and political risk associated with the uncertainties of the health care enterprise is borne by the provinces. The federal government must contribute more financially and assume more of the risk to maintain the political and moral right to play the policy role it has historically played.

But the amount of money is not the only issue. The way in which the two orders of government relate to one another on fiscal matters is inconsistent with the kind of intergovermental partnership arrangement on health care that Ottawa appears to want and the Canadian public expects. Therefore most of our proposals are aimed at outlining the framework of a renewed intergovernmental fiscal relationship in relation to health care. This framework is based on four general principles: (1) establishing what would be deemed by both orders of government and the Canadian public to be a "fair share" federal contribution; (2) ensuring transparency in any new fiscal arrangements for health; (3) ensuring a measure of predictability that will allow the provinces to undertake the necessary long-range planning and reforms; and (4) moving toward a more collaborative form of intergovernmental partnership.

For the most part these four principles apply across the range of federal financing options presented in this chapter, irrespective of whether the future direction for health care is focused on consolidating and improving the existing system or involves expanding the range of services and insurance coverage. The following paragraphs highlight the implications of this new framework, focusing on the dual sharing model of the federation, which relates most closely to our current system.

To begin with, the federal financial contribution to the provinces for health care purposes should be re-based through a process of federal/provincial/territorial negotiation. Given the large tax transfer that Ottawa provided to

Table 5

SUMMARY OF FEDERAL FINANCING OPTIONS

Sharing community	Predominantly Provincial Sharing (PPS)	Dual Sharing (DS)		Predominantly Canada-Wide Sharing (PCWS)	
Scenario	Maintenance	Maintenance	Transformation	Maintenance	Transformation
Form and nature of transfer	Could be effected either through a transfer of tax room to provinces or a revenue-sharing scheme. Revenue sharing is preferable due to possible adverse effects on tax harmonization and increased potential pressure on Equalization with tax transfer. If tax room transfer preferred, a small cash transfer is also needed to protect portability and mobility (with reduction in size of tax transfer).	Equal per capita cash transfer. Separate block fund for health, Canada Health Transfer (CHT).	New equal per capita block fund for newly covered services in addition to separate CHT.	Equal per capita cash transfer. Separate CHT block fund.	New adjusted equal per capita block fund for newly covered services in addition to CHT. New fund to be folded into CHT once program is mature.
Condition of transfer	No conditions except portability and mobility	Minimum is continuation of current CHA conditions. Might seek to modernize and improve conditions but conditions remain general. Not standards.	Conditions for extended services to be similar to current CHA conditions. Otherwise same as in DS maintenance scenario.	Conditions entail same health care services across country. Much more onerous than today. More like standards.	As in PCWS maintenance scenario with standards. Conditions for extended services to be similar to hospital and medical standards.
Size of transfer	Up to $4 billion on top of existing notional $10 billion for 2001/02 and escalated forward.	With current CHA conditions, add $4 billion to existing notional $10 billion (2001/02). With added conditions that impose costs on provinces, $4 billion would increase, up to maximum of $6 billion.	Hypothetical $4 billion for new services on top of $14-16 billion from maintenance scenario.	Re-base federal cash contribution at 25% of provincial health care costs ($17 billion in 2001/02).	Hypothetical $4 billion on top of $17 billion from maintenance scenario. Result might move Ottawa's contribution to slightly over 25% of provincial costs.

Table 5 (continued)

Escalator	Tax transfer or revenue sharing means that escalator is not an issue	Escalator that reflects growth in national health care costs.	Separate escalator for new programs to reflect their cost pattern until folded into CHT. Otherwise same as in DS maintenance scenario.	Escalator that reflects growth in national health care costs.	Separate escalator for new programs to reflect their cost pattern until folded into CHT. Otherwise same as in PCWS maintenance scenario.
Equalization considerations	Tax room is equalized on basis of current Equalization formula but possibly with needs component. If revenue sharing is preferred, it could be designed to provide equal per capita revenues to provinces, with a possible needs adjustment.	CHT equalized, with needs taken into account in CHT. Case for needs-based adjustment stronger than in PPS.	Same as in DS maintenance option.	Same as in DS model but case for needs-based adjustment even stronger.	Same as in PCWS maintenance scenario.
Other considerations	Possible for federal government to play larger direct role in health via spending on research and information, public health, and Aboriginal service delivery.	Federal government will require *quid pro quo* for added funds, including accepting that new funding deal is "permanent." Larger direct federal role still possible.	Federal government may levy a health tax. Otherwise as in DS maintenance scenario.	Same *quid pro quo* as in DS model. Would require minimum level of provincial support (7/50 rule)	Federal government may levy a health tax. Otherwise same as in PCWS maintenance scenario. This scenario would also require firm commitments from Ottawa on funding (might have to assume the bulk of the cost). Proposed Canada Pension Plan decision model. Similar provincial commitments through model health care act.

the provinces in the 1970s for health care and post-secondary education, a fair and reasonable federal cash contribution for health care should be in the range of 20-25 percent of total provincial health care costs, with the actual share to be determined through a process that takes certain factors into account, such as the nature of the conditions associated with the transfer and the amount of direct federal spending. Our best estimate of the current federal cash contribution is in the order of 15 percent.

The federal cash contribution should be in the form of a separate block fund for health care (the Canada Health Transfer) allocated on an equal per capita basis. We propose this approach in part because of its equalizing properties. It should not be an explicit cost-sharing arrangement. The new transfer should be visible and understood by all Canadians to be the federal contribution for health. The current CHST arrangements make it impossible to know, and to agree on, what the federal contribution is, and the ongoing dispute between the two orders of government on that issue is not only counterproductive but has become detrimental to the health care reform process and the functioning of the federation.

This federal health transfer should have a built-in growth formula (an escalator) that is designed to reflect the growth in national health care costs. It should be predictable and transparent. Consideration should also be given to adjusting the equal per capita transfer on the basis of differences in need among provinces and territories as determined by measurable demographic and geographic factors. While such a needs-related adjustment can be justified in all scenarios, it is strongest in the case of the predominantly Canada-wide sharing model.

If the federal government decides to propose Canada-wide legislation for newly insured services, the federal-provincial/territorial negotiations should be guided by the principles set out in the Social Union Framework Agreement, but with seven or more provinces representing 50 percent of the population as the minimum threshold for extending the Canada-wide health care programs. In this scenario of a broader range of insured services, consideration should be given to the kind of fiscal leverage that the federal government might use to encourage provincial support. Given the provinces' current concerns over escalating health care costs and their view that there is a vertical fiscal imbalance that favours Ottawa, it appears that the incremental costs of the added coverage to the provinces may have to initially be borne by the federal government. An interim measure that could be considered would be for the funding allocated to the new national health care programs to be placed in a separate block fund (separate from the CHT), with a separate escalator that reflects anticipated cost increases in the new programs without being an explicit cost-sharing instrument. The funding for new programs should be folded into the CHT when they become mature.

More generally, whatever direction governments choose to take regarding the future of the Canadian health system, the fiscal relationship between the federal and provincial/territorial governments must be re-examined with a view to establishing a new partnership. The model of federal-provincial fiscal relations that prevailed for more than two decades from the 1950s to the 1970s was characterized by tough negotiations but with a determination to reach agreement. Returning to the earlier model or finding an alternative that gives provinces more influence over outcomes is highly desirable. This requires that the federal government become more collaborative. It also requires that provinces and territories negotiate in good faith with Ottawa whether the federal treasury is in serious difficulty or in strong surplus.

Finally, consideration should be given to ways in which the federal government could cooperate strategically with the provinces and territories in order to help them overcome some of the difficult political obstacles they face in moving forward with health care reform. As a general proposition, both orders of government support the idea that comprehensive reform is necessary. Yet they do relatively little together to overcome the barriers to such reform. We understand that provinces may be nervous that "partnership," in this kind of situation, risks becoming "intrusion." But given the pace of progress so far, it is hard to believe that some form of intergovernmental cooperation would not help advance the common agenda.

NOTES

1   The Premiers' Council on Canadian Health Awareness was created by the premiers as part of their multi-media campaign to disseminate information about health financing challenges to citizens and put pressure on the federal government to increase its share of funding. Their print and television advertisements can be viewed on their website: http://premiersforhealth.ca/communicate.php.

2   We realize that there is also a requirement for comprehensiveness but there is so much uncertainty about the meaning of this term that we chose to exclude it here.

3   See the first chapter of this volume by Keith Banting and Robin Boadway.

4   See, for example, Provincial and Territorial Ministers of Health (2000). See also Commission on Fiscal Imbalance (2002, 33-37).

5   For a summary of public opinion, see Standing Senate Committee on Social Affairs, Science and Technology (2001a, 45-50).

6   For example, see Morgan and Hurley (2002).

7   We say "most" provincial governments because some provinces had implemented hospital insurance before national legislation was introduced by the federal government, and one province had also done so in respect of insured medical services.

8   The cost-sharing formulas were somewhat more complex but this description is adequate at this stage of the analysis.

9   At the time of the 1977 legislation, the federal government also introduced a new program to cover extended health services, such as nursing home intermediate care, lower-level residential care for adults, aspects of home care and ambulatory health services not covered by the hospital insurance agreements. The payments were initially $20 per capita and

were intended to escalate by the rate of growth of per capita GDP. Some of these expenses had previously been covered under the Canada Assistance Plan.

10   EPF was a block transfer that was intended to replace federal cost sharing for hospital and medical insurance and for post-secondary education operating costs. Thus, these are notional estimates only. See Commission on the Future of Health Care in Canada, (2002, Appendix E2, 313).

11   Some provinces might argue that the lower taxes were required due to competitive economic pressures and that they were faster out of the gate than the federal government.

12   According to Proposals of the Government of Canada to the Dominion-Provincial Conference on Reconstruction, (August 1945, 29), in "both federal and provincial circles, health insurance has been under active consideration since the last war."

13   The quotations are from the letter of transmittal of the report, dated February 17, 1943, from Leonard C. Marsh to the Chairman of the Advisory Committee on Reconstruction, F. Cyril James.

14   Ibid.

15   Ibid, 28.

16   Donald Smiley quoted Prime Minister Mackenzie King to the effect that these grants were in aid of several health functions as "fundamental pre-requisites of a nation-wide scheme of health insurance." See Smiley (1963, 29).

17   For a snapshot of how provinces financed their share of costs, see Canadian Tax Foundation (1965, 115-17).

18   Canadian Tax Foundation (1972, 136).

19   In the 1972 amendments to the opting-out arrangements, the tax abatement for HIDSA was increased to 16 percent of the federal individual income tax.

20   Carter cites an Ontario proposal at a 1955 federal-provincial committee to the effect that Ottawa should pay for 60 percent of a wider scheme, Carter (1971, ftn 32).

21   The numbers cited here are derived from Canadian Tax Foundation (1978, 23, Table 2-11).

22   Canadian Tax Foundation (1976, 112-13).

23   For a good discussion of this issue, see Standing Senate Committee on Social Affairs, Science and Technology (2001a, 7-10). We are aware that, from a theoretical viewpoint, individual provinces could not significantly increase their access to federal funding simply by increasing their expenses on insurable items, since the greater part of the funding formula was linked to national average per capita costs and not the costs of individual provinces. At the same time, in a setting where all provinces are experiencing rapidly rising costs, this consideration may not be as important as theory would suggest.

24   The federal government vacated 9.143 points of the personal income tax at the time. Revenues from these points and the 4.357 points that had been vacated earlier, plus 1 point of corporate income tax under previous post-secondary education arrangements were to replace part of the former cash payments.

25   For a good factual discussion of these issues, see Perry (1997, chapter 17). The cash transfers were also augmented to include both transitional and, for some provinces, leveling payments. The latter was a provision under which the cash contributions were to become equal per capita over a five-year phase-in period.

26   This figure was initially estimated using Table 11-1 from the Canadian Tax Foundation (1979, 202). It shows gross provincial expenditures at $9.73 billion for health (excluding a small amount paid for by local government without provincial transfers). It shows federal conditional transfers to provinces at $3 billion. However, only $246 million for Quebec is included in this $3 billion. We have assumed the value of the Quebec transfer, including the abatement, to be equal to 85 percent of the Ontario transfer, which increases it by $987 million. This raises the amount of the federal conditional transfer from $3 billion to $4 billion. The latter number is around 41.5 percent of provincial health spending. Note that we subsequently located data from the federal Department of Finance. The Finance number was almost identical to our initial estimate.

27   Based on transfer data from the federal Department of Finance and provincial expenditure data from CIHI.

28   Provincial and Territorial Ministers of Health (2000, 19).

29   On this point, there are two contrary arguments. On the one hand, given the rapidly deteriorating state of federal finances by the early 1980s (discussed in some detail in chapter 3), it is unrealistic to think that the escalator could have been improved. On the other hand, provinces argued that the rate of increase in health costs would exceed the growth rate of GNP and that the escalator would therefore be inadequate. With the benefits of hindsight, the former argument seems to have more weight (although both can be supported). As it turned out, federal finances were badly out of control in the 1980s and Ottawa found it necessary to lower the escalator. Had a more generous escalator been in place, the structural fiscal imbalance of the federal government would have been even worse. The conclusion that we draw from this is simply that if one is going to use a 1970s benchmark as one input into the determination of a "fair" share for federal cash contributions to provinces for health, the 26 percent number is at the upper end of a range.

30   This comment is not intended to pass any judgment on the efficacy or fairness of such fees.

31   These data are drawn from both federal and provincial sources. They do not seem to be in dispute.

32   See Provincial and Territorial Ministers of Health (2000, 10-13).

33   For example, the 50:50 cost-sharing argument was put forward by the Ontario Minister of Health in an interview on Newsworld following the F/P/T Meeting of Finance Ministers in Corner Brook, Newfoundland, on 25 April 2002. In late 2002, provincial premiers undertook an advertising campaign that compared federal CHST cash contributions for health care to the 50 percent figure that had prevailed prior to EPF.

34   Note that the 68 percent figure represents provincial health care expenditures as a share of provincial expenditure on health care, post-secondary education, and social assistance/services, using FMS data for post-secondary education based on "general" provincial and territorial expenditures. If "total" expenditures for post-secondary education had been used, the 68 percent number would have dropped to 62 percent.

35   Presented at the conference on "Canadian Fiscal Arrangements: What Works, What Might Work Better," 17 May 2002, Winnipeg, Manitoba, by Louis Levesque, a PCO official.

36   The legislation might also increase federal flexibility even further in the event of war.

37   In principle, the provinces could take the initiative and seek to expand coverage of insured health care services. And in practice individual provinces have selectively expanded coverage. To the extent that the expanded services are targeted at provincial populations, then the coverage will differ in scope and nature from province to province. And this does not raise any issues related to fiscal federalism. As for the possibility of provinces acting collectively to create a Canada-wide program, there is no persuasive historical evidence that we are aware of that suggests that provinces are likely to wish to choose to follow this course. Indeed, in the past, provinces that played a leadership role in introducing public health insurance looked to the federal government to turn their initiatives into Canada-wide programs.

38   According to CIHI, the public sector share of prescribed drugs in 2001 was likely to be equal to 49.2 percent. See Canadian Institute for Health Information (2002).

39   Commentary presented at the conference on "Canadian Fiscal Arrangements: What Works, What Might Work Better", 16-17 May 2002, Winnipeg, Manitoba.

CHAPTER 5

FEDERAL-PROVINCIAL RELATIONS AND HEALTH CARE: RECONSTRUCTING THE PARTNERSHIP

HARVEY LAZAR, KEITH BANTING, ROBIN BOADWAY, DAVID CAMERON, AND FRANCE ST-HILAIRE

F ederal and provincial governments have been jointly involved in the provision of universal, publicly insured and administered health care to Canadians for decades. In the early postwar decades, federal and provincial governments agreed on the use of conditional intergovernmental grants as the means to build the system of health care that exists in Canada today. What was done in the 1950s, 1960s, and 1970s was a considerable achievement both in policy and fiscal terms and from the viewpoint of cooperative intergovernmental relations.

Today, however, there is a series of "disconnects" between the federal government's approach to health care financing and intergovernmental relations, on the one hand, and its policy role in promoting a countrywide system of health care for Canadians, on the other. These disconnects are contributing to the difficulties provinces face in reforming their health care systems and are serious irritants in intergovernmental relations.

The main purpose of this final chapter is to lay out a range of possible reforms to the federal financial contribution to provincially operated health care systems. The second and related object is to shed light on ways of improving intergovernmental relations, in particular the process for federal-provincial dispute resolution in the area of health care policy and its financing. These ideas and proposals, which are based on conclusions from the earlier chapters, are intended as contributions to the wider debate about sustaining and improving health care for Canadians. While these issues are fairly technical in nature, they also raise broader political questions about the appropriate role for the federal government in Canadian health care.

To foreshadow our conclusions, we suggest that certain broad principles should guide the federal government's position on these issues. We do not consider, however, that there is a single correct approach to future fiscal arrangements for health care or to intergovernmental relations more generally. Rather, different visions of the federation embody different values, and, depending on which vision is espoused, certain approaches to funding and dispute resolution make better sense than others. Thus, we conclude this chapter with a set of proposals for using the tools of fiscal federalism to sustain and improve Canadian health care in ways that are consistent with three different models of the sharing community and the Canadian federation. We also lay out alternative dispute resolution models that could be used to resolve intergovernmental conflicts or disagreements in health care.

THE CONSTITUTIONAL AND POLITICAL SETTING

T he *Constitution Act, 1867* reflected nineteenth-century ideas about the appropriate role of government. The health and social needs of Canadians were seen then as the responsibility of individuals, families, churches and charities; the state offered only basic forms of poor relief through local agencies. With the expansion of the social role of the state in the twentieth century, Canada had to rethink the intergovernmental division of roles in new areas of state intervention.

Although the Constitution did not assign jurisdiction over health exclusively to one level of government, section 92 of the *Constitution Act, 1867* did give the provinces the primary role in the field. Section 92(7) specifically grants them authority over hospitals. In addition, their jurisdiction over health was inferred from other broader provincial powers, in particular by section 92(13) dealing with property and civil rights and section 92(16) dealing with matters of "local or private nature." In the early decades of the twentieth century, the courts held that these sections empowered provincial governments to regulate the medical professions and private insurance plans. This authority was extended to the new instrument of social insurance during the late 1930s.

In chapter 1, Keith Banting and Robin Boadway set out the constitutional basis for a federal government presence in health care. While several constitutional heads of power are cited, they make clear that Ottawa's largest role has been through the use of conditional intergovernmental transfers. In turn, these transfers have their basis in the principles set out in section 36(1) of the *Constitution Act, 1982* on equalization as well as in the doctrine of the federal spending power.

The principle of the spending power holds that the federal government "may spend or lend its funds to any government or institution or individual it chooses, for any purpose it chooses; and that it may attach to any grant or loan any conditions it chooses, including conditions it could not directly legislate" (Hogg 2000, 6.8a). The use of the spending power has been controversial and has been challenged politically by both the Tremblay Commission (1956) and the Séguin Commission (2002) as well as in the courts. To date, at least, the courts have upheld the concept, although it is probably also true that it has not been tested fully.

The Evolving Federal Role in Funding Provincial Health Care

During the war years, the federal government developed ambitious proposals for a postwar system of social security, including public health insurance. Many of these proposals were linked to the court decisions regarding the powers of the two orders of government. But this package of federal proposals was rejected at the postwar Dominion-Provincial Conference on Reconstruction in 1945, with Ontario and Quebec as the principal opponents. Some other provinces, however, favoured quick action on the hospital insurance component. Thus, in 1947, Saskatchewan introduced public hospital insurance, and, to varying degrees, British Columbia and Alberta followed in rapid succession. Newfoundland also had some form of public health insurance when it entered Confederation in 1949. With the support of a majority of provinces, which by this time included Ontario, the House of Commons unanimously enacted the *Hospital Insurance and Diagnostic Services Act, 1957* (HIDSA).

To qualify for federal cost sharing under the 1957 legislation, provincial plans had to cover each provincial resident on uniform terms and conditions, provide for specified diagnostic services, and limit co-insurance or "deterrent" charges so as to avoid placing an excessive financial burden on patients. All provinces had agreed to join the federal plan by 1961.

The introduction of medicare, extending coverage to include physicians' services, was more controversial. The medical profession and the insurance industry adamantly opposed it. Saskatchewan again took the lead, by introducing a universal model in the early 1960s and urging federal support. But this time governments in Alberta, British Columbia, and Ontario were initially opposed, at least in part because they preferred a system of private health insurance for the majority of the population. In 1965 the federal government opted for the universal model of public health care pioneered in Saskatchewan. It undertook to cover half the costs of provincial expenses for physicians' services, although at the July 1965 federal-provincial conference the prime minister suggested that this need not be a formal cost-sharing arrangement, as was in place for hospital insurance. Following intergovernmental negotiations, the *Medical Care Act* of 1966 did, however, include a formal cost-sharing mechanism. For provinces to qualify for their share of federal financial support, they had to meet several conditions. Their medical plans had to provide for: administration and operation on a non-profit basis by a public authority; coverage of "all services rendered by medical practitioners that are medically required"; universal coverage of all provincial residents (at least 95 percent of eligible population) on equal terms and conditions; and portability of benefits. There are doubts as to whether "access" was viewed then as a co-equal fifth principle or condition, but the federal legislation did explicitly require that insured persons not be charged fees that might impede or preclude "reasonable access" to insured services. This provision for reasonable access was apparently intended to exclude *provincial* charges for physicians' services to patients but may not have applied to extra-billings by *physicians* that impeded or precluded reasonable access. In any case, to the extent that access may not have been a co-equal fifth principle then (the Prime Minister's speech to the July 19-20, 1965 federal-provincial conference had not treated "reasonable access" as a formal principle), it gradually evolved to that status. And despite the initial resistance of some provincial governments, all provinces had joined by 1970.

While the instrument of cost sharing was highly effective in creating a Canada-wide system of public hospital and medical insurance, it also had its downsides. Thus, by the early 1970s, the federal government had become very worried that its open-ended commitment to pay for half of provincial expenditures in a number of social programs, including hospital and medical care, was eroding its capacity to control its own expenditures. And by the mid-1970s provincial governments were also expressing frustration with the cost-sharing model, and in particular the extensive annual negotiations about eligibility issues (for example, which hospital beds were eligible for cost sharing). Provinces also argued that this form of cost-sharing was distorting their resource allocation process and priorities.

After extensive federal-provincial negotiations, a compromise emerged in the form of the *Federal-Provincial Fiscal Arrangements and Established Programs*

Financing Act, 1977. The transfers for hospital and medical services, as well as those for post-secondary education, were combined in one block grant. The initial EPF transfer was intended as an equal per capita payment to each province. Roughly half was initially paid as an equal per capita cash transfer. The other half was made available to provinces as a tax-point transfer. It included 13.5 personal income tax points and one corporate income tax point. The value of the tax points was equalized to the national average on the basis of the then prevailing federal equalization formula. In addition, levelling payments were involved. As a result, over a five-year transition period, the tax points (with equalization and levelling payments) were to be worth as much on a per capita basis to equalization-receiving provinces as they were to wealthier provinces. The federal government gained greater predictability in its financial commitment. Ottawa's cash outlays would grow according to a formula based on the rate of growth in the economy, not provincial spending. The provinces gained a reduction in federal administrative controls. Although the conditions attached to medicare remained in place, federal officials no longer had to rule on whether particular provincial expenditures were eligible for cost sharing.

Today, there is controversy as to whether the end of cost sharing in health care was "a good thing." Most of the arguments, on both sides of this issue, were understood in 1977. (See, for example, Perry 1997.) For some, the shift to block funding was "good" because it removed the federal government from the business of determining the eligibility of provincial expenditures for cost sharing and auditing those expenses. This distancing was thought to be desirable because it was more respectful of provincial constitutional authority in relation to health care. For others, the shift to block funding broke the explicit link between federal cash contributions and provincial health care spending. This was perceived as "bad" because it had the potential to weaken Ottawa's ability to enforce the pan-Canadian principles associated with the hospital and medical insurance legislation (*Toronto Star,* 19 February 1977, A5). What was not anticipated then was the emergence of a serious federal-provincial dispute as to whether the federal tax-point transfer should continue to be "counted" as an ongoing federal contribution, even twenty-five years after the transfer occurred. This issue has since become a political football in the federal-provincial quarrel regarding the adequacy of the federal financial contribution to health care. And the ambiguities surrounding this question have served in recent years to confuse and obfuscate public deliberations about the adequacy of federal funding.

The early 1980s were marked by an increase in extra-billing by some doctors and facility fees by hospitals in some provinces. The federal government opposed both practices on the grounds that they prevented equal access to health care, but it lacked the legislative tools to enforce its view. Parliament therefore unanimously passed the *Canada Health Act, 1984* (CHA) to discourage such practices. The legislation amalgamated the previously separate hospital and medical insurance legislation. To qualify for federal financial support, provincial plans had to satisfy the conditions and principles set out in the 1966 legislation, including access. To facilitate enforcement of the " reasonable access" principle, the legislation also determined that such provincial charges would lead to dollar-for-dollar reductions in the federal transfer. Although all provincial governments had opposed and were angered by the legislation, they generally moved to compliance within a few years, recognizing perhaps that the federal government had broad public support for its action.

With the *Canada Health Act* on the statute books, questions arose about how it was to be interpreted and enforced. For the most part, especially after the election of a new federal government in 1984, senior officials did much of this necessary work on a cooperative intergovernmental basis behind closed doors. And by the late 1980s federal-provincial disagreements about user fees were, at least for the moment, largely on the back burner. During the 1993 election campaign, however, the federal Liberals campaigned on a platform that included the statement: We "will not accept user fees or other attempts to gut the medicare system" (Liberal Party of Canada 1993, 78). With the subsequent change in government in Ottawa and the re-emergence of the user fee issue, the interpretation and enforcement of the CHA again became contentious. And since then, the process through which the federal government has interpreted and enforced the legislation has become a serious concern of provinces in and of itself. As David Cameron and Jennifer McCrea-Logie point out in chapter 2, Ottawa is acting as both a prosecutor and judge when disagreements arise.

Had federal-provincial/territorial fiscal relations been harmonious during these years, dispute resolution might not have become such a substantive issue in intergovernmental health care relations. However, the federal government unilaterally tightened EPF and other transfers on several occasions in the 1980s and early 1990s, culminating in the 1995 announcement of a new blockfunding arrangement under the Canada Health and Social Transfer (CHST). The CHST combined EPF and CAP (the previously separate cost-sharing transfer for social welfare) into a single block transfer and substantially reduced the size of the cash transfers to provinces (beginning in 1996) relative to what the previous legislation had anticipated. The impetus for this change was overwhelmingly fiscal. The federal government found itself in an untenable deficit and debt situation and engaged in a major expenditure-reduction plan, which included, among other things, these especially large cuts in transfers to the provinces.

We discuss below the tensions that resulted from the CHST cuts. Suffice it here to note that there is today a fundamental disagreement between the two orders of government about the adequacy of the federal financial contribution to rapidly growing provincial health care budgets. Related to this are the difficulties associated with the dispute resolution process itself, in relation to both fiscal issues and policy matters. As a result, the sense of federal-provincial political partnership that was so fundamental to the early days of public health insurance has eroded badly since the early 1980s. While the Canadian public continues to believe that intergovernmental cooperation is important to the future of universal public health insurance, governments have been in an adversarial mode for at least two decades, having engaged in too little interactive decision-making on the issues that really matter (Adams 2001).

Given this level of intergovernmental conflict and misunderstanding, it is useful to reflect on how we reached the current situation and what might be done to overcome it. As an initial step in examining these matters, we return to first principles by posing two questions. What are the reasons for a government role in health care? And what is the basis for the federal government role?

CONSIDERATIONS RELATED TO THE PUBLIC ROLE IN HEALTH CARE

Two critical characteristics set many forms of health care apart from other products and services: first, the need for health care is typically uncertain; second, the risk of ill health is unevenly distributed among the population as a whole. Markets can often be established to pool risk among members of the population at large, especially when outcomes are randomly distributed among the population. But good health is not randomly distributed. Some individuals or groups of individuals have a systematically higher risk of illness than do others. Private insurance companies can therefore appropriately be expected to offer different insurance terms to persons with different levels of insurability, and those with a high risk of illness will only be insured at relatively high costs. Indeed, some people may be virtually uninsurable because their chances of becoming seriously ill are so high. Moreover, an individual's insurability can also change over time, especially with aging. Good health and illness are to a great extent determined by the luck of the draw, namely, genetic inheritance at birth.

The institution of social insurance is based on the idea that the fairest way to insure against the misfortune of having a predisposition toward bad health is by pooling this risk among all citizens. It reflects the value that individuals have some responsibility for one another and this can best be implemented through sharing this risk on a society-wide basis. Thus, the case for public health insurance is primarily based on an equity argument.

Efficiency considerations supplement the equity reasons for a public role in health care. Health care providers, especially physicians, have much better information than people who require their services. Physicians also control the supply of health care. As a result, they have a kind of monopoly power. To avoid inappropriately high prices for services a counterweight is required, and the public sector is the obvious choice. For instance, as a single-payer system, the public sector can negotiate effectively to control costs. A single-payer system is also administratively more efficient than a multi-payer system. Thus, as Banting and Boadway conclude in chapter 1, the equity case for public health insurance is supported by a powerful efficiency case.

At the same time, the logic of social insurance itself does not rule out a dual private-public system. As long as a public system is financed out of general revenues and makes health services uniformly available, the coexistence of a private system serving those who wish to opt out is not inconsistent with the principles of social insurance. Arguments to the contrary stem rather from judgments on political feasibility and the sustainability of a public system in the face of a parallel private one (Flood, Stabile, and Tuohy 2002).

The Rationale for a Federal Role in Health Care

Assuming agreement on the principle of social insurance, the question of the precise dimensions of the community within which sharing and redistribution take place still remains open. In a *unitary* nation, a common standard of redistributive equity and sharing is presumed to apply to all citizens across the country, there being no particular reason to discriminate against citizens in one region relative to those in another. In a *federation*, matters are complicated by the fact that individuals are members of two political communities – the community of citizens across the country as a whole, and the community of residents within each province. The role of the federal government, in the context of health care, is thus defined by whether one takes the entire country or the province as the primary sharing community. In this context, it is useful to distinguish, as Banting and Boadway have done in chapter 1, among three versions of the relevant sharing community along a spectrum of possibilities.

Predominantly Canada-wide Sharing

The *predominantly Canada-wide* version takes the country as a whole as the primary sharing community and defines the extent of redistribution in health care in national terms. This vision of countrywide sharing requires sufficient fiscal redistribution among regions to enable all provinces to provide levels of services up to a national average without having to resort to tax rates that are above the national average. It also requires strong, detailed countrywide standards with respect to the kinds of services and redistribution policies that should be available in all provinces. It is difficult to envisage this kind of countrywide sharing without a strong leadership role from Ottawa.

Predominantly Provincial Sharing

The *predominantly provincial* version of the sharing community reflects the idea that the province is the principal community for redistribution. In this context, one province may choose to provide a highly redistributive system of public health insurance, and another may decide to rely more on private insurance. Notwithstanding the distinct possibility of significantly different approaches among provinces, because of constitutional provisions relating to equalization, this model nevertheless preserves the possibility of provinces implementing comparable health care standards across the country if they so wish. In this case, however, the vehicle for such a decision would probably be an interprovincial pact.

Dual Sharing

An intermediate conception of the sharing community is one in which a countrywide framework defines some basic parameters of major social programs including health care, but which leaves room for provincial variation in program design and delivery mechanisms that are consistent with the framework. According to this intermediate position, which is labelled here the *dual sharing community*, citizens across the country are assured of comparable, rather than identical, health care services. The possibility of differences among regions in the sense of attachment to community also raises the possibility of asymmetrical relationships between the federal government, on the one hand, and different provincial and territorial governments, on the other.

Interestingly, most economically advanced federations in practice give substantial weight to the idea of countrywide sharing in health policy, choosing to engage both the federal government and provincial or state governments in health care (Banting and Corbett 2002). In some of these countries, the central government administers important health care programs itself, dealing directly with citizens and service providers. Moreover, where state or provincial governments manage elements of the system, they typically do so within broad parameters defined for the country as a whole and normally rely on the federal government for a significant part of their financing. These intergovernmental transfers incorporate a significant element of interregional redistribution. Although the balance between orders of government differs significantly from one federation to another, the federal government in most economically advanced federal democracies plays a much larger role than is the case in Canada (Watts 1999a).

Surveys of public attitudes and values indicate that Canadians have a sense of attachment or belonging to multiple communities, including Canada and their province. They see no reason to choose one definitively over others. Surveys also regularly find that Canadians see health care as a countrywide program, and overwhelmingly support the engagement of both orders of government in sustaining it. They are thus uneasy about cuts in federal transfers to provinces (Mendelsohn 2001). Public attitudes towards the Equalization program also suggest reasonably strong support for the idea of pan-Canadian sharing. These findings are consistent with the idea of a dual sharing community and a modified conception of social citizenship in health care.

This concept of a dual sharing community seems also to be consistent with the realities of social policy as conducted by the federal government and the provinces/territories up to the present time. In the case of health care, elements of a countrywide framework have existed for several decades. The five principles of the *Canada Health Act* and the interregional transfers embedded in our fiscal arrangements do sustain reasonably comparable standards in key health services across the country as a whole. At the same time, it also has to be recognized that in Canada interregional variation in health services is greater than in many other federations.

There is some variation across provinces in core hospital and physician services, which fall within the framework of the CHA. There are much more substantial regional differences, however, in services that fall beyond the ambit of the *Canada Health Act*, such as pharmaceutical therapy outside of hospitals and home care. Prescription drug insurance differs sharply across the country. Provincial programs tend to cover low-income senior citizens and social assistance recipients in all regions, but coverage of other citizens varies considerably. In the case of home care, although each province and territory offers some coverage, there are major differences in eligibility, the proportion of those needing care that is covered, the range of services provided, and the level of user fees. When the countrywide framework was established in the postwar decades, hospital and physician services were the core elements in health care. In the current context, however, drug therapies and home care are rapidly growing components of the sector. The fact that they also fall outside the scope of the *Canada Health Act* means that the extent of Canada-wide sharing that applies in health care is being reduced with each passing year.

The preceding discussion of different visions of the sharing community provides a perspective on the equity considerations that are relevant in defining the federal role in health care. With regard to efficiency, there are arguments for and against centralization and decentralization that are also linked to arguments for and against different forms of intergovernmental relations. On both these matters (centralization/decentralization and forms of intergovernmental relations), the arguments (addressing spillovers, exploiting economies of scale and administrative efficiencies, on the one hand, and greater ability to reflect local preferences and tastes, and greater opportunity for innovation, on the other) are nicely balanced. If the efficiency arguments pointed powerfully toward centralization and a more federally dominated federalism, or toward decentralization and a more provincially dominated federalism, they might have a major influence in defining the federal role. But given that efficiency arguments balance out, the federal role has in fact been determined mainly by the extent to which the country as a whole rather than the province is seen as the appropriate community for insuring against ill health. That is, redistributive equity considerations dominate.

At the same time, the manner in which the federal government fulfills this role can contribute to the efficiency of the federation rather than detract from it. Provincial governments (or regional authorities) are best placed to understand local needs and preferences. Having several jurisdictions involved in the design and delivery of health care services also improves the possibility of useful innovation. The efficiency advantages of decentralizing health care can therefore be best achieved by following the constitutional norms concerning the provinces' role in providing health care. Predominantly provincial sharing can be achieved with a carefully designed equalization system that attends to both the different revenue-raising abilities and the different needs of the provinces, while leaving them free to design and deliver their own programs. The dual sharing model can be achieved by establishing pan-Canadian norms in a system of block transfers from the federal government to the provinces in support of health care. Such norms, which can be arrived at with provincial participation, need not be so intrusive as to interfere unduly with the detailed aspects of efficient provincial delivery of health care. Moreover, the norms themselves might address efficiency issues such as the portability of health benefits across provincial borders. While the efficiency advantages of provincial program delivery may be harder to achieve in a predominantly Canada-wide sharing system, the intergovernmental transfers associated with such a system can be designed to mitigate any distortions in provincial resource allocation. And the conditions attached to such transfers can be established so that they leave the provinces much scope for innovation in the ways they meet the national standards within their jurisdiction.

The Choice of Federal Instruments

There are several different types of instruments that can be employed by the federal government to sustain and improve health care for Canadians. Some instruments are relevant to all versions of the sharing community, whereas others are more appropriate for a particular version of the sharing community.

Direct Federal Delivery

The main feature of direct federal provision of health insurance is that the same program would apply in all provinces. One benefit of this approach is that the efficiencies of the single-payer system would apply Canada-wide rather than at the provincial level only. The main case for direct federal provision, however, is equity-related. The country as a whole becomes the sharing community for health care, and Canadians are able to enjoy the same health care services no matter which province they live in.

This approach would represent a major departure in Canada. A federal health program such as pharmacare might survive judicial challenge if it were funded through general revenues rather than contributions or premiums. But it would also challenge deeply held political conventions about the division of powers in health care, and in operational terms it might fragment what should be an integrated and seamless system.

Direct Federal Transfers to Citizens

Canada-wide sharing objectives might also be achieved through a system of direct federal transfers to citizens. Moreover, different degrees of Canada-wide versus provincial sharing could be accomplished by co-provision of transfers by both orders of government. Such an approach has been used in other areas of social policy, such as the federal program of refundable tax credits. The question is whether this approach could sensibly be made to fit the case of health insurance.

Direct transfers to citizens could be used to introduce some incentives into the use of health services by citizens by offering, for example, only partial reimbursement of expenses incurred. One advantage over direct user fees would be that if it was offered as a government program, reimbursement might be readily tied to ability to pay. This might be a way for the federal government to actually implement a countrywide income-contingent user fee system, given that health services are provincial programs. An alternative, more direct way might be to include some proportion of health expenses as taxable benefits for income tax purposes. Yet another proposal for injecting individual incentives into health insurance that has attracted some debate is the use of so-called *Medical Savings Accounts* (Ramsay 1998; Forget, Deber, and Roos 2002).

All of these options focus to some extent on strengthening incentives to avoid abuse of the system by patients or providers. Perhaps the reason they have not played a major role in Canadian health care to date is that there is a lack of convincing evidence that the current emphasis on social insurance is in fact associated with a high level of abuse. In other words, these options could undermine the essential purpose of social insurance without sufficient offsetting benefits.

Federal Transfers to Provincial Governments

Should Canadians wish to maintain some form of dual sharing community in health care or adopt a predominantly Canada-wide sharing system, transfers to provinces are highly likely to remain a central instrument. To be effective, this approach ideally requires a clear definition of relevant standards, sufficient levels and predictability of federal funding to ensure that federal policy parameters are credible and effective, and a suitable procedure for resolving disputes between the federal government and the provinces. However, Canada has never fully met this ideal and has over time fallen further away from some aspects of it.

It is useful to distinguish between the level, form, and predictability of the federal transfer. The moral and political authority of the federal government to sustain a meaningful countrywide framework through the CHA is clearly correlated with the level of its financial commitment. The federal government has to be a serious financial partner to be credible. Moreover, the more exacting the countrywide framework, the greater the level of federal support presumably needed.

As for form, it is doubtful that a return to cost sharing as existed under the federal hospital insurance and medical care legislations is the best way forward. Given past experience, that traditional form of cost sharing would presumably apply to aggregate provincial expenditures rather than to expenditures of individual provinces. Even in that case, however, the federal government would have to determine the eligibility of provincial expenditures for cost sharing, and this process would necessarily therefore reintroduce administrative complexities and costs and add to potential intergovernmental frictions. The advantages of this approach over a simple increase in the block transfer are doubtful, although we recognize that some form of cost sharing might initially play a role if the coverage of the CHA were to be broadened.

There are some within the federal government and elsewhere who would prefer to make any further increases in the federal CHST contribution conditional on achieving specific health reform goals, whether related to primary care reform, home care improvements, hospital rationalization, or some other chosen objective. There will be others in provinces and elsewhere who wish to see larger federal transfers for health care but only within the framework of the current broadly defined set of conditions. The second group considers block funding to be the appropriate form of transfer in our federation, as it leaves provinces with the freedom to assume their constitutional responsibilities within the parameters of the CHA. To the extent that this debate is joined, a possible compromise approach worth pursuing is the earmarked transfer; that is, new federal funding to be spent exclusively by provinces for certain designated health care reforms, but with the earmarking for a limited time only (say five years) and the increased funding subsequently being folded into the block fund.

The predictability of federal support is also a crucial issue. As in the case of interpersonal trust, nurturing intergovernmental trust requires transparency and predictability in relationships. Given the propensity of the federal government to make unilateral changes to the transfer system, the case for an automatic escalator that bases growth in the CHST on a formula rather than on federal discretion is strong. Possible escalators include those based on economic indicators such as GDP growth or the rate of growth in all or some federal revenue bases. The escalator that may make the most sense, however, is the rate of growth in health care spending for all provinces and territories, as measured by Statistics Canada. If the two orders of government were able to agree on an appropriate federal contribution at a point in time, and then have it grow based on such an indicator, then the federal share would remain constant (and without the intrusiveness of traditional federal cost sharing). We refer to this approach as "non-traditional cost sharing".

Other proposals focus primarily on making the federal contribution more visible by separating the block transfer for health from those for social assistance and post-secondary education. The main argument in favour of this reform is that a separate transfer would enhance the transparency and visibility of the federal role in health care. At the same time, such a transfer would remain fully fungible in the hands of the provinces.

At the other end of the spectrum are proposals that would reduce the commitment to a Canada-wide system by converting the CHST into a straight tax-point transfer to the provinces. This approach makes most sense under a predominantly provincial conception of the sharing community. It would thus entail an end to Canada-wide norms except in the unlikely event of an interprovincial pact to maintain and enforce them (Courchene 1996).

Equalization Considerations

To the extent that the federal government continues to make transfer payments to the provinces through an equal per capita CHST-like instrument, these payments will have the effect of equalizing fiscal resources available to the provinces. The CHST is funded from general revenues, and wealthier provinces pay more per capita into general revenues than less affluent provinces. The result is a redistribution that favours the less wealthy regions and thus helps to reinforce the Equalization program.

These forms of revenue equalization alone, however, do not satisfy fully the principle of equalization as set out in section 36(2) of the Constitution (see chapter 1 for a more detailed discussion). Although revenue equalization goes part way toward enabling provinces to provide reasonably comparable levels of public services at reasonably comparable levels of taxation, provinces may also face different "needs" for public services. In the case of health care, there is a systematic difference in the costs of providing services to persons of different ages and other socio-economic characteristics. It can therefore be argued that some or all of the federal Equalization payments should be adjusted to reflect needs. And with regard to the CHST, it can also argued that needs ought to be taken into account in its allocation. Needs equalization could be based on the cost of a national standard level of care for different demographic groups, where the costs could represent some average of actual provincial costs. As with revenue equalization, the idea would be to base the entitlement to needs-based equalization on objective measures that are outside the direct control of the recipient provinces.

FEDERAL-PROVINCIAL POLITICAL DISPUTES RELATING TO HEALTH CARE

The current federal-provincial dispute regarding the adequacy of federal funding for health care was triggered by the CHST announcement in the 1995 federal budget. That debate is familiar. It is sufficient here to note that from the outset the provinces have argued that the cuts in transfers associated with the CHST were grossly unfair. And since the late 1990s they have also insisted that a vertical fiscal imbalance favouring Ottawa has come to characterize federal-provincial fiscal relations.

Despite subsequent increases in federal CHST contributions, provinces remain of the view that the current amount of federal cash transfers for health, post-secondary education, and social assistance and services is neither adequate nor fair.

The substance of the provincial position on vertical fiscal imbalance has been stated in various documents prepared by the provincial and territorial finance ministers. Their argument is simple. First, the structure of federal finances today is stronger than that of the provinces and territories. The federal government enjoys substantial and recurrent budgetary surpluses; provinces and territories do not. Second, federal revenues are expected to grow faster than those of the provinces and territories, given the extent to which the two orders of governments occupy the different tax bases. Third, provincial and territorial expenditures can be expected to increase at a more rapid pace than Ottawa's. This is in part because of the relative importance that the public attaches to provincial programs such as health care and education and the cost drivers associated with them, especially health care (Standing Senate Committee on Social Affairs, Science and Technology 2001b).

The issue of vertical fiscal imbalance has also received much attention in Quebec. In 2001 the Government of Quebec formed the Commission on Fiscal Imbalance, headed by Yves Séguin. In order to restore fiscal balance and eliminate the use of the federal spending power, the Commission recommended an end to CHST, and proposed that the federal government transfer the GST to the provinces. It also recommended several improvements to Equalization (Commission of Fiscal Imbalance 2002).

The federal government has all along disputed provincial arguments, citing several considerations. First, public debt is much higher at the federal than the provincial level. Second, both orders of government have access to all the major tax bases and can set their own tax rates. Third, provinces have been simultaneously cutting taxes and claiming revenue shortages. Fourth, federal cash transfers to provinces are expected to grow at a faster rate (6.1 percent) between 2000/01 and 2005/06 than federal revenues (1.9 percent) over the same period. The federal government's general response to provincial arguments is that fiscal imbalance is a "myth" (Privy Council of Canada 2002). (For a more detailed analysis of vertical fiscal imbalance and the related concept of vertical fiscal gap, see Lazar, St-Hilaire, and Tremblay's discussion in chapter 3.)

The dispute regarding the adequacy of federal funding is compounded by disagreements between Ottawa and some provinces over the appropriateness of various forms of private funding for services covered by the *Canada Health Act*. With the federal government opposed to this source of financing, provinces that favour this approach find themselves doubly frustrated. They believe not only that the federal government is contributing insufficiently to health care but also that Ottawa is effectively depriving them of other potential funding sources. Moreover, they contest the federal government's exclusive power, *de jure*, to interpret and enforce the provisions of the CHA. This long-standing issue recently resurfaced on the agenda and led to the introduction of a new dispute avoidance and resolution process by the federal minister of health that reflects ideas that provincial governments have been advocating.

The Issue of Dispute Resolution

Conflict and cooperation are inevitable in federal systems, and their consequences can be noxious or beneficial depending on the circumstances. An indicator of a mature form of government is its capacity to challenge non-beneficial cooperation, to accommodate useful conflict, and to resolve disputes that impede the effective functioning of the system. The importance of a dispute settlement mechanism in a particular policy field such as health depends on the tenor of intergovernmental relations more generally. *Dispute avoidance* is most likely to be an attractive option when the parties involved have shared policy goals and are engaged in a relationship characterized by a high level of trust and ongoing dialogue and negotiation. Parties may need to resort to formal and informal *dispute resolution* approaches when they have entrenched disagreements and when considerations of turf, status, credit-claiming, and blame avoidance take precedence over substantive policy concerns.

Canada has historically lacked an effective dispute resolution mechanism in the health care field. Instead, it has relied on a system of intergovernmental relations that is weakly institutionalized, with no decision-making rules and no settled processes for tackling the resolution of disputes. Ottawa has used its spending power to uphold national standards in health care in areas of provincial jurisdiction that it could not directly regulate, given constitutional requirements. The provinces have protested that Ottawa does not transfer sufficient resources to them to give it the moral and political authority it needs to encourage them to uphold CHA principles over the long term. Thus, at least as seen from the provincial perspective, the crux of the conflict has been the hierarchy implicit in the unilateral federal control over health care funding and over enforcement of the CHA conditions.

We do not question the legal right of the federal government to determine the amount of revenues it transfers to the provinces or to determine the conditions associated with such transfers. But the federal-provincial relationship in respect of health care is not mainly legal; it is political. And when Ottawa acts unilaterally on such matters it erodes the trust that is essential to a functional political partnership. In this regard, we acknowledge that, over the years, the relationship between Health Canada and the provincial health ministries in respect of *Canada Health Act* interpretation and enforcement has been mainly collegial. The record shows a history of collaboration and quiet, effective conflict management that has served Canadians well. However, for issues that cannot be resolved in that way, a formal dispute resolution mechanism would be beneficial, since it could provide a channel for easing tensions in the health and fiscal systems when intergovernmental disputes break out at the political level.

In a federal state, one's view of the sharing community is likely to shape one's conception of the appropriate site for authoritative decision-making in the health care field and therefore structures one's understanding about how conflicts and disputes can most appropriately be resolved. If, for example, Canada is understood as composed of predominantly provincial sharing communities, where the federal government withdraws substantially from the health care field, there would be fewer points of conflict between the two orders of government because there would be fewer points of contact. Hence, the absence of an explicit dispute settlement mechanism would not be felt as a significant institutional lack. If Canada is understood as composed of dual sharing communities in which both federal and provincial governments have equal status and equally valid roles and responsibilities, then a dispute settlement process that respects the authority and autonomy of the two orders of government is appropriate. In the predominantly Canada-wide sharing community, where the Government of Canada emerges as the dominant authoritative decision-maker, the model logically calls for a well-developed dispute settlement mechanism, since the relationship between the two orders of government is intense. Nevertheless, the practical reality is that Canada is weakly endowed with such mechanisms in the health care field. This may be in part because the federal government has doubted the benefits of an impartial, equitable dispute settlement mechanism to govern its relationship with the provinces – and it has had the power to avoid it. It may also be because the federal government has objected to the idea of another order of government being involved in the interpretation of federal law and deciding on the appropriateness of federal expenditures.

In some respects, this situation is similar to that which applies to Canada's trade relations with the United States. Canada prefers to have a legal basis for resolving trade disputes because if disputes are settled mainly through the exercise of raw power, then Canada is not likely to fare well very often. For similar reasons, provinces may have a somewhat stronger interest in a formal dispute resolution mechanism in respect of health care than does Ottawa because of disparities in power.

In other respects, however, the analogy with the United States is less appropriate. The American and Canadian governments have obligations to different groups of citizens, whereas Canadian federal, provincial, and territorial governments (collectively) have the same constituents. The two orders of government do therefore have an incentive to cooperate in establishing a dispute resolution mechanism in order to avoid the many unproductive and destructive traps that can stall and jeopardize intergovernmental agreements that are designed to serve these constituents.

Ideally, an "effective" dispute resolution mechanism in this field would meet the criteria proposed by Cameron and McCrea-Logie in chapter 2. It would be authoritative; hence the public and the disputing governments would accept its pronouncements as definitive and legitimate. It would be compatible with values of federalism, since it would recognize that both orders of government have constitutional status and have their own competences and policy-making capacities. Both orders of government would agree to participate in the design of the dispute mechanism, choose representatives to be a part of the body, and follow its procedures to bring an end to the destructive conflicts that sometimes impede the proper functioning of the health care system. It would be guided by clear rules, be perceived as transparent and impartial, and be accessible to all those who have a legitimate interest in the outcomes. It would also facilitate clear, efficacious, and timely settlement of a broad range of disputes, including those regarding federal fiscal transfers, since, as we have seen, this is an area where disagreements have been particularly intense.

Cameron and McCrea-Logie describe six dispute settlement models, organized from the least to the most highly developed:

> Model 1, *federal withdrawal,* is consistent with the notion of predominantly provincial sharing communities and envisions Ottawa transferring tax room to the provinces, abrogating the *Canada Health Act,* and leaving it to the provinces to manage the health care system in accordance with the aspirations of their regional communities. This model would address the problem of destructive intergovernmental disputes by reducing the extent to which the two orders of government are in relationship with each other.

> Model 2, the *base-case model,* is the status quo situation where no explicit conflict resolution regime applies to the fiscal and policy dimensions of the intergovernmental relationship. By most standards of conflict resolution, it would be judged deficient on several grounds: the relationship between the actors is paternalistic rather than egalitarian; only one party has recourse to the instrument; one of the parties acts as both prosecutor and judge; as a consequence, the process and the decisions, while they may be effective, are not regarded as legitimate by all of the government participants.

> Model 3, the *Social Union Framework Agreement,* seeks to place the conflictual and cooperative behaviour of governments in an orderly frame of reference and to expose both forms of conduct to the fuller scrutiny of the public. Its provisions for dispute avoidance and resolution outlined in section 6 of the agreement are clearly intended to apply to the broad range of intergovernmental social policy matters, and not just to a particular program. The scope explicitly includes federal transfers. Although the provisions refer to dispute avoidance, fact-finding, mediation, third-party involvement, and public reporting, the details are not developed.

> Model 4, the *McLellan dispute settlement process,* encourages the two orders of government to avoid disputes and, in cases where they do not, makes provisions for a third-party panel to release a public report with recommendations for resolving disputes. However, it does not fundamentally alter the play of intergovernmental forces, since the panel's report would be non-binding, and the federal government would retain the dominant role in enforcing the *Canada Health Act.* The procedure would be used exclusively to resolve disputes over interpretations of the *Canada Health Act;* it is not intended to apply to federal fiscal transfers.

Citizens and interest groups would be excluded as potential participants in the dispute resolution process.

> Model 5, *interlocking legislation*, an approach mooted by Richard Zuker, effectively ties together the policy and fiscal components of the intergovernmental health care regime and imposes reciprocal obligations on all the actors in the system. It envisions the parties agreeing to a funding formula for a set period of time, which could not be changed without the approval of a certain number of provinces, and the provincial and territorial governments passing the equivalent of the CHA, with the provision that the legislation could not be amended without federal government approval. This model clearly reflects the underlying philosophy of dual sharing communities, in which representatives of the two orders of government find the means to work together on the basis of equality.

> Model 6, *bringing the public in*, suggested by Richard Simeon, involves the creation of a jointly appointed advisory body, the Canadian Health Care Commission, which would review the federal government's decisions to withhold funds for CHA violations before they could go into effect. Similarly, no provincial health care legislation with significant implications for other provinces or for the national system as a whole could go into effect without the commission's review. The public would have the opportunity to be involved in its hearings and deliberations and could scrutinize its recommendations. The advantage of this model is that it would elevate the quality and expand the scope of public debate. Moreover, it would focus greater attention on citizens' needs in their health care system, and less on political considerations.

A shift to a federal-provincial partnership approach would involve all parties assuming joint responsibility for the functioning of the system and accepting the risks and benefits that go along with it. As we discuss below, it would also involve working together to ensure that the fiscal strength of the two orders of government is relatively balanced.

The Issue of Fiscal Imbalance

The larger political dispute between the two orders of government relates to the magnitude of federal cash transfers for provincial health care programs. This issue is linked in turn to the broader question of whether there is indeed a vertical fiscal imbalance that favours the federal government, and to related concerns from less affluent provinces about horizontal imbalances. The concept of vertical fiscal imbalance entails the idea that one order of government has more revenue than it requires relative to its expenditure responsibilities, whereas the other order of government has less. To turn this concept into an operational tool for assessing whether the current allocation of revenues between the two orders of government is appropriate, it is necessary to form a view about the weight to be attached to their respective expenditure responsibilities. Since such a weighting task is value-laden, a largely political, rather than scientific, element necessarily attaches to the idea of vertical fiscal imbalance. Thus, it is not surprising that there are divided views within the research community about whether – and to what extent – a vertical fiscal imbalance now exists in Canada.

In this regard, over recent years, three major studies have been published that purport to document or disprove the existence of a vertical fiscal imbalance in the Canadian federation. In chapter 3 Harvey Lazar, France St-Hilaire, and Jean-François Tremblay carefully review these analyses. It is important to note that these studies differ in their conclusions; two argue that a vertical fiscal imbalance now exists, whereas the third makes a different assessment. And the two studies that argue that such an imbalance exists differ significantly from one another in their estimates. Although all three studies take as given the taxation and expenditure structure in place in the base year and assume steady economic growth and no policy change, they differ significantly in their treatment of interest payments on the debt and in their definition of fiscal imbalance. The variation in the results is also due in large part to the different assumptions made about the rate of growth of particular revenue sources and spending categories in projecting the fiscal balances of both orders of government over a twenty-year horizon. Of course, the results of long-term fiscal projections such as these are only of limited value, since governments must adjust to both economic and fiscal circumstances on an ongoing basis. This means that the relative fiscal position of the two orders of government in any given year is inevitably the outcome of cumulative fiscal effects and adjustments over time and therefore may not necessarily constitute a firm basis from which to assess what the situation might be in the future.

Indeed, a retrospective look at the relative strength of federal and provincial fiscal balances over several decades reveals a pattern of ebb and flow with important consequences for intergovernmental fiscal relations, which have been in a constant state of flux. As a result, it is not clear that a state of vertical fiscal balance was ever achieved that could reasonably be seen as a benchmark or standard to be attained. For instance, coming out of the Second World War, the federal financial position was stronger than that of the provinces, notwithstanding large accumulated war-time debts. Ottawa chose not to give up the revenue bases it had occupied during the war. Instead, among other things, it used its fiscal power, through cost-sharing transfers, to encourage provinces to create or expand provincial programs for health care, post-secondary education, and social assistance and services. The growth in federal transfer payments to the provinces did not necessarily improve provincial finances, however, as provinces were concurrently assuming major new expenditure responsibilities. In retrospect, it can be argued that the relatively strong federal fiscal position of the early postwar decades was used to help provide Canadians with the kind of economic and social security that they wanted at the time. During this period, governments created the modern welfare state to ensure that there would be no return to the massive hardships of the Great Depression.

But by the 1970s Ottawa had become increasingly concerned that, as a result of cost sharing, provincial expenditure decisions were determining too much of its own spending. As was discussed above, this situation helped to motivate EPF. And although both orders of government encountered fiscal difficulties in the early 1980s, at that time the federal position was by far the weaker. If there was a vertical fiscal imbalance then, it favoured the provinces. Thus, the tide had shifted.

Ottawa's deteriorating financial position led in turn to several increases in federal taxes and a growing emphasis on expenditure restraint through the 1980s and early 1990s, including substantial cuts in planned levels of transfer payments to provinces. Following the implementation of the 1995 federal budget measures and a return to a more favourable fiscal environment (in terms of economic growth and interest rates), the federal government was able to turn the fiscal corner, and by the end of the century Ottawa was once again in a strong financial position relative to the provinces. All of this is to say that the current fiscal strength of the federal government relative to the provinces follows a period in which their positions were reversed on two occasions.

Based on their analysis of these fiscal trends in chapter 3, Lazar, St-Hilaire and Tremblay conclude that, whether or not the term "vertical fiscal imbalance" is used to characterize the current situation, there are good grounds to be publicly debating alternative uses of the substantial federal surplus. Should it be used to pay down federal debt or reduce taxes? Should it be used to enhance spending on children, on the military, or on other forms of security? Or should it be used to improve health care in partnership with the provinces?

Calculating the Federal Share of Health Care Funding

The latter question in turn leads to two related queries and long-standing objects of dispute. How much is the federal government now contributing annually to the provinces for health? And how much should it be contributing? Although the second question involves normative judgments, the first question, at least at first blush, appears simple. As was demonstrated in chapter 4, however, the answer to both queries is anything but simple. To understand why this is so, we need to look again at some of the history of the federal role in funding health care, including the controversy as to whether the federal tax transfer to the provinces in 1977 can and should be reasonably counted as part of the current federal contribution.

During the first year of EPF, the notional value of the federal cash transfer for health, as a share of total provincial health expenditures, has been estimated by Lazar, St-Hilaire, and Tremblay at 26 percent (see chapter 4). While the federal share at that transition point (1977) may not have been "fair" based on some objective measure of fairness, it did reflect thirty years of intergovernmental bargaining that dated back to the federal government's postwar planning. From this perspective, therefore, a federal cash contribution equal to 26 percent of total provincial health care spending would have some rationale. It is, however, a much larger percentage than Ottawa's recent contribution and also well beyond what provinces are now demanding. In fact, provinces have argued that Ottawa should now be paying an amount in cash (or equivalency) equal to its cash share of provincial costs for health care, post-secondary education, and social assistance and services in 1994/95, the year just prior to the announcement of CHST. According to provincial governments, the federal share in that year was 18 percent. For health care alone, Lazar, St-Hilaire, and Tremblay have estimated the federal share at 16 percent. This is another possible benchmark for the federal cash contribution. In short, the 26 percent and 16 percent figures might be considered an appropriate maximum-minimum range for the federal contribution to provincial health care programs.

As for reckoning how much of provincial health care costs Ottawa is currently bearing with its CHST cash contribution, this calculation entails a number of steps. The first involves forming a view about what percentage of CHST cash can reasonably be attributed to health care. On this matter, unfortunately, there are at least five possible perspectives. These differing perspectives were laid out in chapter 4 and are not repeated here. As Lazar et al. point out, however, only three of them can be used as a way of estimating the number of federal dollars directed to provincial health care programs. Based on these three perspectives, the estimated health component of CHST cash varies quite considerably. The results are 43 percent, 50 percent, and 68 percent, respectively. If we then apply these percentages to the $18.3 billion spent on CHST for 2001/02, we generate estimates of the federal contribution ranging from 11.6 to 18.2 percent of the $68 billion in provincial health care spending in that year (see chapter 4, Table 3). The key conclusion from this analysis of different, and each partially valid, perspectives is that under the current transfer system *there is no single or correct number that objectively represents the federal CHST cash contribution for health*. Thus a number close to halfway between the high and low of these percentages — that is, 15 percent, or around $10 billion for 2001/02 — is adopted as "no worse than any other estimate." It is used as the starting point in discussing federal finance options for the future.

A number of other observations that flow from the analysis of the federal financial contribution to health care in chapter 4 and are central to our overall message are summarized here. First, there is clearly an imbalance between the federal government's cash contribution to provincial health care and the amount of policy influence it seeks to exert. The 15 percent federal cash share is low relative to previous levels of federal support and clearly low also in relation to the influence Ottawa seeks to exercise.

Second, there is a need to secure intergovernmental agreement on what would constitute a "fair" federal contribution to provincial health care. Unless the parties agree on what Ottawa's share of provincial health care spending actually is, what it should be, and also how it is to be measured, within months of a new fiscal arrangement, provinces will claim the new federal cash contribution is too small and the federal government will argue the opposite. In that event, the best that can be hoped for is a series of brief ceasefires in an ongoing federal-provincial fiscal quarrel.

Third, there is a disconnect between the expressed public desire for federal-provincial cooperation on public health insurance, on the one hand, and the way in which the federal government has made decisions regarding its financial contribution, on the other. The cost-sharing agreements of the 1950s and 1960s, as well as the 1977 EPF arrangements, were the result of prolonged and often difficult federal-provincial dialogue and negotiations. They were not arbitrarily and unilaterally imposed by the federal government. Since the early 1980s, however, we have seen much more unilateralism ("take it or leave it") on Ottawa's part.

This last point is related to the issue of predictability of funding and the absence of built-in growth provisions (escalator) for federal transfers. Under current law, the size of the CHST is set year by year until 2006 but with no indication as to what is to come after 2006. Nor is there a set of principles that would guide the provinces as to what they might expect. This uncertainty regarding the longer-term federal contribution unnecessarily complicates the task of the provinces (and hospitals) in long-range planning at a time when major health care reforms are required.

Fifth, the current intergovernmental impasse regarding health care financing and how to calculate the federal contribution erodes the quality of Canadian governance. The public has no idea how much Ottawa contributes to provincial health care because of the multiplicity of ways of calculating the contribution. Transparency is absent and accountability is confused.

Given these observations, the normative question about what amount the federal government *should* be contributing to the provinces for health care remains. In answering this question we draw a distinction between what might be an appropriate federal contribution under current *Canada Health Act* conditions and what might be appropriate in the event of more substantial provisions that limit the flexibility of the provinces and impose additional costs on them. As indicated in chapter 4, under current conditions, a 20 percent figure strikes us as a reasonable and politically sustainable compromise. In making this judgment, we take account of the fact that this percentage is much closer to the 25 percent figure notionally associated with the 1977 EPF cash transfer and that the tax room transferred at that time was expected to grow at a faster rate than GNP. The 20 percent benchmark also appears to exceed current provincial demands, although whether it would do so in practice would also depend on the growth in federal cash transfers for post-secondary education and social assistance and services, including early childhood development.

There would be a stronger case for setting the federal contribution above the 20 percent figure if the conditions attached to the transfer were to become more restrictive on the provinces (even if they were to agree to these conditions). Moving toward, or even to, a 25 percent benchmark might be appropriate in that situation. At the same time, other factors might come into consideration in deciding on the "right" number. For example, direct federal spending on health research and health information, and on public health, should have pay-offs in terms of the improved quality and efficiency of Canada's health care systems. It can be argued that these kinds of federal spending should be taken into account in any negotiation of the benchmark federal financial contribution to provincial health care. Similarly, consideration would also need to be given to the relevance of federal expenditures on Aboriginal health.

In summary, a 20-25 percent federal cash contribution strikes us as reasonable, given the large tax transfer from Ottawa to the provinces in 1977. The financial implications of a federal contribution within this range are significant, as shown in Table 1.

Assuming a federal cash contribution in this range (and, as will be discussed below, there are financing options that do not entail continued cash transfers), the question of an escalator arises. An escalator should have the following characteristics. First, it should provide provinces with a reasonable measure of predictability regarding the growth in transfers. Second, it should be set out in law and be based on an indicator that is expected to grow at a rate similar to the anticipated growth rate in Canada-wide health care costs. Third, if the trend in the rate of growth in provincial health care costs changes, then, with appropriate notice (say two or three years), it should be possible to adjust the escalator. Fourth, the legislation should allow Ottawa a necessary degree of flexibility in the face of an unexpected financial crisis.

There may be some within the federal government who will be concerned that an escalator with the above characteristics would weaken Ottawa's capacity to control the growth of its expenditures. Given the federal government's long experience with deficits, such a concern is understandable. Yet, if Ottawa chooses to continue to participate as a player in setting Canada-wide health care policy, it seems only reasonable that it assume some of the related financial risks. Provinces would still have a considerable interest in managing health costs effi-

Table 1

SCENARIOS FOR THE FEDERAL CONTRIBUTION TO PROVINCIAL HEALTH CARE, 2001/02

Federal Share of Provincial Health Care Costs	Under Current CHA Conditions - 20 percent	Under More Demanding CHA Conditions - Up to 25 percent
Required federal contribution	$14 billion	$14.5-$17 billion
Additional federal contribution in 2001/02 above notional $10 billion in CHST health cash	$4 billion	$4.5-$7 billion

Source: Based on authors' calculations in chapter 4.

ciently, given that, under all conceivable fiscal arrangements, provinces would pay the lion's share of costs.

It also seems clear that the federal government is worried that further increases in federal transfers may do too little to improve either the quality of care or the fiscal sustainability of provincial health care systems. The concern is that the additional funds will flow in large measure into the compensation package of current health care providers without contributing to the health care reforms that provinces are trying to achieve but are having political difficulty putting in place. To reduce this risk, further federal funding should be accompanied by other actions that enhance the probability that provinces will be successful in their reform efforts. In particular, Ottawa has extensive research, communications, and political resources that can be mobilized to help provinces overcome resistance to needed change. We recognize that it may be easier for the federal government to create these political partnerships with some provincial governments than with others.

The federal government has, in recent years, made some of its transfers to the provinces conditional on certain end uses, such as the purchases of particular categories of equipment. It would not be surprising if Ottawa were to try to insist that future transfer increases also be earmarked for specific purposes, such as primary care reform. To the extent that this is done, it would be preferable if such special purpose funds were designated for their stated purposes for a limited time period only, say five years, and then were folded into the general transfer for health care. This could be a useful middle ground between conditional and unconditional transfers.

OPTIONS FOR THE FUTURE

How does the normative analysis presented above inform decisions to be made regarding the future of Canadian health care? In this regard, there are two sets of variables that need to be considered. One relates to whether the scope of Canada's countrywide universal publicly insured and administered health care system is to be expanded to include services that are not currently covered. We describe the case in which the health system might be broadened to cover items like prescription drugs and home care as the *transformation* scenario. We distinguish it from the *maintenance* scenario, where future reforms would focus more on improving the quality of care and the fiscal sustainability of currently insured hospital and medical services. If the scope of coverage is expanded, the political and fiscal dynamics will change markedly.

The second set of variables has to do with one's views on the different conceptions of the sharing community described earlier. There is no objective basis for asserting that any one of these is intrinsically superior to the other. While each has advantages and disadvantages relative to the other, deciding among them is much more a matter of societal consensus about values than it is about technical merit. What is relevant here, of course, is that each of these conceptions has significantly different implications for federal funding, with the largest difference being between the predominantly provincial sharing community and the other two models.

Taking account of these two sets of variables, the following points highlight key elements of the federal financing options outlined in chapter 4.

> While a continuation of block funding with an equal per capita cash transfer for health care is appropriate under both the dual sharing and the predominantly Canada-wide sharing models of the federation, a revenue-sharing arrangement or tax transfer makes more sense in the predominantly provincial sharing model.

> Under the predominantly provincial version of the sharing community, the conditions of the *Canada Health Act* should be dropped except for

those related to portability and mobility. The current CHA conditions (or an appropriately modernized version of them), are consistent with the other two models. Indeed, in the Canada-wide sharing version, the conditions would need to be buttressed with countrywide standards to assure similar levels of services across the country.

> In the case of a maintenance scenario the federal cash transfer should be equal to at least 20 percent of provincial health care costs. The transfer should be closer to 25 percent in the Canada-wide sharing model, where more substantial countrywide conditions add to provincial costs. This option would entail increases in the federal contribution in the order of $3.6-$7 billion annually. For the predominantly provincial sharing model, the appropriate shift of resources would be at the bottom end of this range or slightly lower, as provinces would have fewer costs and constraints associated with a conditional federal transfer.

> In options that entail a continued cash transfer, there are more advantages than disadvantages in having a separate block fund for health care alone – a Canada Health Transfer (CHT). In any case, assuming that the federal cash contribution is re-based at 20-25 percent of provincial health care expenses, it would be very desirable for the federal government to do away with the notion that the 1977 tax room transfer under EPF remains a part of current CHST funding for health care.

> In options that entail continued cash transfers, there is also a strong case for adjusting the equal per capita payment on the basis of need. The same case can also be made, but less strongly, in the event of revenue sharing or of a tax transfer.

> The transformation scenario would entail several billion dollars of additional public expenditure. The actual magnitude of the increase would depend on the scope of coverage. Given provincial views about the adequacy of current federal cash contributions for hospital and medical costs, it is probable that the federal government would have to commit to cover all, or almost all, of the incremental costs to secure provincial agreement to a much-broadened range of publicly insured health services. While one or more provinces might initially prefer not to participate in the broadened coverage and instead seek financial compensation, the prospects of achieving full provincial and territorial participation may be significant, given that Ottawa would be absorbing most of the additional costs.

> The transformation scenario might be facilitated by the kind of inter-locking federal and provincial legislation referred to above. Fiscal arrangements would be buttressed by statutory commitments not to alter the federal financial commitment without the approval of seven provinces representing at least one-half of the Canadian population. All provinces would pass Canadian health care provisions in provincial statutes, committing themselves to meet countrywide conditions and undertaking not to amend these commitments without the agreement of the federal government.

> Where a cash transfer is the preferred option, it should increase annu-ally according to a transparent and predictable formula (escalator) that is expected to grow at a rate similar to the anticipated growth rate in national per capita health care costs. Using a Statistics Canada index of aggregate provincial and territorial health care costs is the simplest way to meet this standard. There should be an "escape clause" for the feder-al government in cases of national financial emergency.

SUMMARY AND CONCLUSIONS

Our main conclusions are summarized below.

(1) The primary rationale for government involvement in health care arises from the uncertainty of health care needs for any one individual at any point in time coupled with the uneven incidence of illness and injury. People want to insure against these risks. For some, however, private health insurance is either prohibitively expensive or simply unavailable. This cre-ates a strong social insurance rationale for a public role.

(2) The rationale for the federal role in health care is related to the idea of Canada as sharing community. There are different conceptions of the Canadian sharing community and each has different implications in terms of the relative roles of the federal and provincial governments in social shar-ing, including in their provision of health care. The federal role is deter-mined mainly by the extent to which the country as a whole, or the individual province, is seen as the relevant community for insuring against the risks of ill health. Determining what constitutes the appropriate com-munity for social-sharing purposes is a matter of societal values, not scien-

tific principle. At present, in the case of health care in Canada, we have a dual sharing community. As the relative importance of services not covered by the *Canada Health Act* grows, however, countrywide sharing declines in importance relative to province-based sharing.

(3) A predominantly Canada-wide vision of sharing would entail ensuring that common health care services, provided according to common standards, were available in all provinces and territories. A predominantly provincial sharing community model does not require that any services be insured on a countrywide basis. It does, however, require that all provinces have adequate fiscal capacity to provide some given basket of health care services on a Canada-wide basis at comparable levels of taxation, if they so choose. A dual sharing community includes elements of both Canada-wide sharing and provincial sharing.

(4) While the case for public and federal involvement in health care relates mainly to equity considerations, the manner in which the federal government fulfills its role can contribute to the efficiency of the federation (for example, by removing barriers to mobility). Under the three visions of the sharing community outlined above, there are efficiency advantages in retaining provincial delivery (such as the ability to reflect local conditions and preferences and a greater potential for innovation). These advantages are consistent with the constitutional division of powers.

(5) There is a range of instruments through which the federal government can fulfill its role. While the choice of instruments will be affected by the societal consensus on sharing, under all versions of the sharing community there is a strong case for equalization payments. Such instruments include direct federal delivery (which on the whole we consider to be unwise), transfers to individuals (possibly through the tax system), transfers to provinces, revenue sharing, and tax-point transfers. Federal transfers to provinces have been a key instrument in the past and are likely to remain so under dual sharing and Canada-wide sharing models. If Canadians prefer a predominantly provincial model of sharing, revenue sharing is an attractive instrument.

(6) The adequacy of the federal financial contribution to Canada-wide health care is a matter of dispute between the two orders of government, as is the broader question of fiscal imbalance. In our judgment, the structure of federal public finances is at present stronger than that of almost all provinces

and territories. This has been the case since the late 1990s. In the preceding couple of decades, the opposite was true. These shifts are integral to the history of Canadian federalism. They occur with changing economic circumstances and the evolving revenue and expenditure policies of both orders of government.

(7) The prospect of ongoing fiscal dividends at the federal level and ever-rising health care costs at the provincial and territorial level inevitably raises issues of resource allocation. This in turn, however, opens up a much larger debate regarding appropriate debt levels, tax burdens, and other competing claims on the public purse. Improving the federal financial contribution to provincial and territorial health care programs and expanding the coverage of Canada-wide health care services under the *Canada Health Act* are two options that merit careful consideration in this broader public debate.

(8) There is at present an imbalance between the role the federal government appears to want to play in respect of the Canada-wide dimensions of health care and the magnitude of its financial contribution. The federal government simply contributes insufficient funding to sustain the ability and right to play the role it has historically played. Assuming we are correct about Ottawa's wish to sustain its role, the federal contribution needs to be re-based through a process of federal-provincial/territorial negotiation. We consider a fair federal contribution to be in the order of 20-25 percent of provincial costs based on factors discussed above. Ottawa should also share more fully in the fiscal and political risks associated with the future of the health care system.

(9) Ottawa's largely unilateral approach to fiscal relations with the provinces since the early 1980s is also inconsistent with the kind of intergovernmental partnership arrangement in health care that the federal government appears to want and that the Canadian public clearly expects. At the same time, a return to a more collaborative approach to fiscal decision-making would require that provinces also engage constructively and realistically in financial negotiations with federal counterparts.

(10) Further considerations that should guide the fiscal relationship between federal and provincial governments include the following:

    a) If Canada were to move toward a predominantly provincial sharing community vision, a federal-provincial/territorial revenue-sharing arrangement would be the preferred option, with a transfer of tax room as second best. In either case, the revenues allocated should be equalized. Under this model, the conditions associated with the *Canada Health Act* should be dropped, except those related to portability and mobility.

b) Under either alternative models (dual sharing or predominantly Canada-wide sharing), a federal cash transfer should be maintained. The transfer should be visible and understood by all Canadians to be the federal contribution for provincial health care programs. In this case, it would be appropriate to maintain conditions along the lines of those now in the *Canada Health Act* or some modernized version of them.

c) The 20-25 percent federal-share contribution should be provided in the form of a separate equal per capita block transfer for health care (CHT), in part because of its equalizing properties. It should not be a formal cost-sharing arrangement.

d) Any federal health transfer should grow based on a formula that reflects growth in Canada-wide health care costs. It should be predictable and transparent.

e) Consideration should also be given to adjusting the equal per capita transfer on the basis of differences in need among provinces and territories as determined by measurable demographic and geographic factors. While such a needs-related adjustment can be justified in all scenarios, it is strongest in the case of the predominantly Canada-wide sharing model.

(11) Insured hospital and medical services are declining as a share of total health care expenditures. To the extent that there is interest in broadened public insurance coverage, and given our conclusions in items 6-8 above, it appears that all, or almost all, of the incremental costs of the added coverage would have to be borne by the federal government. Determining the amount of funding involved would require very detailed provincial information on current program costs and a careful assessment of the expected costs of the proposed programs. Assuming it does absorb the incremental costs, Ottawa may wish to be fiscally prudent and finance this initiative through a dedicated tax. Additional features of broadened coverage could include:

a) As an interim measure, federal funding for the new Canada-wide health care programs should be provided through a separate block fund(s) (separate from the CHT).

b) The separate fund(s) should have its own escalator reflecting anticipated cost increases in the new programs (based on a Statistics Canada measure of relevant cost increases).

c) The funding for new programs should be folded into the CHT when they become mature, with an appropriate adjustment, if necessary, to the CHT escalator.

(12) The fiscal relations between the two orders of government should be rethought and adjusted to better reflect a partnership relationship. The model of federal-provincial fiscal relations from the 1950-70s era was characterized by tough negotiations but with a determination to reach agreement. Returning to the earlier model, or finding an alternative that provides provinces and territories with a greater say in the outcomes, is highly desirable.

(13) Consideration should also be given to ways in which the federal government can become the political partner of the provinces and territories with a view to helping them overcome some of the difficult political obstacles they face in moving forward with health care reform.

(14) In the context of reconstructing the fiscal and political partnership between orders of government, arrangements for handling disputes that cannot be avoided must be considered. The need for improved dispute resolution mechanisms is not as great in the context of a predominantly provincial sharing model as it is under the dual and predominantly Canada-wide models of the sharing community. And to the extent that future policy changes in effect broaden the scope of countrywide health care coverage or make the federal conditions attached to the *Canada Health Act* more onerous for the provinces, there will be a greater need to ensure that dispute resolution mechanisms are seen as authoritative and legitimate by the public and both orders of government. This will require new institutional developments. Under the latter two versions of the Canadian sharing community, dispute resolution provisions should encompass a number of elements. They should:

> apply to a broad range of disputes, both fiscal and programmatic;

> embody the core values guiding health care in Canada;

> provide citizens a role in the dispute settlement process;

> make provisions for the use of third parties as appropriate for advisory, mediatory, and facilitative functions, in a fashion consistent with the preservation of the democratic accountability of elected officials;

> encourage the development of shared language and relationships by providing a forum for consultation involving representatives of the two orders of government; and
> include the public release of fact-finding reports that would inform citizens and apply moral suasion on the parties.

There is no single "right" approach to defining the future role of the federal government in Canadian health care. Finding viable solutions will first require reconciling competing views about the nature of the Canadian sharing community and the Canadian federation through societal debate and consensus. Independent of the outcome of this debate, however, there is clearly a lack of coherence between the vocabulary of partnership that marks Ottawa's policy pronouncements with respect to health care and the way it has used the tools of fiscal federalism and dispute resolution, over the last two decades, to implement its policies.

This lack of coherence needs to be addressed. It is our hope that the framework for renewal proposed in this volume can provide some useful guidelines for improving intergovernmental relations in the field of health care in particular and fiscal relations generally. The federal government in the last few years has taken some steps in regard to both fiscal federalism and dispute resolution that are consistent with the principles we propose. At the same time, our analysis suggests that further steps will be required of all governments if these improvements are to be sustained and the intergovernmental partnership renewed. Reconstructing the partnership is what Canadians want. It is the key to ensuring the quality and sustainability of health care for future generations.

BIBLIOGRAPHY

Aba, Shay, Wolfe D. Goodman, and Jack M. Mintz. 2002. Funding public provision of private health: the case for a copayment contribution through the tax system. *C.D. Howe Institute Commentary* No. 163. Toronto: C.D. Howe Institute (accessed 12 June 2002). http:\www.cdhowe.org/pdf/commentary_163.pdf

Adams, Duane, ed. 2001. *Federalism, Democracy and Health Policy in Canada.* Montreal: McGill-Queen's University Press for the Institute of Intergovernmental Relations, Queen's University.

Alberta. 1995. Letter from the Alberta Minister of Health to the Minister of Health and Welfare Canada, including attachment "Public/Private Health Services: The Alberta Approach," 11 October.

— Federal and Intergovernmental Affairs. 1997. Albertans named to dispute settlement panel roster. News release, May 22. Alberta Federal and Intergovernmental Affairs.

— Premier's Advisory Council on Health. 2001. *A Framework for Reform: Report of the Premier's Advisory Council on Health* (accessed 6 June 2002). http://www.premiersadvisory.com/reform.html

Andersen, Steven K. 2000. NAFTA: mediation and the North American free trade agreement. *Dispute Resolution Journal* 55(2), 56-64.

Appleton, Barry. 1999. International agreements and national health plans: NAFTA, in *Market Limits in Health Reform: Public Success, Private Failure,* edited by Daniel Drache and Terrence Sullivan. London: Routledge, 87-104.

Arnett, Ronald C. 1986. *Communication and Community: Implications of Martin Buber's Dialogue.* Carbondale: Southern Illinois University Press.

Asselin, Robert B. 2001. The Canadian social union: questions about the division of powers and fiscal federalism. Working paper PRB00-31E, Library of Parliament, Parliamentary Research Branch Ottawa (accessed 20 January 2002). http://www.parl.gc.ca/information/library/PRBpubs/prb0031-e.htm

Auditor General of Canada. 1999. *Report of the Auditor General of Canada.* Ottawa: Office of the Auditor General (accessed 5 February 2002). http://www.oagbvg.gc.ca/domino/reports.nsf/html/99menu_e.html

Australia. Parliament of Victoria. Federal-State Relations Committee. 1999. *Federalism and the Role of the States: Comparisons and Recommendations.* Victoria: Federal-State Relations Committee (accessed 2 February 2002). http://www.parliament.vic.gov.au/fsrc/Report3/contents.htm

Azfar, Omar, Satu Kähkönen, Anthony Lanyi, Patrick Meagher, and Diana Rutherford. 1999. *Decentralization, Governance and Public Services: The Impact of Institutional Arrangements: A Review of the Literature.* Center for Institutional Reform and the Informal Sector (IRIS Center), University of Maryland (accessed 2 February 2002). http://www1.worldbank.org/publicsector/decentralization/LitReview0999%20final.doc

Baker, Michael, Abigail Payne, and Michael Smart. 1998. The impact of federal fiscal arrangements: evidence from the "cap on CAP." *Policy Options* 19(9), 56-8. Montreal: Institute for Research on Public Policy.

Bakvis, Herman. 2002. Checkerboard federalism? Labour market development policy in Canada, in *Canadian Federalism: Performance, Effectiveness, and Legitimacy*, edited by Herman Bakvis and Grace Skogstad. Don Mills: Oxford University Press, 197-220.

Bakvis, Herman, and Grace Skogstad. 2002. Canadian federalism: performance, effectiveness and legitimacy, in *Canadian Federalism: Performance, Effectiveness and Legitimacy*, edited by Herman Bakvis and Grace Skogstad. Don Mills: Oxford University Press, 3-23.

Bankes, Nigel. 1991. Co-operative federalism: third parties and intergovernmental agreements and arrangements in Canada and Australia. *Alberta Law Review* 29(4), 792-838.

Banting, Keith. 1998. The past speaks to the future: lessons from the postwar social union, in *Canada: The State of the Federation 1997*, edited by Harvey Lazar. Kingston: Institute of Intergovernmental Relations, 3-32. http://www.iiigr.ca/pdf/publications/33_Canada_The_State_of_the_F.pdf

— 1998. Social citizenship and the social union in Canada. *Policy Options* 19 (9), 33-6. Montreal: Institute for Research on Public Policy.

Banting, Keith, Douglas M. Brown, and Thomas J. Courchene, eds. 1994. *The Future of Fiscal Federalism*. Kingston: School of Policy Studies.

Banting, Keith, and Stan Corbett. 2002. Health policy and federalism, in *Health Policy and Federalism: A Comparative Perspective on Multi-Level Governance*. Montreal: McGill-Queen's University Press, for the Institute of Intergovernmental Relations, School of Policy Studies, Queen's University, 2002, 1-38.

Barker, Paul. 1998. Disentangling the federation: social policy and fiscal federalism, in *Challenges to Canadian Federalism*, edited by Martin Westmacott and Hugh Mellon. Scarborough: Prentice Hall Canada, 144-57.

Bégin, Clermont, Pierre Bergeron, Pierre-Gerlier Forest, and Vincent Lemieux. 1999. *Le Système de santé québécois: Un modèle en transformation*. Montreal: Les Presses de l'Université de Montréal.

Bégin, Monique. 1987. *Medicare: Canada's Right to Health*. Translated by David Homel and Lucille Nelson. Ottawa: Optimum Publishing.

— 1999. *The Future of Medicare: Recovering the Canada Health Act*. Ottawa: Canadian Centre for Policy Alternatives, September (accessed 22 January 2002). http://www.policyalternatives.ca/publications/medicare.pdf

Belgium. The Chamber of Representatives. 1999. The Court of Arbitrage. Information sheet. The House of Representatives (accessed August 13, 2002). http://www.lachambre.be/pri/fiche/pdfE/31.pdf

— 2002a. Cooperation and settlement of conflicts within the federal State of Belgium. Information sheet. The House of Representatives (accessed August 13, 2002). http://www.lachambre.be/pri/fiche/pdfE/30.pdf

— 2002b. The Council of State. Information sheet. The House of Representatives. (accessed August 13, 2002). http://www.lachambre.be/pri/fiche/pdfE/11_08.pdf

— 2002c. The dividing up of competences. Information sheet. The House of Representatives (accessed August 13, 2002). http://www.lachambre.be/pri/fiche/pdfE/05.pdf

— 2002d. Schematic presentation of the levels of authority in federal Belgium. Information sheet. The House of Representatives (accessed August 13, 2002). http://www.lachambre.be/pri/fiche/pdfE/06.pdf

Bhagwati, Jagdish. 2001. After Seattle: free trade and the WTO. *International Affairs* 1, 15-29.

Biggs, Margaret. 1996. Highlights of the research findings of building blocks for Canada's new social union. Backgrounder.

Ottawa: Canadian Policy Research Networks. Working paper no. F02, 30-43 (accessed 20 January 2002). http://www.cprn.com/cprn.html

Bird, Richard M. 1999. Transfers and incentives in intergovernmental fiscal relations, in *Decentralization and Accountability of the Public Sector*. Proceedings of the Annual World Bank Conference on Development in Latin America and the Caribbean, held in Valdivia, Chile, June 20-22, 1999, edited by Shahid Javed Burki and Guillermo E. Perry. Washington, D.C.: The World Bank, 111-27 (accessed 3 February 2002). http://www.worldbank.org

— 2000. Fiscal decentralization and competitive governments, in *Competition and structure: The Political Economy of Collective Decisions*. Essays in honor of Albert Breton, edited by Gianluigi Galeotti, Pierre Salmon, and Ronald Wintrobe. Cambridge: Cambridge University Press, 129-49.

Bird, Richard M., and Audrey Tarasov. 2002. Closing the gap: fiscal imbalances and intergovernmental transfers in developed federations. Working paper no. 02-2. Andrew Young School of Policy Studies, Georgia State University, March (accessed 6 June 2002). http://isp-aysps.gsu.edu/papers/ispwp0202.pdf

Bird, Richard M., and Duanjie Chen. 1998. Fiscal federalism and federal finance: the two worlds of Canadian public finance. *Canadian Public Administration* 41, 51-74.

Boadway, Robin W. 1996. The folly of decentralizing the Canadian federation. *Dalhousie Review* 75(3), 313-49.

— 1998. Delivering the social union: some thoughts on the federal role. *Policy Options* 19(9), 37. Montreal: Institute for Research on Public Policy. Accessed 20 November, 2003. www.irpp.org/po/archive/nov98/boadway.pdf

— 2000. Recent developments in the economics of federalism, in *Canada: The State of the Federation 1999-2000: Toward a New Mission Statement for Canadian Fiscal Federalism*, edited by Harvey Lazar. Kingston: Institute of Intergovernmental Relations, 41-78. http://www.iigr.ca/pdf/publications/16_Canada_The_State_of_the_F.pdf

— 2001. The imperative of fiscal sharing transfers. *International Social Science Journal* 53(1), 103-10.

Boadway, Robin W., and Paul A.R. Hobson. 1993. *Intergovernmental Fiscal Relations in Canada*. Toronto: Canadian Tax Foundation.

Boadway, Robin W., and Michael Keen. 2000. Redistribution, in *Handbook of Income Distribution*, edited by Anthony Atkinson and François Bourguignon. New York: Elvesier, 677-789.

Boadway, Robin W., and Ronald Watts. 2000. Fiscal federalism in Canada. A paper prepared for the Russia Project on Federalism. Kingston: Institute of Intergovernmental Relations, Queen's University.

Boadway, Robin W., and Paul A.R. Hobson, eds. 1998. *Equalization: Its Contribution to Canada's Economic and Fiscal Progress*. Kingston: John Deutsch Institute for the Study of Economic Policy, Queen's University.

Boase, Joan Price. 2001. Federalism and the health facility fees challenge, in *Federalism, Democracy and Health Policy in Canada*, edited by Duane Adams. Montreal: Institute of Intergovernmental Relations, 179-207.

Boessenkool, Kenneth J. 1998. Clearly Canadian: improving equity and accountability with an overarching equalization program. *C.D. Howe Commentary* 114. Toronto: C.D. Howe Institute (accessed 15 February 2002). http://www.cdhowe.org/pdf/kbkool-3.pdf

Boothe, Paul. 1998a. *Finding a Balance: Renewing Canadian Fiscal Federalism*. C.D. Howe Benefactors Lecture. Toronto: C.D. Howe Institute (accessed 20 January 2002). http://www.cdhowe.org/english/publications/currentpubs.html

— 1998b. Is it time to reform fiscal transfers. *Policy Options* 19(9), 53-55. Montreal: Institute for Research on Public Policy.

Boothe, Paul, and Derek Hermanutz. 1998. *Paying for ACCESS: Province by Province.* (3 February 2002). http://www.ualberta.ca/~econweb/IPE/pubs/bhdw.pdf

— 1999. Simply sharing: an interprovincial equalization scheme for Canada. *C.D. Howe Institute Commentary* 128. Toronto: C.D. Howe Institute (accessed 8 January 2002). http://www.cdhowe.org/english/publications/currentpubs.htmlB

Boothe, Paul, ed. 1996. *Reforming Fiscal Federalism for Global Competition: A Canada-Australia Comparison.* Edmonton: University of Alberta Press.

Breton, Albert. 1985. Supplementary Statement, *Report of the Royal Commission on the Economic Union and Development Prospects for Canada* (Macdonald Commission), vol. 3. Ottawa: Supply and Services Canada, 486–526.

Brimacombe, Glenn G. 2001. *The First Ministers' Accord on Health Care: Can the Discussion Move to Structure from Money?* Ottawa: The Conference Board of Canada, May (accessed 21 March 2002). http://www.conferenceboard.ca/Health/documents/318-01mb.pdf

British Columbia. Ministry of Finance and Corporate Relations. 1998. Report F: Federal spending power, fiscal imbalance and risks to health care and education. (accessed 2 March 2002). http://www.fin.gov.bc.ca/archive/budget98/bgt_rptf.html

Brzinski, Joanne Bay. 1999. Changing forms of federalism and party electoral strategies: Belgium and the European Union. *Publius* 29(1), 45-70.

Buchanan, James M. 1975. The Samaritan's dilemma, in *Altruism, Morality, and Economic Theory*, edited by Edmund S. Phelps. New York: Russell Sage Foundation.

Cahn, Dudley D. 1997. Conflict communication: an emerging communication theory of interpersonal conflict, in *Emerging Theories of Human Communication*, edited by Branislav Kovacic. Albany: State University Press, 45-64.

Cameron, David. 1994. Half-eaten carrot, bent stick: decentralization in an era of fiscal restraint. *Canadian Public Administration* 37(3), 431-44.

— 1997. *Assessing ACCESS: Towards a New Social Union.* Kingston: Institute of Intergovernmental Relations, Queen's University.

— 2001. The structures of intergovernmental relations. *International Social Science Journal* 53(1), 121-7.

Cameron, David, and Fraser Valentine. 2001. Comparing policy-making in federal systems: the case of disability policy and programs – an introduction, in *Disability and Federalism: Comparing Different Approaches to Full Participation*, edited by David Cameron and Fraser Valentine. Montreal: McGill-Queen's University Press, for the Institute of Intergovernmental Relations, School of Policy Studies, Queen's University, 1-45.

Cameron, David, and Richard Simeon. 2000. Intergovernmental relations and democratic citizenship, in *Governance in the Twenty-First Century: Revitalizing the Public Service*, edited by B.G. Peters and D. Savoie. Montreal: McGill-Queen's University Press and the Canadian Centre for Management Development.

— 2002. Intergovernmental relations and democracy: an oxymoron if there ever was one? in *Canadian Federalism: Performance, Effectiveness, and Legitimacy*, edited by Herman Bakvis and Grace Skogstad. Don Mills: Oxford University Press, 278-96.

Campbell, Robert M., and Leslie A. Pal. 1991. *The Real Worlds of Canadian Politics: Cases in Process and Policy.* Peterborough: Broadview Press.

Canada. 1956-57. *Hospital Insurance and Diagnostic Services Act. S.C.*, c. 28.

Canadian Institute for Health Information. 2002. *Drug Expenditures in Canada, 1985-2001.* Ottawa: Canadian Institute for Health Information (accessed 10 June 2002). http://ecomm.cihi.ca/ec/product.asp?sku=DRUGEXP8501PDF

Canadian Intergovernmental Conference Secretariat. 1999. *A Framework to Improve the Social Union for Canadians.* First Ministers' Meeting. Ottawa (accessed 8 February 2002). http://www.scics.gc.ca/cinfo99/80003701_e.html

Canadian Tax Foundation. 1965. *Provincial and Municipal Finances, 1965.* Toronto: Canadian Tax Foundation.

— 1972. *The National Finances, 1972-73: An Analysis of the Revenues and Expenditures of the Government of Canada.* Toronto: Canadian Tax Foundation.

— 1976. *The National Finances, 1975-76: An Analysis of the Revenues and Expenditures of the Government of Canada.* Toronto: Canadian Tax Foundation.

— 1978. *The National Finances, 1977-78: An Analysis of the Revenues and Expenditures of the Government of Canada.* Toronto: Canadian Tax Foundation.

— 1979. *Provincial and Municipal Finances, 1979.* Toronto: Canadian Tax Foundation.

Carter, George E. 1971. *Canadian Conditional Grants Since World War II.* Canadian Tax Paper 054. Toronto: Canadian Tax Foundation.

Caulfield, Timothy A., Colleen Flood, and Barbara von Tigerstrom. 2002. *Comment: Bill 11: Health Care Protection Act.* Edmonton: Health Law Institute.

Centre for Research and Information on Canada. 2001. Federalism: intergovernmental cooperation: a priority for Canadians, in *Portraits of Canada - 2001.* Ottawa: Centre for Research and Information on Canada (accessed 20 January 2002). http://www.ccu-cuc.ca/pdf/portraits/portraits2001_federalism.pdf

Certified General Accountants. 2001. *Canada's Agreement on Internal Trade: It Can Work if We Want it to.* Vancouver: Certified General Accountants Association of Canada.

Charlottetown Accord. 1992 (accessed 21 February 2002). http://www.uni.ca/charlottetown.html

Choudhry, Sujit. 1996. The enforcement of the *Canada Health Act. McGill Law Journal* 41(2), 461-93.

— 2000. Bill 11, the *Canada Health Act* and the social union: the need for institutions. *Osgoode Hall Law Journal* 39(1), 39-76.

Clendenning, E. Wayne. 1997. *Analysis of International Trade Dispute Settlement Mechanisms and Implications for Canada's Agreement on Internal Trade.* Ottawa: Industry Canada.

Cohn, Daniel. 1996. The Canada Health and Social Transfer: transferring resources or moral authority between levels of government? in *Canada: The State of the Federation 1996,* edited by Patrick C. Fafard and Douglas M. Brown. Kingston: Institute of Intergovernmental Relations, 167-89.

Coleman, William D. 2002. Federalism and financial services, in *Canadian Federalism: Performance, Effectiveness, and Legitimacy,* edited by Herman Bakvis and Grace Skogstad. Don Mills: Oxford University Press, 178-97.

Commission on Fiscal Imbalance. 2001a. *Fiscal Imbalance: Problems and Issues.* Québec, Commission on Fiscal Imbalance. http://www.desequilibrefiscal.gouv.qc.ca/en/pdf/fiscal_imbalance.pdf (accessed 15 February 2002).

— 2001b. *Intergovernmental Fiscal Arrangements: Germany, Australia, Belgium, Spain, United States, Switzerland.* Background paper for the International Symposium on Fiscal Imbalance. Sept. 13-14 (accessed 15 February 2002). http://www.desquilibrefiscal.gouv.qc.ca/en/pdf/internationnal_ang.pdf-

—2002. *A New Division of Canada's Financial Resources. Final Report* (accessed 19 March 2002). http://www.desequilibrefiscal.gouv.qc.ca

Commission on the Future of Health Care in Canada. 2002. *Building on Values: The Future of Health Care in Canada.* Saskatoon: The Commission on the Future of Health Care in Canada.

Conference Board of Canada. 2002a. *Fiscal Prospects for the Federal and Québec Governments.* Report prepared for the Commission on Fiscal Imbalance. Ottawa: Conference Board of Canada. http://www.desequilibrefiscal.gouv.qc.ca/en/pdf/board_en.pdf

—2002b. *Fiscal Prospects for the Federal and Provincial/Territorial Governments.* Ottawa: Conference Board of Canada (accessed August 2002). http://www.conferenceboard.ca/pdfs/fiscalimbalance.pdf

Conrad, Alexis Jonathan. 1999. Assessing the adequacy of intergovernmental collaboration as an organizing principle for environmental protection: a case study of the Canada-wide accord on environmental harmonization's environmental standards sub-agreement. MA thesis, Queen's University, Kingston.

Cotter, John. 2002. Ottawa agrees to set up medicare dispute panel. *Toronto Star,* 12 April, A8.

Coulombe, Serge, and Marcel Mérette. 2000. Fiscal needs and the CHST per capita division rule. *Canadian Tax Foundation Journal* 28, 2, 340-55.

Council of Canadians. 1999. *Power Game: Five Problems With the Current Social Union Talks.* Ottawa: Council of Canadians (accessed 20 January 2002). http://www.canadians.org.

Courchene, Thomas J. 1984. *Equalization Payments: Past, Present, and Future.* Toronto: Ontario Economic Council.

—1991. *In Praise of Renewed Federalism.* The Canada Round: A Series on the Economics of Constitutional Renewal 2. Toronto: C.D. Howe Institute.

—1995a. *Celebrating Flexibility.* C.D. Howe Benefactors Lecture. Toronto: C.D. Howe Institute.

—1995b. *Redistributing Money and Power: Analysis of the Canada Health and Social Transfer.* Toronto: C.D. Howe Institute.

—1996. ACCESS: A convention on the canadian economic and social system. *Canadian Business Economics* 4(4), 3-26.

—1998a. In praise of provincial ascendancy. *Policy Options* 19(9), 30-3. Montreal: Institute for Research on Public Policy.

—1998b. *Renegotiating Equalization: National Polity, Federal State, International Economy.* Toronto: C.D. Howe Institute, September (accessed 20 January 2002). http://qsilver.queensu.ca/~courchen/papers.html

—2002. Half-way home: Canada's remarkable fiscal turnaround and the Paul Martin legacy. *IRPP Policy Matters* 3(8). Montreal: Institute for Research on Public Policy (accessed 20 August 2002). http://www.irpp.org/pm/archive/pmvol3no8.pdf

Courchene, Thomas J., David W. Conklin, and Gail C.A. Cook, eds. 1985. *Ottawa and the Provinces: The Distribution of Money and Power,* vol. 2. Toronto: Ontario Economic Council.

Coyne, Deborah. 1989. The Meech Lake Accord and the spending power proposals: fundamentally flawed, in *The Meech Lake Primer: Conflicting Views of the 1987 Constitutional Accord,* edited by M.D. Behiels. Ottawa: University of Ottawa Press, 245-67.

Crommelin, Michael. 2001. Dispute resolution in federal systems. *International Social Science Journal* 53(1), 139-44.

Cunningham, Dianne. 1998. Ontario's approach to improving Canada's social union. *Policy Options* 19(9), 14-17. Montreal: Institute for Research on Public Policy (accessed 20 January 2002). http://www.irpp.org/archive/policyop/no98sume.htm

Cutler, David M. 2002. Health care and the public sector, in *Handbook of Public*

Economics, edited by Alan J. Auerbach and Martin Feldstein. Volume 4. Amsterdam: North-Holland.

Cutler, Fred, and Matthew Mendelsohn. 2001. What kind of federalism do Canadians (outside Quebec) want? *Policy Options*, 23-9. Montreal: Institute for Research on Public Policy (accessed 12 March 2002). http://www.lrpp.org/po/index.htm

Dahlby, Bev. 1999. Taxing choices. Background paper, International Conference on Federalism, Mont Tremblant. Ottawa: Forum of Federation (accessed 28 July 2003). http://www.forumfed.org/federal/IIviewpapers.asp#

Dahlby, Bev, and L.S. Wilson. 1994. Fiscal capacity, tax effort, and optimal equalization grants. *Canadian Journal of Economics* 26(3), 657.

Davey, William J. 2000. Supporting the World Trade Organization dispute settlement system. *Journal of World Trade* 34(1), 167-70.

Deber, Raisa B. 2000. Who wants to pay for health care? *Canadian Medical Association Journal* 163(1), 43-4.

Decter, Michael B. 1994. *Healing Medicare: Managing Health System Change the Canadian Way*. Toronto: McGilligan Books.

— 2000. *Four Strong Winds: Understanding the Growing Challenges to Health Care*. Toronto: Stoddart.

Delacourt, Susan, and Donald G. Lenihan, eds. 1999. *Collaborative Government: Is There a Canadian Way?* New Directions, Number 6. Toronto: Institute of Public Administration of Canada.

Department of Finance Canada. 1995a. *Budget Speech 1995*. Ottawa: Department of Finance.

— 1995b. *Budget in Brief*. Department of Finance Canada (accessed 24 July 2003). http://www.fin.gc.ca/budget95/binb/BINBE.html

— 2000. Backgrounder on federal support for health in Canada (March 29).

— 2001. Securing progress in an uncertain world: the budget speech, 2001. Department of Finance Canada (accessed 6 June 2002). www.fin.gc.ca/budget01/pdf/speeche.pdf

— 2002a. A brief history of the Canada Health and Social Transfer (CHST). Department of Finance Canada. www.fin.gc.ca/FEDPROV/hise.html

— 2002b. Federal support for health care: the facts. Department of Finance Canada, April (accessed 10 June 2002). http://www.fin.gc.ca/facts/fshc_e.html

— 2002c. The economic and fiscal update. Ottawa, Department of Finance, October (accessed October 30, 2002). www.chamber.ca/public_info/2002/lynch.pdf

Department of Foreign Affairs and International Trade. 2001. *WTO Consultations: Dispute Settlement System (DSU) - Information Paper*. Consultations with Canadians. Ottawa (accessed 3 June 2002). http://www.dfait-maeci.gc.ca/tna-nac/dsu-info-en.asp

d'Estrée, Tamra Pearson, Larissa A. Fast, Joshua N. Weiss, and Monica S. Jakobsen. 2001. Changing the debate about "success" in conflict resolution efforts. *Negotiation Journal* 17(2), 101-13.

Deutsch, Morton. 1991. Subjective features of conflict resolution: psychological, social and cultural influences, in *New Directions in Conflict Theory: Conflict Resolution and Conflict Transformation*, edited by Raimo Väyrynen. London: Sage Publications, 26-57.

Doern, G. Bruce, and Mark MacDonald. 1999. *Free-Trade Federalism: Negotiating the Canadian Agreement on Internal Trade*. Toronto: University of Toronto Press.

Donaldson, Cam, Craig Mitton, and Gillian Currie. 2002. Managing medicare: the prerequisite to spending or reform. *C.D. Howe Institute Commentary*, 157. (accessed 28 July 2003). Toronto: C.D. Howe Institute. http://www.cdhowe.org/pdf/commentary_157.pdf

Dorse, Kevin. 1998. Sadly off in all directions: the federal/provincial dynamic in postsecondary education policy since the Canada Health and Social Transfer. MA thesis. Carleton University, Ottawa.

Dufour, Christian. 2002. Restoring the federal
principle. *IRPP Policy Matters*. Montreal:
Institute for Research on Public Policy.
3(1) (accessed 21 March 2002).
http://www.irpp.org/pm/index.htm

Dunsmuir, Mollie. 1991. The spending power:
scope and limitations. BP-272E.
Parliamentary Research Branch, Library
of Parliament, Ottawa (accessed 21
February 2002).
http://www.parl.gc.ca/information/library/
PRBpubs/bp272-e.htm

Economic Council of Canada. 1982. *Financing
Confederation, Today and Tomorrow.*
Ottawa.

Epps, Tracey. 2001. Merchants in the temple?
The implications of the GATS and NAFTA
for canada's health care system. Faculty
of Law, University of Toronto.

Facal, Joseph. 1998. Pourquoi le Québec a
adhéré au consensus des provinces sur
l'union sociale. *Policy Options* 19(9), 12-13.
Montreal: Institute for Research on Public
Policy (accessed 20 January 2002).
http://www.irpp.org/archive/policyop/no9
8sume.htm

Fafard, Patrick, and Kathryn Harrison, eds.
2000. *Managing the Environmental
Union: Intergovernmental Relations and
Environmental Policy in Canada.*
Kingston: School of Policy Studies, the
Institute of Intergovernmental Relations
and the Saskatchewan Institute of Public
Policy, Queen's University.

Fierlbeck, Katherine. 1997. Canadian health care
reform and the politics of decentralization, in
*Health Policy Reform, National Variations
and Globalization*, edited by Christa
Altenstetter. London: Macmillan Press, 17-39.

— 2002. Cost containment in health care: the
federal context, in *Federalism, Democracy
and Health Policy in Canada*, edited by
Duane Adams. Montreal: McGill-Queen's
University Press, for the Institute of
Intergovernmental Relations, School of
Policy Studies, Queen's University, 131-79.

First Ministers. 1997. Joint communiqué. News
release, ref: 800-036/06, Ottawa, Ontario,
12 December (accessed 10 June 2002).

http://www.scics.gc.ca/cinfo/80003606_e.
html

— 2000a. Communiqué on health. News
release, ref: 800-038/004, Ottawa,
Ontario, 11 September 2000 (accessed 10
June 2002).
http://www.scics.gc.ca/cinfo00/8000380
04_e.html

— 2000b. Funding commitment of the
Government of Canada. News release,
September 11 ref: 800-038/006. Ontario,
11 September 2000 (accessed 10 June
2002).
http://www.scics.gc.ca/cinfo00/8000380
6_e.html

Fitz-James, Michael. 2001. Medicare not reim-
bursing for uninsured. *The Medical Post*,
37(21) 5 June.

Flood, Colleen M. 1999. The structure and
dynamics of Canada's health care system,
in *Canadian Health Law and Policy*, edited
by J. Downie and T. Caulfield. Markham:
Butterworths Canada, 11-50.

— 1999. Contracting for health care services in
the public sector. *Canadian Business Law
Journal* 31(2), 175-208.

Flood, Colleen M., Mark Stabile, and Carolyn
Hughes Tuohy. 2002. The borders of solidarity: how countries determine the
public/private mix in spending and the
impact on health care. *Health Matrix* 12(2)
(accessed 24 February 2002).
http://www.law.utoronto.ca/healthlaw/HEALT
HMATRIX.SEPTEMBERFINALPUBPRIV.doc

Forest, Pierre-Gerlier. 2000. Du neuf avec du
vieux? L'union sociale et la santé. *Policy
Options*, 41-2. Montreal: Institute for
Research on Public Policy (accessed 20
January 2002).
http://www.irpp.org/po/archive/po0400.htm.

Forget, Claude E. 2001. Success, omissions and
challenges in harmonizing Canada's social
programs, in *The Dynamics of
Decentralization: Canadian Federalism
and British Devolution*, edited by Trevor
C. Salmon and Michael Keating. Kingston:
School of Policy Studies, 125-35.

Forget, E.L., R. Deber, and L.L. Roos. 2002.
Medical savings accounts: will they reduce

costs? *Canadian Medical Association Journal*, 167(2), 143-47.

Friendlander, Lara. 1994. Constitutionalizing intergovernmental agreements. *National Journal of Constitutional Law*, 4, 153-67.

Ganguly, Samrat. 2000. The investor-state dispute mechanism (ISDM) and a sovereign's power to protect public health. *Columbia Journal of Transnational Law* 38(113), 112.

Garman, Julie, and Louise Hilditch. 1998. Behind the scenes: an examination of the importance of the informal processes at work in conciliation. *Journal of European Public Policy* 5(2), 271-84.

Gershberg, Alec Ian. 1998. Decentralisation, recentralisation and performance accountability: building an operationally useful framework for analysis. *Development Policy Review* 16(4), 405-31.

Gibbins, Roger. 2001. Shifting sands: exploring the political foundations of SUFA. *IRPP Policy Matters*, 2(3), 1-20. Montreal: Institute for Research on Public Policy (accessed 20 January 2002). http://www.irpp.org/pm/archive/pmvol2no3.pdf

Gormley, William T. Jr., and Cristina Boccuti. 2001. HCFA and the states: politics and intergovernmental leverage. *Journal of Health Politics, Policy and Law* 26(3), 557.

Gottlieb & Pearson. 1999. *International trade standards and the regulatory powers of Governments and the Canadian public health system.* Prepared for Canadian Health Coalition, Ottawa (accessed 23 January 2002). http://www.healthcoalition.ca/gottlieb.html

Grané, Patricio. 2001. Remedies under WTO law. *Journal of International Economic Law*, 4,4, 755-72.

Gray, Gwendolyn. 1991. *Federalism and Health Policy: The Development of Health Systems in Canada and Australia.* Toronto: University of Toronto Press.

Gregory, Robin, Tim McDaniels, and Daryl Fields. 2001. Decision aiding, not dispute resolution: creating insights through structured environmental decisions.

Journal of Policy Analysis and Management 20(3), 415-32.

Hancock, Dave, in cooperation with officials from Alberta Intergovernmental and Aboriginal Affairs. 1998. Designing a new social framework for Canadians. *Policy Options* 19(9), 17-20. Montreal: Institute for Research on Public Policy (accessed 20 January 2002). http://www.irpp.org/archive/policyop/no98sume.htm

Hanson, Karl E. 1999. New trends in executive federalism: on the road to asymmetry. M.A. thesis. Dalhousie University, Halifax.

Harrison, Kathryn. 1996. *Passing the Buck: Federalism and Canadian Environmental Policy.* Vancouver: University of British Columbia Press.

Health Canada. 2001. 1999-2000 Canada Health Act annual report. Ottawa, Health Canada, February (accessed 20 January 2002). http://www.hcsc.gc.ca/medicare/AnnualReports.htm

— 2002. *Canada Health Act Overview.* Ottawa, Health Canada (accessed 30 May 2002). http://www.hc-sc.gc.ca/datapcb/datahins/chaover.htm

Heisey, D. Ray. 1991. Defining peace communication, in *Peacemaking Through Communication*, edited by R. Troester and C. Kelley. Annandale, VA: Speech Communications Association, 19-20.

Herperger, Dwight. 1991. Distribution of powers and functions in federal systems. Ottawa, Minister of Supply and Services Canada (accessed 1 April 2002). http://www.pco-bcp.gc.ca/aia/

Hoberg, George, and Paul Howe. 1999. Law, knowledge, and national interests In trade disputes: the softwood lumber case. Working paper no. 29. Vancouver: Institute of International Relations, University of British Columbia.

Hobson, Paul A.R., and France St-Hilaire. 1993. *Toward Sustainable Federalism: Reforming Federal-Provincial Fiscal Arrangements.* Montreal: Institute for Research on Public Policy.

— 2000. The evolution of federal-provincial fis-
cal arrangements: putting Humpty toge-
ther again, in *Canada: The State of the
Federation, 1999-2000: Toward a New
Mission Statement for Canadian Fiscal
Federalism*, edited by Harvey Lazar.
Kingston: Institute of Intergovernmental
Relations, Queen's University, 159-88
(accessed 20 January 2002).
http://iigr.ca/pdf/publications/16_Canada_
The_State_of_the_F.pdf

Hogg, Peter. 1999. Spending power.
Constitutional Law of Canada.
Scarborough: Carswell, 159-63.

— 2000. *Constitutional Law of Canada.*
Scarborough: Carswell.

Howse, Robert J. 1995. Between anarchy and
the rule of law: dispute settlement and
related implementation issues in the
Agreement on Internal Trade, in *Getting
There: An Assessment of the Agreement
on Internal Trade*, edited by M.J.
Trebilcock and D. Schwanen. Toronto: C.D.
Howe Institute, 171-86.

— 1996. Securing the Canadian economic
union: legal and constitutional options for
the federal government. *C.D. Howe
Institute Commentary* 81. Toronto: C. D.
Howe Institute.

Institute of Intergovernmental Relations. 1996.
*Assessing Access: Towards a New Social
Union.* Proceedings of the symposium on
the Courchene proposal. Kingston:
Institute of Intergovernmental Relations,
Queen's University.

Internal Trade Secretariat. 1994. The agreement on internal trade. Ottawa (accessed
3 June 2002).
http://www.intrasec.mb.ca/eng/main.htm

— 2001. CGA/Ontario panel report, October 5
(accessed 3 June 2002).
http://www.intrasec.mb.ca/pdf/cga_on_e.pdf.

Jackson, Robert, Doreen Jackson, and Nicolas
Baxter-Moore. 1986. *Politics in Canada:
Culture, Institutions, Behaviour and
Public Policy.* Scarborough: Prentice-Hall
Canada.

Jérôme-Forget, Monique. 1998. Canada's social
union: staking out the future of federalism.

Policy Options 19(9), 3-4. Montreal:
Institute for Research on Public Policy.

Johns, Carolyn. 2001. Pressures on Canada's
"environmental" federation from inside
and out. *Federations* 1(4) (accessed 3
June 2002).
http://www.ciff.on.ca/Publications/bv1n4/
bri.htm

Johnston, Larry. 1999. Behind the "social
union." *Backgrounder* 29. Toronto,
Ontario Legislative Library, Legislative
Research Service (accessed 10 March
2002).
http://www.ontla.on.ca/library/reposito-
ry/mon/1000/10278503.htm.

Keen, Michael. 1998. Vertical tax externalities in
the theory of fiscal federalism. *IMF Staff
Papers* 45(3), 454 (accessed 2 February
2002).
http://www.imf.org.

Kellett, Peter, and Diana Dalton. 2001. *Managing
Conflict in a Negotiated World: A
Narrative Approach to Achieving
Dialogue and Change.* Thousand Oaks:
Sage Publications.

Kennett, Steven A. 1998. *Securing the Social
Union: A Commentary on the
Decentralized Approach.* Kingston:
Institute of Intergovernmental Relations
and the School of Policy Studies, Queen's
University.

Kent, Tom. 1997. Medicare: how to keep and
improve it, especially for children. Ottawa,
Caledon Institute (accessed 23 January
2002).
http://www.caledoninst.org/full83.htm

Keohane, Robert O., Andrew Moravcsik, and
Anne-Marie Slaughter. 2000. Legalized
dispute resolution: interstate and transnational. *International Organization* 54(3),
457-88.

Kernaghan, Kenneth and David Siegel. 1995.
Public Administration in Canada: A Text.
3rd edition. Scarborough: Nelson Canada.

Kincaid, John. 2001. Economic policy-making:
advantages and disadvantages of the federal model. *International Social Science
Journal* 53(1), 85-92.

Kitchen, Harry. 2000. Provinces and municipalities, universities, schools and hospitals: recent trends and funding issues, in *Canada: The State of the Federation 1999/2000: Toward a New Mission Statement for Canadian Fiscal Federalism*, edited by Harvey Lazar. Kingston: Institute of Intergovernmental Relations, copublished by the School of Policy Studies, Queen's University, 295-336 (accessed 20 January 2002). http://www.iigr.ca/pdf/publications/16_Canada_The_State_of_the_F.pdf

Klassen, Thomas R. 2000. The federal-provincial Labour Market Development Agreements: brave new model of collaboration? in *Federalism, Democracy and Labour Market Policy in Canada*, edited by Tom McIntosh. Montreal: McGill-Queen's University Press for the School of Policy Studies, copublished by the Institute of Intergovernmental Relations, Queen's University, 159-205.

Knop, Karen, Sylvia Ostry, Richard Simeon, and Katherine Swinton. 1995. *Rethinking Federalism: Citizens, Markets and Governments in a Changing World*. Vancouver: University of British Columbia Press.

Konisky, David M. 1998. The United Nations dispute settlement system and international environmental disputes. *Journal of Public and International Affairs* (accessed 25 July 2003). http://www.princeton.edu/~jpia/past_articles_98.html

Lajoie, Andrée, and Patrick A. Molinari. 1978. Partage constitutionnel des compétences en matière de santé au Canada. *Canadian Bar Review* 56, 579.

Lan, Zhiyong.1997. A conflict resolution approach to public administration. *Public Administration Review* 57(1), 27-35.

Lazar, Harvey. 1998. The social union: taking the time to do it right. *Policy Options* 19(9), 43-6. Montreal: Institute for Research on Public Policy (accessed 20 January 2002). http://www.irpp.org/archive/policyop/no98sume.htm

— 2000. The Social Union Framework Agreement: lost opportunity or new beginning? Working paper 3, Kingston, School of Policy Studies (accessed 22 January 2002). http://qsilver.queensu.ca/sps/WorkingPapers/files/sps_wp_03.pdf

— 2000a. In search of a new mission statement for Canadian fiscal federalism, in *Canada: The State of the Federation 1999/2000: Toward a New Mission Statement for Canadian Fiscal Federalism*, edited by Harvey Lazar. Kingston: Institute of Intergovernmental Relations, copublished by the School of Policy Studies, Queen's University, 3-40 (accessed 20 January 2002). http://www.iigr.ca/pdf/publications/16_Canada_The_State_of_the_F.pdf

— 2000b. The Social Union Framework Agreement and the future of fiscal federalism in *Canada: The State of the Federation 1999/2000: Toward a New Mission Statement for Canadian Fiscal Federalism*, edited by Harvey Lazar. Kingston: Institute of Intergovernmental Relations, copublished by the School of Policy Studies, Queen's University, 99-128 (accessed 20 January 2002). http://www.iigr.ca/pdf/publications/16_Canada_The_State_of_the_F.pdf

Lazar, Harvey, and Peter Stoyko. 2001. Canadian labour market policies: the changing role of government and the extent of decentralization, in *The Dynamics of Decentralization: Canadian Federalism and British Devolution*, edited by Trevor C. Salmon and Michael Keating. Kingston: McGill Queen's University Press for the School of Policy Studies, Queen's University, 137-63.

Leeson, Howard. 2000. *The Agreement on Internal Trade: An Institutional Response to Changing Conceptions, Roles and Functions in Canadian Federalism*. Kingston: Institute of Intergovernmental Relations (accessed 10 April 2002). http://www.iigr.ca/pdf/publications/206_The_Agreement_on_Interna.pdf

Legowski, Barbara, and Lindsey McKay. 2000. Health beyond health care: twenty-five years of federal health policy development. Discussion paper no. H/04, Canadian Policy Research Networks, Ottawa (accessed 20 January 2002). http://www.cprn.com/cprn.html

Leslie, Peter M., Kenneth Norrie, and Irene K. Ip. 1993. *Partnership in Trouble: Renegotiating Fiscal Federalism.* Policy study no. 18, Toronto: C.D. Howe Institute.

Lexchin, Joel. 2001. *A National Pharmacare Plan: Combining Efficiency and Equity.* Ottawa: Canadian Centre for Policy Alternatives.

Liberal Party of Canada. 1993. *Creating Opportunity: The Liberal Plan for Canada.* ("The Red Book") Ottawa: Liberal Party of Canada.

Liebfried, Stephan, and Paul Pierson, eds. 1995. *European Social Policy: Between Fragmentation and Integration.* Washington, D.C.: The Brookings Institution.

Lin, Vivian, and Cathy King. 2000. Intergovernmental reforms in public health, in *Health Reform in Australia and New Zealand*, edited by Abby L. Bloom. South Melbourne: Oxford University Press, 251-63.

Lucas, Adetokunbo O. 2001. *Reconciling Decentralisation and Equity: Health.* Ottawa, Forum of Federations (accessed 2 February 2002). http://www.ciff.on.ca/Reference/documents/bg_paper/docbg_lucas.html

Lynch, Scott, Wade Locke, and Paul Hobson. 1997. *Should Our Concern Be the Gift Horse or the Ideological Bull? A Critical Assessment of "Looking the Gift Horse in the Mouth: The Impact of Federal Transfers on Atlantic Canada."* Moncton: Canadian Institute for Research on Regional Development.

MacDonald, Mark R. 2002. The Agreement on Internal Trade: trade-offs for economic union and federalism, in *Canadian Federalism: Performance, Effectiveness, and Legitimacy,* edited by Herman Bakvis and Grace Skogstad. Don Mills: Oxford University Press, 138-59.

Madore, Odette. 2000. The Canada Health Act: overview and options, 94-4e, Parliamentary Research Branch. Library of Parliament, Ottawa (accessed 20 January 2002). http://www.parl.gc.ca/information/library/prbpubs/944-e.htm

Maguire, L.A., and L.G. Boiney. 1994. Resolving environmental disputes: a framework incorporating decision analysis and dispute resolution techniques. *Journal of Environmental Management* 42(1), 31-48.

Maioni, Antonia. 1997. Decentralization in health policy: comments on a convention on Canadian economic and social systems. Prepared for the conference on "Decentralization: Dimensions and Prospects in Canada," Political Economy Research Group, University of Western Ontario, London, October 23-24.

— 2000. Assessing the Social Union Framework Agreement/Évaluer l'entente-cadre sur l'union sociale. *Policy Options*, 38-41. Montreal: Institute for Research on Public Policy (accessed 20 January 2002). http://www.irpp.org/po/archive/po0400.htm

— 2001. Emerging solutions: Quebec's Clair Commission Report and health care reform. *Backgrounder*. Canadian Policy Research Networks, Ottawa (accessed 20 January 2002). http://www.cprn.com/cprn.htm

— 2002. Health care in the new millennium, in *Canadian Federalism: Performance, Effectiveness, and Legitimacy,* edited by Herman Bakvis and Grace Skogstad. Don Mills, Oxford University Press, 87-105.

Mahoney, Jill, and Brian Laghi. 2002. Ottawa wants medicare mediation panel. *Globe and Mail*, 13 April, A9.

Manfredi, Christopher P., and Antonia Maioni. 2002. Courts and health policy: judicial policy making and publicly funded health care in Canada. *Journal of Health Politics, Policy and Law* 27(2), 213-32.

Marshall, T.H. 1992. Citizenship and social class, in *Citizenship and Social Class*, edited by

T.H. Marshall and T. Bottomore. London: Pluto Press.

Maslove, Allan M. 1997. The Canadian Health and Social Transfer: forcing issues, in *How Ottawa Spends, 1996-97: Life Under the Knife*, edited by Gene Swimmer, Ottawa: Carleton University Press, 283-303.

— 1998. National goals and the federal role in health care, in *Striking a Balance: Health Care Systems in Canada and Elsewhere*, vol. 4, Canada Health Action: Building on the Legacy. Papers commissioned by the National Forum on Health, Ottawa: Éditions MultiMondes, 371-99.

Matier, Chris, Lisa Wu, and Harriet Jackson. 2001. Analysing vertical fiscal imbalance in a framework of fiscal sustainability. Working paper 2001-23, Department of Finance Canada. http://www.fin.gc.ca./wp/2001-23e.html

Maxwell, Judith. 1998. More decentralization dangerous if not well managed. Ottawa: Canadian Policy Research Networks (accessed 3 June 2002). http://www.cprn.com/jmaxwell/files/cmdd_e.htm

McArthur, William, Cynthia Ramsay, and Michael Walker. 1996. *Healthy Incentives: Canadian Health Reform in an International Context*. Vancouver: Fraser Institute.

McGiffen, Steven P. 2001. *The European Union: A Critical Guide*. London: Pluto Press.

McKay, Lindsey. 2001. Changing approaches to health: the history of a Federal/Provincial Territorial Advisory Committee. Background paper to *Health Beyond Health Care: Twenty-five Years of Federal Health Policy Development*. Ottawa: Canadian Policy Research Networks (accessed 20 January 2002). http://www.cprn.com/cprn.html

McLellan, Anne. 1998. Modernizing Canada's social union: a new partnership among governments and citizens. *Policy Options* 19(9), 6-8. Montreal: Institute for Research on Public Policy (accessed 20 January 2002). http://www.irpp.org/archive/po/archive/po1198.htm

— 2002. Letter from Federal Health Minister Anne McLellan to Alberta Health Minister Gary Mar regarding dispute settlement mechanisms (accessed 9 August 2002). http://www.healthcoalition.ca/Mar-McLellan.pdf.

McMahon, Fred. 1996. *Looking the Gift Horse in the Mouth: The Impact of Federal Transfers on Atlantic Canada*. Halifax: Atlantic Institute for Market Studies (accessed 20 January 2002). http://www.aims.ca

Mendelsohn, Matthew. 2001. Canadians' thoughts on their health care system: pre serving the Canadian model through innovation. Submission to the Commission on the Future of Health Care in Canada (accessed 23 January 2002). http://www.healthcarecommission.ca.

Mendelsohn, Matthew, and John McLean. 2000. SUFA's double vision: citizen engagement and intergovernmental collaboration. *Policy Options*. 43-5. Montreal: Institute for Research on Public Policy (accessed 20 January 2002). http://www.irpp.org/po/archive/po0400.htm.

— 2002. Reconcilable differences: public partic-ipation and intergovernmentalism in Canada, in *Federalism and Democracy*, edited by Paul Thomas and David Stewart. University of Manitoba Press, forthcoming (accessed 28 July 2003). http://qsilver.queensu.ca/~mattmen/papers/Manitoba.doc

Milne, David. 1986. *Tug of War: Ottawa and the Provinces Under Trudeau and Mulroney*. Toronto: James Lorimer.

Moravcsik, Andrew. 1993. Preferences and power in the European Community: A lib-eral intergovernmentalist approach. *Journal of Common Market Studies* 31(4), 473.

Morgan, Steve, and Jeremiah Hurley. 2002. Influences on the "health care technology cost-driver." Discussion paper no. 14, Centre for Health Services and Policy Research, University of British Columbia, August.

http://www.chspr.ubc.ca/hpru/pdf/hrpu02-8R-CFHC-En.pdf

Murray, Heather L. 1998. The asymmetrical alternative: is asymmetrical federalism a viable option for the future? MA thesis, Carleton University, Ottawa.

Myles, John, and Paul Pierson. 1997. *Friedman's Revenge: The Reform of "Liberal" Welfare States in Canada and the United States*. Ottawa: Caledon Institute of Social Policy.

National Forum on Health. 1997. *Canada Health Action: Building on the Legacy*, vol. 1. Papers commissioned by the National Forum on Health. Ottawa. St. Foy: Éditions MultiMondes

—1997. *Canada Health Action: Building on the Legacy*, vol. 2. Papers commissioned by the National Forum on Health, Ottawa. St. Foy: Éditions MultiMondes

Neumann, Ronald, and T. Russell Robinson. 2001. The structures and conduct of intergovernmental relations with special reference to fiscal relations in Canada. Prepared for the World Bank Institute (accessed 3 June 2002). http://www.worldbank.org/wbi/publicfinance/documents/fiscalfederalism_Russia/neuman.pdf.

Ng, Kelvin, and David R. Sloan. 1998. Reforming Canada's social union: the territorial perspective. *Policy Options* 19(9), 23-6. Montreal: Institute for Research on Public Policy (accessed 20 January 2002). http://www.irpp.org/archive/policyop/no98sume.htm

Noël, Alain. 1998. Les trois unions sociales. *Policy Options* 19(9), 26-9. Montreal: Institute for Research on Public Policy (accessed 20 January 2002). http://www.irpp.org/archive/policyop/no98sume.htm

—2000. Without Quebec: collaborative federalism with a footnote? *IRPP Policy Matters* 1(2). Montreal: Institute for Research on Public Policy (accessed 21 March 2002). http://www.irpp.org/pm/index.htm.

—2001. Power and purpose in intergovernmental relations. *IRPP Policy Matters* 2(6), 1-27.

Montreal: Institute for Research on Public Policy (accessed 20 January 2002). http://www.irpp.org/pm/archive/pmvol2no6.pdf.

Norrie, Kenneth. 2002. On fiscal balance in the Canadian federation, in Robert Brown ed., *Canadian Conundrums: Views from the Clifford Clark Visiting Economists: C.D. Howe Institute Observation* 43. Toronto: C.D. Howe Institute, 23-34.

Norrie, Kenneth, and L.S. Wilson. 2000. On re-balancing Canadian fiscal federalism, in *Canada: The State of the Federation, 1999-2000: Toward a New Mission Statement for Canadian Fiscal Federalism*, edited by Harvey Lazar. Kingston: Institute of Intergovernmental Relations, copublished by the School of Policy Studies, Queen's University. http://www.iigr.ca/pdf/publications/16_Canada_The_State_of_the_F.pdf

O'Hara, K. with the assistance of S. Cox. 1998. Securing the social union. Study no. 2, Canadian Policy Research Networks, Ottawa (accessed 20 January 2002). http://www.cprn.com/cprn.html.

O'Leary, Rosemary, and Susan Summers. 2001. Lessons learned from two decades of alternative dispute resolution programs and processes at the U.S. Environmental Protection Agency. *Public Administration Review* 61(6), 682-95.

O'Leary, Rosemary, and Tracy Yandle. 2000. Environmental management at the millennium: the use of environmental dispute resolution by state governments. *Journal of Public Administration Research and Theory* 20(1), 137-55.

Opeskin, Brian R. March 2001. Mechanisms for intergovernmental relations in federations. *International Social Science Journal* 53(1), 129-39.

O'Reilly, Patricia. 2001. The federal/provincial/territorial health conference system, in *Federalism, Democracy and Health Policy in Canada*, edited by Duane Adams. Montreal: McGill-Queen's University Press, 107-31.

Painter, Martin. 1996. The Council of Australian Governments and intergovernmental relations: A case of cooperative federalism. *Publius* 26(2), 101-21.

— 1998. *Collaborative Federalism: Economic Reform in Australia in the 1990s.* New York: Cambridge University Press.

— 2001. Multi-level governance and the emergence of collaborative federal institutions in Australia. *Policy and Politics* 29(2), 137-50.

Palley, Howard D. 1987. Canadian federalism and the Canadian health care program: a comparison of Ontario and Quebec. *International Journal of Health Services* 17(4), 595-616.

Parliamentary Task Force on Federal-Provincial Fiscal Arrangements. 1981. *Fiscal Federalism in Canada.* Report of the Parliamentary Task Force on Federal-Provincial Relations. Ottawa: Supply and Services Canada.

Parson, Edward A. 2000. Environmental trends and environmental governance in Canada. *Canadian Public Policy* 26 (Supplement 2), S130-35. http://economics.ca/cgi/jab?journal=cpp&view=v26s2/Parson.pdf

Perry, David B. 1997. *Financing the Canadian Federation, 1867 to 1995: Setting the Stage for Change.* Toronto: Canadian Tax Foundation.

Persson, Torsten, and Guido Tabellini. 1996. Federal fiscal constitutions: risk sharing and redistribution. *Journal of Political Economy* 104(5), 979.

Petter. A. 1989. Federalism and the myth of the federal spending power. *Canadian Bar Review,* 68, 448-79.

Pfingsten, Andreas, and Andreas Wagener. 1997. Centralized vs. decentralized redistribution: a case for interregional transfer mechanisms. *International Tax and Public Finance* 4(3), 429-51.

Phillips, Susan D. 1995. The Canada Health and Social Transfer: fiscal federalism in search of a vision, in *Canada: The State of the Federation 1995,* edited by Douglas M. Brown and Jonathan W. Rose. Kingston: Institute of Intergovernmental Relations, 65-97.

— 2000. *Canada's Social Union Framework Agreement: Implications and Opportunities for the Voluntary Sector.* Ottawa: The Coalition of National Voluntary Organizations.

— 2001. SUFA and citizen engagement: fake or genuine masterpiece? *IRPP Policy Matters* 2(7). Montreal: Institute for Research on Public Policy (accessed 20 January 2002). http://www.irpp.org/

Prince, Michael J. 1999. From health and welfare to stealth and farewell: federal social policy, 1980-2000, in *How Ottawa Spends, 1999-2000, Shape Shifting: Canadian Governance Toward the 21st Century,* edited by Leslie A. Pal. Don Mills: Oxford University Press, 151-97.

Privy Council Office. 2002. *Fiscal Balance and Fiscal Relations Between Governments in Canada.* http://www.pco-bcp.gc.ca/aia/docs/financial/FiscalBalance/fiscalbalance2_e.pdf

Provincial and Territorial Finance Ministers. 1997. *Redesigning Fiscal Federalism – Issues and Options. Part One.* Background paper.

— 1998. News release, February 13, ref. 860-368/11. Fredericton, New Brunswick, 13 February (accessed 10 June 2002). http://www.scics.gc.ca/cinfo98/86036811_e.html

— 2001. Addressing fiscal imbalance: report of provincial and territorial finance ministers. Annual Premiers' Conference, Victoria, British Columbia, August 1-3, 2001 (accessed 3 March 2002). http://www.apc2001.gov.bc.ca/fiscal_e.pdf

— 2002. Canada's fiscal imbalance: resolving this issue is key to sustaining health care and other social programs. Fact sheet, 26 April.

Provincial and Territorial Ministers of Health. 2000. Understanding Canada's health care costs: final report (accessed 10 June 2002). http://www.gov.on.ca/health/english/pub/ministry/ptcd/ptcd_doc_e.pdf

Provincial and Territorial Premiers. 1995. Final communiqué. 36th Annual Premiers Conference, St. Johns, Newfoundland, 23-25 August.

— 1998. Health care funding. News release, ref: 850-070/16. 39th Annual Premiers' Conference, Saskatoon, Saskatchewan, 5-7 August (accessed 10 June 2002). http://www.scics.gc.ca/cinfo98/85007016_e.html

— 2000. Fiscal imbalance in Canada. News release, ref. 850-080/014. 41st Annual Premiers' Conference, Winnipeg, Manitoba, 9-11 August (accessed 10 June 2002). http://www.scics.gc.ca/cinfo00/850080014_e.html

— 2001. Canadian federalism and disability policy making. *Canadian Journal of Political Science* 34(4), 791-817.

Quebec. Commission d'étude sur les services de santé et les services sociaux. 2000. *Emerging Solutions – Report and Recommendations* (Clair Commission). Ministère de la Santé et des Services sociaux du Québec (accessed 23 January 2002). http://www.cessss.gouv.qc.ca/pdf/en/01-109-01a.pdf

Québec. Secrétariat aux affaires intergouvernementales canadiennes. 1998. *Position historique du Québec sur le pouvoir fédéral de dépenser, 1944-1998* (accessed 8 January 2002). http://www.cex.gouv.qc.ca/saic/position.htm

Radin, Beryl A., and Joan Price Boase. 2000. Federalism, political structure, and public policy in the United States and Canada. *Journal of Comparative Policy Analysis* 2(1), 65-89.

Ramsay, Cynthia. 1998. *Medical Savings Accounts: Universal, Accessible, Portable and Comprehensive Health Care for Canadians.* Vancouver: Fraser Institute, May (accessed 12 June 2002). http://www.fraserinstitute.ca/admin/books/files/MedicalSavingsAccounts.pdf

Rapoport, Anatol. 1992. *Peace: An Idea Whose Time Has Come.* Ann Arbor: University of Michigan Press.

Redden, Candace. 1998. *Through the Looking Glass: Federal and Provincial Decision Making for Health Policy.* Kingston: Institute of Intergovernmental Relations (accessed January 2003). http://www.iigr.ca/pdf/publications/149_Through_the_Looking_Glas.pdf

Richards, John. 1998. The "unholy alliance" versus "securing our future together." *Policy Options* 19(9), 40-3. Montreal: Institute for Research on Public Policy (accessed 20 January 2002). http://www.irpp.org/archive/policyop/no98sume.htm.

Robertson, Gordon. 1988. The role of interministerial conferences in the decision-making process, in *Perspectives on Canadian Federalism*, edited by R.D. Olling and M.W. Westmacott. Scarborough: Prentice-Hall Canada, 224-32.

Robson, William B. 2000. How federal tax cuts can improve your health. *Financial Post* 2(86), 3 February, C7.

Robson, William B., and D. Schwanen. 1999. Social Union Agreement: Too flawed to last. *Backgrounder*, February 8. Toronto: C.D. Howe Institute (accessed 20 January 2002). http://www.cdhowe.org/pdf/rob-sch.pdf

Robson, William B., Daniel Schwanen, and Finn Poschmann. 1999. Who gets what? The 1999 federal budget and the Canada Health and Social Transfer. *Backgrounder*. Toronto: C.D. Howe Institute (accessed 24 February 2002). http://www.cdhowe.org/pdf/posch-6.pdf

Rocher, Francois, and Miriam Smith. 1995. *New Trends in Canadian Federalism.* Peterborough: Broadview Press.

Roemer, John E. 1998. *Equality of Opportunity.* Cambridge, MA: Harvard University Press.

Romanow, Roy. 1998. Reinforcing "the ties that bind." *Policy Options* 19(9), 9-11. Montreal: Institute for Research on Public Policy (accessed 20 January 2002). http://www.irpp.org/archive/policyop/no98sume.htm

Rosa, Andrew Kayumi. 1993. Old wine, new skins: NAFTA and the evolution of international trade dispute resolution. *Michigan Journal of International Law* 15, 225.

Royal Commission on Constitutional Problems. 1956. *Report of the Royal Commission on Constitutional Problems*. Chaired by Judge Thomas Tremblay. Ottawa: Queen's Printer.

Royal Commission on Health Services. 1964. *Report of the Royal Commission on Health Services*. Chaired by Justice Emmett Hall. Ottawa: Queen's Printer.

Ruggeri, Giuseppe C. 1998. Vertical fiscal imbalances and renewed federalism. *Policy Options* 19(9), 47-9. Montreal: Institute for Research on Public Policy (accessed 20 January 2002). http://www.irpp.org/archive/policyop/no9 8sume.htm

— 2001. A Federation out of balance: update. Department of Economics, University of New Brunswick, Fredericton (accessed 15 February 2002). http://www.scics.gc.ca/pdf/860430004.p df

Ruggeri, Giuseppe C., and Robert Howard. 2000. On the concept and measurement of vertical fiscal imbalances. Paper presented at the conference "Fiscal Federalism: Working Out the Future," Saskatchewan Institute of Public Policy, Regina, October.

Ruggeri, Giuseppe C., Robert Howard, and Donald Van Wart. 1993a. Structural imbalances in the Canadian fiscal system. *Canadian Tax Journal* 41(3), 454-72.

Ruggeri, Giuseppe C., Donald Van Wart, Grant K. Robertson, and Robert Howard. 1993b. Vertical fiscal imbalance and the reallocation of tax fields in Canada. *Canadian Public Policy* 19(2), 194-215.

Ruggeri, Giuseppe C., Donald Van Wart, and Robert Howard. 1995. Reassignment of tax fields and the changing federal role. *Canadian Journal of Regional Science* 18(2).

Ruggeri, Joe, and Frank Strain. 2001. Equalization: Let's stick to the principles. *Caledon Commentary*. Ottawa: Caledon Institute of Social Policy (accessed 23 January 2002). http://www.caledoninst.org/PDF/5538200 10.pdf

Sacks, Michael Alan, Karaleah S. Reichart, and W. Trexler Proffitt, Jr. 1999. Broadening the evaluation of dispute resolution: context and relationships over time. *Negotiation Journal*, 15, 4, 339-45, October.

Sanger, Matt. 2001. Reckless abandon: Canada, the GATS and the future of health care. Executive summary. Ottawa: Canadian Centre for Policy Alternatives (accessed 20 January 2002). http://www.policyalternatives.ca

Saskatchewan. Commission on Medicare. 2001. *Caring for Medicare: Sustaining a Quality System*. Chaired by Kenneth J. Fyke. Regina: The Commission on Medicare, Policy and Planning Branch, Saskatchewan Health (accessed 23 January 2002). http://www.health.gov.sk.ca/info_center_p ub_commission_on_medicare-bw.pdf

Savoie, Donald. 1999. *Governing From the Centre: The Concentration of Power in Canadian Politics*. Toronto: University of Toronto Press.

Scharpf, Fritz W. 1988. The joint-decision trap: lessons from German federalism and European integration. *Public Administration* 66(3), 239-78.

—1997. *Games Real Actors Play: Actor-Centred Institutionalism in Policy Research*. Boulder: Westview Press.

Schwanen, Daniel. 1999. More than the sum of our parts: improving the mechanisms of Canada's social union. *C.D. Howe Commentary* 120. Toronto: C.D. Howe Institute (accessed 8 January 2002). http://www.cdhowe.org/pdf/sch-06.pdf

Schwartz, Bryan. 1995. Assessing the Agreement on Internal Trade: the case for a "more perfect union," in *Canada: The State of the Federation 1995*, edited by Douglas Brown and Jonathan Rose. Kingston: Institute of Intergovernmental Relations, 189-221.

Segal, Hugh. 2000. Beyond the vertical and horizontal hold: the challenge of practical collaboration. Speech presented at the Saskatchewan Institute of Public Policy Forum/Conference on the Social Union, February (accessed 20 January 2002). http://www.irpp.org/archive/020700e.pdf

Shaul, Randi Zlotnik. 2000. The implications of Canadian law for economic approaches to allocating health care resources: the round hole and the square peg. Ph.D. thesis, University of Toronto.

Silver, Susan. 1996. The struggle for national standards: lessons from the federal role in health care, in *Remaking Canadian Social Policy: Social Security in the Late 1990s*, edited by Jane Pulkingham and Gordon Ternowetsky. Halifax: Fernwood, 67-80.

Simeon, Richard. 2001. Making federalism work: intergovernmental coordination and institutional capacity. Notes for a presentation to the Forum of Federations. International seminar on Modernization and Fiscal Federalism: Alternatives to Tax Wars: Sustainable Economic Development in Brazil, Sao Paulo, Brazil, June 21-22 (accessed 2 February 2002). http://www.ciff.on.ca/Reference/documents/docm10.doc

Simeon, Richard, and David Cameron. 2002. Intergovernmental relations and democracy: an oxymoron if there ever was one? in *Canadian Federalism: Performance, Effectiveness, and Legitimacy*, edited by Herman Bakvis and Grace Skogstad. Don Mills: Oxford University Press, 278-96.

Simeon, Richard, ed. 1979. *Confrontation and Collaboration - Intergovernmental Relations In Canada Today*. Toronto: The Institute of Public Administration of Canada.

Simeon, Richard, research coordinator. 1985. *Division of Powers and Public Policy*. Royal Commission on the Economic Union and Development Prospects for Canada, vol. 61. Toronto and Ottawa: University of Toronto Press and Ministry of Supply and Services.

Simeon, Richard, and Mary Janigan, eds. 1991. *Toolkits and Building Blocks: Constructing a New Canada*. Toronto: C.D. Howe Institute.

Skogstad, Grace. 2000. Canada: dual and executive federalism, ineffective problem-solving, in *Public Policy and Federalism*, edited by Dietmar Braun. Aldershot: Ashgate, 57-77.

Skogstad, Grace, and Paul Kopas. 1992. Environmental policy in a federal system: Ottawa and the provinces, in *Canadian Environmental Policy: Ecosystems, Politics, and Process*, edited by Robert Boardman. Toronto: Oxford University Press, 43-60.

Smiley, Donald V. 1962. The Rowell-Sirois Report, provincial autonomy, and post-war Canadian federalism. *Canadian Journal of Economics and Political Science*, 28, 54.

— 1963. *Conditional Grants and Canadian Federalism*. Toronto: Canadian Tax Foundation.

Smith, Denis. 1977. President and parliament: the transformation of parliamentary government in Canada, in *Apex of Power: The Prime Minister and Political Leadership in Canada*, edited by Thomas A. Hockin. 2nd edition. Scarborough: Prentice-Hall, 308-25.

Smith, Jennifer. 1998. The meaning of provincial equality in Canadian federalism. Working paper, Institute of Intergovernmental Relations, Kingston (accessed 20 January 2002). http://iigr.ca/pdf/publications/144_The_M eaning_of_Provincia.pdf

Snodden, Tracy R. 1998. The impact of the CHST on interprovincial redistribution in Canada. *Canadian Public Policy* 4(1), 49-67. http://economics.ca/cgi/jab?journal=cpp& view=v24n1/Snod.pdf

Sparer, Michael S. 1999. Myths and misunderstandings: health policy, the devolution revolution, and the push for privatization. *American Behavioral Scientist* 43(1), 138-54.

Standing Senate Committee on Social Affairs, Science and Technology. 2001a. *The Story So Far*. Vol 2 of *The Health of Canadians – The Federal Role. Interim Report*. Chaired by Michael J.L. Kirby. Ottawa: Queen's Printer for Canada, March.

— 2001b. *Issues and Options*. Vol. 4 of *The Health of Canadians – The Federal Role. Interim Report*. Chaired by Michael J.L. Kirby. Ottawa: Queen's Printer for Canada.

— 2002. *Recommendations for Reform*. Vol. 6 of *The Health of Canadians – The Federal Role. Final Report*. Chaired by Michael J.L. Kirby. Ottawa: Queen's Printer for Canada.

Stewart, Terence P., and Amy Ann Karpel. 2000. Review of the dispute settlement understanding: operation of panels. *Law and Policy in International Business* 31(3), 593.

Stilborn, Jack. 1997. National standards and social programs: what the federal government can do. BP-379E. Ottawa, Library of Parliament, Parliamentary Research Branch (accessed 20 January 2002). http://www.parl.gc.ca/information/library/prbpubs/bp379-e.htm

Strick, J. 1992. Critical limits to taxation. *Canadian Tax Journal* 40(6), 1314-31.

Supreme Court of Canada. 1991. *Reference Re Canada Assistance Plan (B.C.)*. 2 S.C.R (accessed 30 May 2002). http://www.lexum.umontreal.ca/csc-scc/en/pub/1991/vol2/html/1991scr2_0525.html

Swacker, Frank, Kenneth Redden, and Larry Wenger. 1995. *World Trade Without Barriers: The World Trade Organization (WTO) and Dispute Resolution*. Vol. 1, Charlottesville, VA: The Michie Company.

— 1996. *World Trade Without Barriers: Comparative Dispute Resolution – Public and Private*. Vol. 2, Charlottesville, VA: The Michie Company.

Sweet, Alec Stone, and Thomas L. Brunnell. 1998. Constructing a supranational constitution: dispute resolution and governance in the European Community. *American Political Science Review* 92(1), 63.

Tavares, Antonio F., and Richard C. Feiock. 2001. Intergovernmental institutions and local environmental policy choices. Paper presented to the American Political Science Association, San Francisco, August 30-September 2 (accessed 3 February 2002). http://pro.harvard.edu/papers/025/025004TavaresAnt.pdf

Taylor, Malcolm. 1987. *Health Insurance and Canadian Public Policy: The Seven Decisions that Created the Canadian Health Insurance System and Their Outcomes*. Toronto: Institute of Public Administration in Canada.

— 1989. Health insurance: the roller-coaster in federal-provincial relations, in *Federalism and Political Community, Essays in Honour of Donald Smiley*, edited by David P. Shugarman and Reg Whitaker. Peterborough: Broadview Press, 73-93.

Telford, Hamish. 1999. The federal spending power in Canada: nation-building or nation-destroying? Working paper 143. Institute of Intergovernmental Relations, Kingston (accessed 20 January 2002). http://www.iigr.ca/pdf/publications/143_The_Federal_Spending_Pow.pdf

Thériault, Camille. 1998. New Brunswick's perspective on the social union. *Policy Options* 19(9), 20-3 (accessed 20 January 2002). http://www.irpp.org/archive/policyop/no98sume.htm.

Thomas, David M. 1993. Turning a blind eye: constitutional abeyances and the Canadian experience. *International Journal of Canadian Studies* 7(8), 63-81.

Torjman, Sherri. 1995. *Can We Have National Standards?* Ottawa: Caledon Institute of Social Policy.

Treasury Board Secretariat. 2001. Social Union Framework Agreement (SUFA): Accountability (accessed 26 July 2002). http://www.tbs-sct.gc.ca/rma/account/sufa-ecus_e.asp

Trebilcock, Michael J., and Robert Howse. 1995. *The Regulation of International Trade*. London: Routledge.

Tremblay, André. 2000. Federal spending power, in *The Canadian Social Union Without Quebec: 8 Critical Analyses.* Introduced by Alain-G. Gagnon and Hugh Segal. Montreal: Institute for Research on Public Policy, 155-86.

Tremblay, Guy. 2000. Dispute avoidance and resolution, in *The Canadian Social Union Without Quebec: 8 Critical Analyses,* introduced by Alain-G. Gagnon and Hugh Segal. Montreal: Institute for Research on Public Policy, 189-209.

Trudeau, Pierre E. 1969. *Federal-Provincial Grants and the Spending Power of Parliament.* Ottawa: Queen's Printer.

Tuohy, Carolyn. 1994a. Federalism and health policy, in *Challenges to Federalism: Policy-Making in Canada and the Federal Republic of Germany,* edited by William M. Chandler and Christian W. Zollner. Kingston: Institute of Intergovernmental Relations.

—1994b. Health policy and fiscal federalism, in *The Future of Fiscal Federalism,* edited by Keith Banting, Douglas Brown, and Thomas Courchene. Kingston: School of Policy Studies, Queen's University, 189-212.

Usher, Dan. 1996. The uneasy case for equalization payments. Vancouver, Fraser Institute.
http://collection.nlc-bcn.ca/100/200/300/fraser/equalization/

Vail, Stephen. 2001. Canadians' values and attitudes on Canada's health care system: a synthesis of survey results. Ottawa: The Conference Board of Canada (accessed 21 March 2002).
http://www.conferenceboard.ca/Health/documents/307-00df.pdf.

Vaillancourt, François. 1998. Alter the federal-provincial powers mix to improve social policy. *Policy Options* 19(9), 50-2. Montreal: Institute for Research on Public Policy (accessed 20 January 2002).
http://www.irpp.org/archive/policyop/no98sume.htm.

Vaillancourt, Yves. 2002. Le modèle québécois de politiques sociales et ses interfaces

avec l'union sociale canadienne. *IRPP Enjeux publics* 3(2). Montreal: Institute for Research on Public Policy (accessed 21 March 2002).
http://www.irpp.org/pm/index.htm.

Van Loon, Richard J., and Michael Whittington. 1987. *The Canadian Political System: Environment, Structure and Process.* Toronto: McGraw-Hill Ryerson.

Walton, Richard E. 1987. *Innovating to Compete: Lessons for Diffusing and Managing Change in the Workplace.* San Francisco: Jossey-Bass.

Watts, Ronald L. 1999a. The Canadian experience with asymmetrical federalism, in *Accommodating Diversity: Asymmetry in Federal States,* edited by Robert Agranoff. Baden-Baden: Nomos Verlagsgesellschaft, 118-36.

—1999b. *Comparing Federal Systems,* 2nd ed. Montreal: McGill Queen's Press, for the Institute of Intergovernmental Relations, Queen's University.

—2001. Models of federal power sharing. *International Social Science Journal* 53(1), 23-32.

Western Premiers' Conference. 2000. Toward fiscal balance: a Western perspective. Paper prepared by the ministers of finance of British Columbia, Alberta, Saskatchewan, Manitoba, Yukon, Northwest Territories, and Nunavut. Brandon, Manitoba (accessed 10 June 2002).
http://www.scics.gc.ca/pdf/850077008_e.pdf

—2001. Revitalizing federal-provincial/territorial fiscal relations: summary and recommendations. A presentation to Western premiers by the finance ministers of Alberta, Saskatchewan, Manitoba, Yukon, Northwest Territories and Nunavut (accessed 15 February 2002).
http://www.scics.gc.ca/pdf/850082014.pdf

Wilson, Kumanan. 2000. Health care, federalism, and the new Social Union. *Canadian Medical Association Journal* 162(8), 1171-4.
http://collection.nlcbnc.ca/100/201/300/cdn_medical_association/cmaj/vol-162/issue-8/1171.htm

Winer, Stanley L. 2000. On the reassignment of fiscal powers in a federal state, in *Competition and Structure: The Political Economy of Collective Decisions. Essays in Honor of Albert Breton*, edited by Gianluigi Galeotti, Pierre Salmon, and Ronald Wintrobe. Cambridge: Cambridge University Press, 150-73.

Winfield, Mark R. 2002. Environmental policy and federalism, in *Canadian Federalism: Performance, Effectiveness, and Legitimacy*, edited by Herman Bakvis and Grace Skogstad. Don Mills: Oxford University Press, 124-38.

World Trade Organization. 1999. The World Trade Organization in brief. Geneva: World Trade Organization (accessed 3 June 2002). http://www.wto.org/english/res_e/doload_ e/inbr_e.pdf

Young, Robert, ed. 1999. *Stretching the Federation: The Art of the State in Canada.* Kingston: Institute of Intergovernmental Relations, Queen's University.

Zekos, Georgios I. 1999. An examination of GATT/WTO arbitration procedures. *Dispute Resolution Journal* 54(4), 72-6.

Zuker, Richard. 2002. Vertical fiscal imnalance Is the produce of vertical political imbal- ance. Paper presented at "Canadian Fiscal Arrangements: What Works, What Might Workd Better," conference held in Winnipeg, Manitoba, 16-17 May (accessed 17 October, 2003). www.iigr.ca/conferences/archive/pdfs2/zu ker.pdf

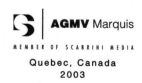

MEMBER OF SCABRINI MEDIA
Quebec, Canada
2003